Liberatory Psychiatry

Liberatory Psychiatry

Philosophy, Politics, and Mental Health

Edited by

Carl I. Cohen, MD

Sami Timimi, MBChB, MRCPsych

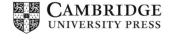
CAMBRIDGE
UNIVERSITY PRESS

CAMBRIDGE UNIVERSITY PRESS
Cambridge, New York, Melbourne, Madrid, Cape Town, Singapore, São Paulo, Delhi

Cambridge University Press
The Edinburgh Building, Cambridge CB2 8RU, UK

Published in the United States of America by Cambridge University Press, New York

www.cambridge.org
Information on this title: www.cambridge.org/9780521689816

First published 2008

Printed in the United Kingdom at the University Press, Cambridge

A catalog record for this publication is available from the British Library

ISBN 978-0-521-68981-6 paperback

Contents

Contributors

Joan Benach
Unitat de Salut Laboral, Dept Ciencis
Experimentals I de la Salut, Universitat
Pompeu Fabra, Barcelona, Spain

Carme Borrell
Agencia de Salut Publica de Barcelona,
Barcelona, Spain

Pat Bracken
Institute for Philosophy, Diversity and
Mental Health, University of Central
Lancashire, UK

Haejoo Chung
Department of Health Policy and
Management, Johns Hopkins School of
Public Health, Baltimore, MD, USA

Carl I. Cohen
Division of Geriatric Psychiatry, SUNY
Downstate Medical Center,
New York, NY, USA
Email: carl.cohen@downstate.edu

Duncan Double
Norfolk and Waveney Mental Health
Partnership NHS Trust and University of
East Anglia, UK

Amjad Hindi
Department of Psychiatry, SUNY Downstate
Medical Center, New York, NY, USA

Bradley Lewis
Gallatin School of Individualized Study,
New York University, New York, NY, USA

Begum Maitra
Child and Adolescent Psychiatry, East
London and the City Mental Health NHS
Trust, London, UK

Kwame McKenzie
Social, Equity and Health Centre, Centre
for Addictions and Mental Health and
University of Toronto, Toronto,
Canada

Joanna Moncrieff
Department of Mental Health Sciences,
University College London, London, UK

Carles Muntaner
Social Equity and Health Centre, Social
Policy and Prevention Department, Centre
for Addictions and Mental Health, Toronto,
Canada

Isaac Prilleltensky
School of Education University of Miami,
Coral Gables Campus, Coral Gables, FL, USA

Ora Prilleltensky
School of Education, University of Miami,
Coral Gables Campus, Coral Gables,
FL, USA

Astrid Rusquellas
Department of Psychiatry, University of
California at San Francisco, Berkeley,
CA, USA

Ramotse Saunders
Department of Psychiatry, SUNY
Downstate Medical Center, New York,
NY, USA

Philip Thomas
Institute for Philosophy, Diversity and
Mental Health, University of Central
Lancashire, UK

Kenneth S. Thompson
University of Pittsburgh School of Medicine,
Pittsburgh, PA, USA

Sami Timimi
Lincolnshire Partnership NHS Trust,
Bracebridge Heath, Lincoln, UK
Email: stimimi@talk21.com

Charles W. Tolman
University of Victoria, North Saanich, BC,
Canada

Ipsit Vahia
SUNY Downstate Medical Center,
New York, NY, USA

Courte Voorhees
Center for Community Studies, Peabody
College of Vanderbilt University,
Nashville, TN, USA

Acknowledgments

We thank Katie Brown for providing the wonderful artwork for the cover. We also thank the staff at Cambridge University Press, including special mention to Richard Marley, Mary Sanders, Laura Wood, and Bethan Jones for shepherding the manuscript to publication, and Pauline Graham and Betty Fulford, both now longer with Cambridge, but who helped launch this endeavor. Carl Cohen thanks SUNY Downstate Medical Center and his chair, Dr. Stephen Goldfinger, for affording him the opportunity to work on this project, Ms Barbara Singh for her administrative assistance, and his family for their love and support – his wife Kate, who is looking forward to dancing in the revolution, his children Sara and Zack, his father Lou, and his new granddaughter, Melanie, who will surely carry the liberatory quest onward. Sami Timimi thanks his employers Lincolnshire Partnership Foundation NHS Trust for its support in the writing and research for this book, his secretaries Susan and Louise for their help, and his wonderful family – his wife, Kitty, and his children Michelle, Lewis and Zoe, for their enduring love and patience.

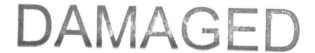

Introduction

Carl I. Cohen and Sami Timimi

Pinel's unchaining of the eighteenth century Parisian insane has been an historical metaphor for the dual liberatory underpinnings of psychiatry: it can free persons from social, physical, and psychological oppression, and it can assist persons to be what they can be (i.e., self-realization), and to lead self-directed lives. Thus, psychiatry can help people to be both "free from" and "free to." These goals not only link psychiatry to medicine and science but also to sociopolitical elements. Hence, two foundational points guide our work: (1) The project of psychiatry has always been one of liberation; (2) Psychiatry's principal object, the mind (i.e., the psychological sphere), is inherently biological and social. If we are to take these two points seriously, it means that psychiatry has a critical and necessary role to play in social struggles that further liberation.

What are the liberatory roles for psychiatry? When we refer to "free from," we mean that psychiatry can help to free persons from the effects of internal biological forces that contribute to mental illness and distress. In addition, because it is also linked to sociopolitical elements, psychiatry can explore the subjective ramifications of living under a particular social formation. For example, the impact of domination, alienation from the products of one's labor or from one's coworkers, of being treated as a commodity, or of being in a particular social class, gender category, ethnic or racial group. Moreover, if the mind is both biological and social, what are the implications of the social world being imbedded within the individual? For example, in a social world in which the self-worth is based on monetary values, those parts of the self that cannot be commodified may be devalued and alienated. Or, what are the effects of social forces on cognition and emotional responses? The structure of the external world contributes to the structure of the internal world. Hence, oppressive social circumstances can hinder psychological development and lead to psychological distress or psychopathology.

From the racism of the mental hygiene movement, the creation of the eugenic movement, through Nazi Germany's quest to create the "master race," to the Soviet's use of psychiatry to help silence dissidents; psychiatry has always been

Liberatory Psychiatry: Philosophy, Politics, and Mental Health, ed. Carl I. Cohen and Sami Timimi.
Published by Cambridge University Press. © Cambridge University Press.

vulnerable to being used as part of the state's tools for social control. The modern neoliberal state is no exception. By individualizing and commodifying mental health, the radical and liberatory potential of psychiatry is neutralized. Neoliberalism has arguably produced more misery and suffering than at any time in the past; however, once this suffering can be reduced to the effects of abnormal molecules, not only are the social dynamics rendered invisible, but enormous new potential markets emerge (such as for the pharmaceutical industry). Why is psychiatry so vulnerable to being used in this way? We may need some forms of social control, but what is benign, humane, just, and "good" and what is oppressive, and who should be involved in social control?

Psychiatry's role in assisting persons to be free to flourish and lead self-directed lives remains to be developed conceptually. Perhaps it will be by assisting persons to identify values and goals that are consistent with their cognitive abilities, emotional framework, and with their biological makeup. However, at this moment, psychiatry's principal function is to address the conditions that impede human development, i.e., the "free-from" sphere.

Traditional Western psychiatry has focused primarily on the biological and individual elements of psychology, and has had a much narrower view of liberation. Thus, freedom from mental illness/distress and self-realization is addressed within the confines of the existing social structure. A smaller group of theorists have focused on the social elements, but they have typically neglected the biological/physical components.

In the twentieth century there were a few attempts to take seriously the liberatory agenda of psychiatry. The Freudian Left, most notably Reich, Fromm, Marcuse, and Kovel, struggled to develop radical theories that incorporated the biological, psychological, and social world. Critical Psychologists in Germany and Leontyev in the former Soviet Union attempted to meld Marxism with a "scientific" psychology that was primarily cognitively focused. Each of these attempts was not fully realized because of their reliance on non-materialist concepts in the case of Freudians, the absence of a biological component (e.g., Fromm, Leontyev, German Critical Psychologists), or the omission of emotional elements and the unconscious (e.g., Leontyev). Moreover, the theories were created by "experts," with little or no conceptual input from other important stakeholders, especially consumers, workers, women, and people of color.

These theorists developed their frameworks between 30 to 75 years ago, considerably predating the dramatic transformations in social structures that have occurred worldwide. The causes of this transformation have included the rapid globalization of the world economy, advances in technology, and alterations in the world's political structure following the demise of the Soviet Union. The psychological ramifications of these changes have been pronounced. The problems of domination, alienation, commodification, class, gender, religion, race, and ethnicity are becoming more universal, although they are not uniform.

The need to confront the psychological impact of these historical changes provides a compelling opportunity to modernize the liberatory psychiatry agenda by incorporating advances in theory and practice that could, in turn, allow for new perspectives on this project. For example, potentially fruitful points of departure include new conceptual frameworks and research data from neuropsychology, psychoanalysis, critical social theory, political economy, and philosophy (particularly postmodernism). Most importantly, we need to develop this project from an international perspective.

Despite these pressing needs, the mental health profession has not responded in any systematic way. The aim of this book will be to lay the groundwork for such a response. The international group of contributors to this volume approaches this undertaking from a variety of perspectives. Indeed, there is no one correct method or theory. At this point in time it is more important to privilege debate over consensus. However, the authors are united by their desire to revitalize the original liberatory project of psychiatry.

In Chapter 1, Carl Cohen begins by conceding that, given the long history of failures by leftist theorist and practitioners at producing a progressive (liberatory) psychiatry, it would be presumptuous to claim that his chapter or this volume can overcome the limitations of earlier efforts. Rather, he proposes a more modest goal of providing an updated version of this project, and to re-open the debate. Cohen uses his chapter to address two issues: (1) To provide an outline of the structure of a progressive psychology that would be compatible with radical sociopolitical theory. He proposes several broad principles that such a psychology must include, and also illustrates how deviations from these principles lead to conceptual distortions. (2) In conjunction with this first aim, he describes new approaches to understanding unconscious process that may assist in explaining why people have failed to act in their "best interests." He concludes with seven key points: (1) Progressives can embrace science if they do not restrict themselves to a limited view of the enterprise. (2) Scientists and scientific theories are separate from real objects and forces. The validity of a theory depends on it being tested against the latter. (3) All scientific theories contain social elements, but it is possible to critique them and take them into account as theory is developed and tested. (4) In developing a progressive psychology we must account for real people within real relations. (5) Failures to develop a progressive psychology have occurred because conceptual models have relied on speculative, untestable theories, or have ignored or minimized the concrete, biological individual or real social relationships. (6) In developing a progressive psychology we must recognize conscious and unconscious cognitive and emotional forces that act on the individual. This entails recognition of biological as well as social elements. An appreciation of neuro-science will be needed to understand how these elements become integrated. (7) Progressives need to embrace science and biology, to radicalize it, and direct it towards the goal of promoting and sustaining human liberation.

In Chapter 2, Philip Thomas and Pat Bracken use a postmodern analysis that revolves around the writing and thinking of Michel Foucault to illustrate the ways in which constraints operate in our social lives. We do not control the ideas, constructions, words, and priorities of the worlds in which we live and grow. Instead, these representations present us with a picture of what it is to be human, to be normal, and indeed to be free. They hold our conduct within certain limits, but also incite us in certain directions and ultimately present us with a vision of what liberation and freedom are all about. They argue that the process of liberation and the state of freedom are simply more complex than allowed for in the thought of the previous generations of radicals from both within and without psychiatry. Further that, whatever it is; liberation is not something that is in the gift of one professional group or another, or something to be defined by one professional discourse or another. Thus, in a critique of arguably the central thesis of this book, they suggest that, whilst psychiatry can offer more help and support to "experts by experience," and can be less controlling and more transparent, it *cannot* offer liberation. The most that we can do as critical psychiatrists is to work towards more openness and honesty, and through this to show how a great deal of psychiatric discourse is nothing more than mythology.

In Chapter 3, Duncan Double looks at the potentially negative effects of the modern concept of "risk" in psychiatry and the creation of a "defensive" form of practice that results from governmental legislation and enquiries that focus on the risk posed by the mentally ill to the public. He first reminds us of the history of the attempts at a more liberatory form of psychiatry particularly in the 1960s and 1970s discussing amongst other things the *Dialectics of Liberation* conference organized by David Cooper and held in London in July 1967, and Franco Basaglia's *Psichiatria Democratica* founded in 1973 and whose campaigning eventually led to the passing of Law 180 by the Italian parliament in May 1978. Double sees the opportunities to take creative risks in theory and practice as being eroded due to the creation of public fear of the mentally ill, consequently making liberatory ideals of community based care ever harder to achieve.

In Chapter 4, Bradley Lewis observes that previous liberatory efforts, e.g., Pinel, Tuke, Freud, Lacan, and Szasz, were created and designed by "experts." However, he argues that liberatory psychiatry cannot be achieved without the input of users of services, who are psychiatry's major stakeholders. Thus, the next wave of liberatory reform must be democratically driven. Informed primarily by a post-modern perspective, Lewis reviews some of the problems of expert driven theory and practice. He then shifts from critique to application. He proposes three steps towards a democratic psychiatry. These steps consist of reforming the American Psychiatric Association, creating a critical psychiatry network, and reconfiguring clinical care with a narrative frame.

In Chapter 5, Charles Tolman introduces readers to the work of German "critical psychology." Notably, Tolman points that it was originally called "critical emancipatory psychology," and it has never lost its emancipatory intent. Tolman describes the critical psychologists' contribution to the early debates in the 1960s concerning the value interest of science, particularly psychological research. He provides several illustrations of the "anti-emancipatory" bias of traditional psychological research such as behaviorism, personality theory, and cognitive psychology. Such theories have provided little room for intentionality, ignored subjectivity, and have isolated the individual. Tolman asserts that all these theories are missing the concreteness of individual life. Tolman believes that an emancipatory psychology can only be attained with a method that is both developmental and historical. He summarizes the critical psychology model that human subjects evolved with the systematic creation and use of tools, and the development of societal mode of existence. The latter meant human existence and action is now dominated by "meaning," and this aspect has been minimized or neglected by mainstream psychology. People now have the choice of action within an historical context, although uneven distribution of power, knowledge, and privilege can restrict people's freedom. Tolman concludes that emancipatory psychology is possible only if it begins with recognition that human subjectivity is constituted in societal relations, and that emancipation is not just a psychological affair, but depends on societal structures of power. He closes with some illustrations of how critical psychologists are striving to make research endeavors more democratic and less objectifying, and striving towards elaborating the interactional context of practice.

In Chapter 6, Isaac Prilleltensky and his coauthors direct their attention to the inability of helping professions to shift from the traditional medical models, with its disempowering, reactive, deficit focused, and individual approaches. They maintain that, despite considerable critique, there has been a huge chasm between critical discourse and concrete action. They build a case for action around the concept of "psychopolitical validity." Psychopolitical validity consists of the level of attention given to the role of power in explaining psychological and political phenomena that impact on the suffering and the well-being of individuals. Most notably, they point to the fact that the term "psychopolitical" underscores the inseparable nature of psychological and political dynamics. They emphasize the interplay of power in affective, behavioral, and cognitive experiences, and the subjective and cultural forces that shape political contexts. Finally, the authors examine the impact of power and oppression at various levels of analysis, and propose concrete applications of a "liberation" approach to counseling and psychotherapy at the community, organizational, and individual level.

In Chapter 7, Carles Muntaner, Carme Borrell, and Haejoo Chung present a novel perspective on the political economy of mental health. They start by reviewing the well-established linkages between social class and psychiatric disorders. The authors contend that it is time to move beyond these elementary associations and begin to elaborate on the mechanisms by which social class impacts on mental functioning. The authors distinguish between social stratification (i.e., social rankings) and social class (i.e., relations of property and control), and then introduce the concept of "exploitation." They posit empirical methods for assessing exploitation. They argue for more sophisticated class insights based on exploitation that will give social psychiatry more depth and allow for alternative models for the social production of psychiatric illness.

In Chapter 8, Kwame McKenzie sets out the case for re-invigorating public health psychiatry. Modern medicine has its roots in epidemiological mapping that could identify specific environmental sources of disease. This eventually led to the hypothesis that infectious diseases were caused by micro-organisms and the discovery of specific bacteria and viruses. The cause of chronic diseases proved more difficult to demonstrate. Rather than catching a disease, you developed it sometimes over a life-course due to multiple exposures. Lifestyle seemed to increase your risk of developing an illness and the risk of it not getting better. Risk factor analysis became the order of the day, and manipulating risk factors became the role of public health. Mirroring changes in the political discourse, the focus had changed from the environment being the primary etiological concern to the individual and his or her lifestyle being most important. More recently several "new" concepts of how societies and health interact have been put forward. One such concept is "social capital", which is a measure of social cohesion. McKenzie calls for greater attention to be paid to this concept. This is because in psychiatry our inability to offer much more than symptom amelioration (rather than effective treatment) argues for giving precedence for prevention over attempts at cure.

In Chapter 9, Sami Timimi notes that prescriptions of psychotropic medication to children and adolescents have shown a dramatic increase in most Western countries and in many non-Western ones. He asks how such a change could have occurred, and he argues that central to understanding this change is an engagement with issues of context: socioeconomic, cultural and political. In approaching the task of trying to understand why this increase is happening, he first contextualizes current theory and practice through reference to the particular conditions within which child psychiatry was born and started to grow, followed by a brief critique of the notion of "development" on which so much child and adolescent mental health theory and practice relies. Following this, Timimi explores how a context rich ecological analysis helps provide new theoretical directions. Finally, he suggests that his analysis, which favors context rich "ecological" paradigms, has some radical implications for both theory and practice in child and adolescent psychiatry.

In Chapter 10, Begum Maitra reflects on her arrival in Britain in the early 1980s where she discovered that she entered a cultural "limbo" of immigrant doctors and nurses from British ex-colonies. Maitra first attempts to unpick the confusion of shame, guilt, and gratitude in order to explore the territory of cultural understanding, and the undeniable potential that misunderstanding has to inflict damage, but also to look at the profound, long-term effects of Britain's colonial past on contemporary practice in psychiatry in the UK. Exploring the effects of multiple hierarchies based on perceptions of superiority/inferiority, she also suggests something more subtle may be occurring "unseen" as a result of the increasing numbers of immigrant doctors from the ex-colonies (like her) practicing within UK psychiatric system. She suggests a quiet cultural revolution within the public sector in UK mental health may be taking place and discusses its unpredictable impact on professional culture and practice more broadly.

In Chapter 11, Amjad Hindi, Ramotse Saunders, and Ipsit Vahia direct their attention towards developing a new psychiatry within the context of postcolonialism. The chapter brings together the authors' perspectives from Syria, West Indies, and India. Moreover, they approach this topic from different conceptual models. Amjad Hindi provides a postmodern analysis of globalization and postcolonialism. Ramotse Saunders tackles the relationship between Western psychiatric theory, Western trained psychiatrists, and indigenous cultures in the early twenty-first century. Finally, Ipsit Vahia speculates about the prospects for melding traditional indigenous practices with modern psychiatry.

In Chapter 12, Joanna Moncrieff explores the relationship between the dominant psychiatric paradigm (biopsychiatry) and the dominant economic system (neoliberalism). She asks whether biologically oriented psychiatry helps to create the social and cultural milieu favored by neoliberal policies, and whether these policies in turn have helped a certain view of psychiatry to become hegemonic. Neuroscience research, which aims to uncover the biological origins of psychiatric disorders, has burgeoned and flourished, gaining a high degree of credibility outside psychiatry as well as within, with psychiatry now plying its wares to a widening proportion of the population. Use of psychiatric drugs has risen dramatically, with a larger proportion of the general population now willing to identify themselves as needing psychiatric help. These developments in psychiatry parallel profound social and economic changes, commonly referred to as "neoliberalism," that have occurred in varying degrees throughout the world. The question she addresses in her chapter is whether these two developments are related.

In Chapter 13, Astrid Rusquellas describes the progressive elements in psycho-analysis drawing from the seminal work of Wilhelm Reich in Germany during the 1920s and 1930s, and the work of Marion Langer, who had a profound influence in Latin America, beginning in the 1960s. Langer was able to integrate Freudian Left with an emerging new Psychoanalytic Left in Latin America. After an elaboration of the theoretical foundations of the Latin American Psychoanalytic Left, Rusquellas describes the contributions of psychoanalysts to the struggles of workers in more than 600 factories in Argentina.

Finally, in Chapter 15, Carl Cohen, Sami Timimi, and Kenneth Thompson review the disparate ideas presented in this volume and suggest ways to create a "new psychiatry" that will more fully incorporate the liberatory project of psychiatry.

We believe that there will be a wide audience for this book because it addresses an area that is at the essence of psychiatry and psychological practice, but one that has been neglected over the past three decades. Importantly, in recent years there have been signs of renewed interest in this topic. For example, the critical psychiatry group in Britain attracts large number of persons to its meetings and they have published in several prestigious journals including the *British Journal of Psychiatry* and *British Medical Journal*. At the 2004 annual meeting of the American Psychiatric Association, we presented an issue workshop on this topic to a nearly filled room, despite it being on the last day of the convention. Several books have emerged that have touched on aspects of this project. These include Patrick Bracken and Philip Thomas' *Postpsychiatry*, Bradley Lewis' *Moving Beyond Prozac, DSM, and the New Psychiatry. The Birth of Postpsychiatry*, and Duncan Double's *Critical Psychiatry: The Limits of Madness*. All of these authors have contributed chapters to this volume.

This volume will be of interest to mental health practitioners across a variety of disciplines (e.g., psychiatry, psychology, social work), to consumers of mental health services, social and political scientists, social activists, and academic audiences, particularly in classes that deal with psychology, philosophy, or social theory. The book should also be of interest to lay audiences with an interest in novel approaches to psychological theory and practice. Finally, the international composition of the contributors should broaden the book's appeal to a global audience.

This volume is the beginning of a long struggle to resurrect the liberatory potential of psychiatry, and in so doing, to develop a liberatory theory and practice. As we work to realize this project, we welcome input and feedback from all readers. We look forward to hearing new voices and sharing ideas.

1

Working towards a liberatory psychiatry? Radicalizing the science of human psychology and behavior

Carl I. Cohen

My family has the revolution blues. My grandparents wondered why there were no radical political changes in the aftermath of World War I. My parents were certain that the Great Depression would spark political revolution. I believed that the 1960s would lead to dramatic transformations in society and culture. And my children wonder why there aren't progressive revolts throughout the developing world. Although radical political change is not easy, it seems that many times there were conditions that made change possible, but nothing happened. Moreover, when "revolutions" occurred, too often these systems reverted to another form of oppression, and the opportunity for liberation was lost. Woody Allen satirized this phenomenon in *Bananas* when, after the revolutionary leader assumed power, his first act was to require everyone to speak Swedish and to wear their underwear on the outside.

In the years after the end of World War I theorists began to examine more seriously whether psychological factors might impede revolutionary change. Specifically, they were interested in whether there were unconscious elements that worked against rational conscious thinking and perpetuated oppression and domination. Despite various problems with Freud's theory, including its conservative elements, many progressives turned to Freud, since at that time, his work provided the only systematic analysis of unconscious processes (Robinson, 1969; Wolfenstein, 1993). These theorists believed that psychoanalysis could be radicalized and that it provided a complement to Marx's analyses of the political and economic system.

Among Western leftists, this patching of psychoanalysis into Marxism has continued to remain the dominant theoretical underpinning for a radical psychology. For example, Jurgen Habermas, following Freud, postulated that social institutions become the manifestation of historically required repression of psychological needs or desires – a compromise between instinctual desires and self-preservation – and therefore the source of distorted communication and non-rational thinking

Liberatory Psychiatry: Philosophy, Politics, and Mental Health, ed. Carl I. Cohen and Sami Timimi.
Published by Cambridge University Press. © Cambridge University Press.

(Held, 1980). Thus, it is likely that human emancipation entails not only overcoming the constraints of nature such as scarcity and disease, but also recognizing those unconscious processes that contribute to ideological distortions and social repression.

Over the years I have participated in countless study groups and attended dozens of lectures, seminars, workshops, conferences, and classes run by Freudo-Marxists and Marxist-Freudians, radical psychiatrists and radical anti-psychiatrists, humanists and anti-humanists, subjectivists and objectivists, structuralists and poststructuralists, deconstructionists and reconstructionists, modernists and postmodernists, and critical theorists and not-so-critical theorists, as well as by Reichians, Pavlovians, Engelsians, existentialists, and various combinations of the above. I developed a great vocabulary, but I found that I was no closer to finding a liberatory psychiatry.

Given this long history of failures, it would be presumptuous of me to claim that in this chapter I can redress the limitations of earlier efforts. If this chapter succeeds at all, it will be in providing an updated version of this project and to re-open the debate.

More specifically, my aims are twofold:

(1) To provide an outline of the structure of a progressive psychology that would be compatible with radical sociopolitical theory. This will entail a prescriptive and proscriptive approach. That is, I will suggest several broad principles that such a psychology must include, and also illustrate how deviations from these principles lead to conceptual distortions.

(2) In conjunction with this first aim, I will describe new approaches to understanding unconscious process that may assist in explaining why people have failed to act in their "best interests."

Several preliminary notes are in order. First, I have more or less used psychology and psychiatry interchangeably, although the latter tends to focus more on psychopathology and clinical practice. Similarly, I use terms such as "progressive," "leftist" and "radical" interchangeably, although historically they have meant different things. I have interspersed these terms, not only to avoid monotony but also to underscore that I am appealing to a variety of interest groups. Second, I do not discuss an emancipatory sociopolitical theory to complement liberatory psychiatry. I believe this sociopolitical theory would probably include Marxist or Neo-Marxist elements; however, it is beyond the scope of this text and my expertise to propose any systematic model. Third, as a politically progressive health practitioner I have always been a bit skeptical about philosophy – I am sympathetic to Marx's dictum that philosophers have merely contemplated the world, the point is to change it – I have been compelled to rely on philosophy for some of my arguments in this chapter. For the reader's sake I have striven to keep it straightforward and to eliminate as much jargon as possible. Finally, this chapter steers clear of clinical issues and practice. Others in this volume address these concerns. Although I believe there are linkages between psychological theory and clinical practice, the former focuses on society and civilization (the "general disorder") and is free to transcend and criticize the current social realm. Individual therapy tends to ignore the whole in order to aid the individual victim. Indeed, several writers suggest that exactly how therapy does this is largely irrelevant to theory. Brown (1959) writes, "technique can be judged only pragmatically. Anything goes if it works ..." (p. 155). However, as Jacoby (1975) pointedly cautions, what "works" must not be mistakenly considered as liberation.

The case for science

In this chapter, I will be bucking several trends among progressives. First, I will advocate for a "scientific" psychology. Beginning in the 1960s and early 1970s with the work of Kuhn (1962) and Feyerabend (1975), and then more aggressively in later decades with the emergence of postmodernism, progressives have pointed to the value biases of science and its inability to provide an anchor of truth. I will argue that this view reflects a narrow perspective on science (that of "positivism") and that we can still feel comfortable with a more nuanced science. Several other writers (Reed, 1996; Young, 1996) working towards a progressive psychology have likewise echoed these sentiments.

Second, I will advocate a more serious consideration of biology. Here again, with the emergence of the emphasis on language (meaning and symbolism) on one hand, or the emphasis on social relations and structure on the other, biology has been seen as being largely transformed and diminished in importance by social being. I will propose an embodied relational perspective, i.e., physical beings within social relations. In so doing, I want to convince progressives that biology is as important as language and sociocultural embeddedness, especially as it impacts on cognition and behavior. As Edward Sampson (1998), a social constructionist psychologist, came to realize, "In recognizing that our words are embodied even as our bodies are enworded and in light of this we cannot stand outside our world but must be invested participants within ..." (p. 31).

Finally, in response to the concern that people do not always act rationally and that they are unaware of unconscious distortions on thinking, I want to broaden the left's attachment to psychoanalysis. I will propose that psychoanalysis has presented an occasionally useful but limited and ideologically tainted conception of the unconscious, and that neuroscience now offers a more extensive view of the unconscious that is necessary for understanding factors that contribute to individual and social change. Moreover, we can use neuroscience to help explain how various perspectives, interests, and desires are created and are affected by socio-cultural as well as by physiological factors.

There is compelling evidence that the scientific enterprise has been the only *systematic* method for obtaining knowledge about the world (Collier, 1979). In arguing for science, I do not mean that other discourses are unimportant. However, I do not believe that the other discourses systematically yield objective knowledge about the world. Art, music, poetry, literature, philosophy, and soccer all have significant places in human affairs; however, they do not regularly yield knowledge. Nor does this mean that non-scientific practices do not stumble upon truths. Indeed, prior to science, our practical daily activities necessitated that we have knowledge of the world; and conversely, out of these activities, new knowl-edge developed. Nonetheless, these truths developed haphazardly out of practical everyday activities. Science, on the other hand, eliminates the anthropocentricity of everyday life. It tests its theories against external reality rather than interpreting findings based on practical experiences and needs: "The immense progress achieved by the human race in the last three hundred years was made possible by this mutation which allowed science to emerge and liberate itself from immediate practical concerns. Of course, this mutation had something to do with the rise of the bourgeoisie, but then the bourgeoisie of that era was carrying out an unpre-cedented development of human liberation" (Collier, 1979, p. 93).

The development and practice of science is consistent with the emancipatory agenda of this book. Rossi (2003) observes that many cultural anthropologists and philosophers of science have accepted the idea of the equivalence of all forms of culture and world pictures. Many contrast the extraordinary possibilities of a magical and spiritual world with the narrow rationality of science. However, historically the former has been dominated by undemocratic systems that depend on secret knowledge, complicated rituals, narrow groups of sages, and extraordinary character of personality of the practitioner. Whereas magic is reserved for the select, science is open to all people. There is a public character to its theories, methods, and results. Freeman Dyson (2007) describes science as an inherently stubborn act. Whether overturning long-standing ideas or received political wisdom, the scientific enterprise follows the data wherever it may lead, and so becomes a threat to establishments of all forms. As a cautionary note, to be sure, this scientific ideal can be distorted, but if scientists are to remain true to its methods, then history has shown that opportunities for correction will ultimately emerge.

My first task is to sort out what we mean by science. Too often, critics of science have used a narrow perspective that has distorted its potential. I use Roy Bhaskar's (1978) notion of "transcendental realism" as the undergirding for my approach to this topic. Bhaskar points out that that we need to distinguish between "transitive" and "intransitive" dimensions. The transitive dimension refers to the activities of scientists, their language, their social relationships, and so forth. The intransitive dimension refers to the real world object that is independent of the scientist. The intransitive dimension can include processes and forces as well as circumscribed objects. Gravity, for example, is not just a concept but a real force in the world. Thus, we begin with the premise that there is a real (material) world that is independent of the observer. Even in the social sciences, there is an "independent" object of study. However, because the object is social, the observer may be part of this object of study. In this way, the analysis may contain an explanation or critique of the observer's methods.

The key point is that science has an object of study that is real and independent from the mind, concepts, and language of the scientist. Failing to recognize this separation produces various forms of "idealism." For example, for the Empiricists such Hume or Berkeley, the outside world can only be sensed, and there is no proof of anything outside of these sensations. For Kant, what is sensed is also acted on by the mind to create various scientific concepts, but these mental procedures conceptualize the world in a human form. The real world cannot be known. These notions produce an inconsistency because, if all knowledge must be sensed, then how can we know that there is a real world separate from us?

Since Kant, a debate has existed between those who believe that the world can be known only through causal experiences and those who believe that it can be known only known through understanding. The updated version is between positivists and hermeneuticists (or subjectivists). As opposed to positivists who see science as value free, subjectivists view all activities as grounded in meanings and values. Several problems arise from this perspective that are relevant with respect to the postmodern critique of science. The first problem concerns what Bhaskar (1978) terms "the epistemic fallacy," in which it is assumed that how we come to know the world (epistemology) is how the world is really structured (ontology). Thus, one version might be a linguistic fallacy (Bhaskar, 1979). For example, Bhaskar (1979) cites the example of one theorist who asserted that "suicides" could not "correctly be said to exist" until a categorization had been made. However, the outer world (including the concrete individual as an object of study) cannot be reduced to a conceptual component. As Held (1980) notes, "this world is part of a complex that, however, symbolically mediated, is also shaped by the constraints of material conditions" (p. 316). Being tortured is not merely possessing an idea of what one is doing; it involves physical isolation and deprivation. Or Morris Zapp, in David Lodge's (1984) *Small World*, when queried about deconstructionists not believing in the individual, responds, "They don't. But death is one concept you can't deconstruct … I can die, therefore I am" (p. 324). He points out that he came to this realization after some would-be assassins "tried to deconstruct me." Thus, because many actions and practices are constructed in discourse does not mean they are wholly constituted by it (Spears & Parker, 1996). Moreover, as I shall discuss below, there are a variety of brain processes that affect emotion and behavior that occur in the absence of concepts. With respect to my case for science, the crucial point is that *there is a real external object and we must be careful to separate scientific activities from the actual object.*

Another important point has been that the opponents of science have used positivist science as a straw man to discredit the entire scientific enterprise. Positivism is based on the notion that for knowledge to be certain there must be a conjunction of events (Bhaskar, 1979). Hence, the world is viewed as atomistic and the person is passive. However, this is a restricted view of science. In the real world, a constant conjunction of events are extremely rare or artificially produced (Bhaskar, 1979). Occasionally, in the natural sciences, positivistic causality can be found where closed systems are possible. But in open systems, laws based on prediction of events are not likely. Rather, theories may point to tendencies and be explanatory. Explanations are needed to account for why a prediction may not occur. Moreover, if one adheres to a realist view, the world is not composed of events but of real structures, e.g., forces, fields, sets of relationships, and objects, and generative mechanisms that form the basis of causal laws. It is the real structures and mechanisms that must be examined. Within open systems, the ways these structures manifest themselves depends on their interaction with a multitude of other structures. Hence, to rely on a conjunction of events as a measure of validity is not supportable from a realist perspective. So, for example, is meteorology less of a science because its predictions are not always correct, although it has good explanatory value?

Postmodernists argue that knowledge is always wrapped up in language and social practices (Lewis, 2006). Therefore, multiple perspectives must be entertained and that multiple truths may exist because knowledge is linguistically mediated (Lewis, 2006). Although postmodernists regularly deny that "anything goes," they typically cast a very wide net with respect to what may go (Parker, 1998, 2000). Indeed, if one believes there is a real world, which is acknowledged by nearly all postmodernists, then some descriptions of parts of this world are better than others, and not all descriptions are equal. Science can overturn perspectives based on appearances, e.g., the Earth revolves around the sun and not vice versa as people had supposed.

As I have described above, we must distinguish between the transitive (where language and practices are involved) and the intransitive dimension (the real objects). Because language and social practices are tied to scientific practice does not mean that there is no longer a real object separate from the scientist. Several writers have underscored that things can at one and the same time be socially constructed and real (Brown *et al.*, 1998; Latour, 1993). Because scientific endeavor is socially situated, it means that we must critically evaluate the role of social forces in scientific practice in order to minimize social distortions (Collier, 1994). Harding (1991) has characterized these strengthened standards as "strong objectivity" (p. 142), and Collier (1994) has called his version "critical realism." Of course, we cannot completely eliminate social influences on scientific thought. However, it should not be "an all or nothing" issue. *Ultimately, each perspective must be tested against the real object.* All perspectives are not equal and that some perspectives have better explanatory or predictive power with respect to the real object. Depending on the object, there may be several useful perspectives.

Finally, to conclude this section, with appropriate caution, I propose that there are least two criteria that establish an activity as scientific. These are based on practices of scientists; what they do within the transitive dimension. First, as argued by Karl Popper (1963), science must have testable hypotheses. It seems reasonable that scientists should be able to frame an object for study, and that theories about this object should be capable of being tested in the real world. On the other hand, Popper's contention that scientists must make risky predictions provides too narrow a view of science because it eliminates practices that deal with open, multivariable systems. A second criterion, first suggested by Louis Althusser (1977), is that science differs from ideology because the former poses questions for study that opens up investigation whereas the latter closes it in advance. Consequently, science enables it to develop, deepen the knowledge it produces, in a process of internal transformations. Science is open to change from within, whereas ideology is a closed system. These propositions do not mean there is a single criterion of truth for use in all sciences. Rather, based on its particular object of study, each science establishes its own appropriate methods for testing its theories against the real object.

In summary, using the criteria described above, it is possible to begin to develop a liberatory psychiatry that is scientifically based. It does not mean that we cannot make choices as to what we wish to study, and it recognizes that the transitive dimension of science always has social influences. However, it is possible to take the latter into account. In so doing, we can radicalize our science, and make it our own.

In the next sections I will lay the groundwork for a progressive or liberatory psychiatry. I propose six elements as the basis for a liberatory psychiatry. The initial three elements follow from the discussion laid out in this section. The last three items will be developed in the next section.

(1) The theory must be consistent with materialist realism.

(2) The transitive dimension must be subject to a critique that recognizes and attempts to minimize the role of ideological elements in its language and methods.

(3) The theory must be tested against the real object.
(4) The object of study must be real persons in real relations.
(5) It must be able to account for the psychology of persons in general as well as being able to account for the psychology of a concrete individual.
(6) It must reflect the impact of the social system and biological processes on psychological development.

Problems with prior attempts at a progressive psychiatry project

In this section, I illustrate some of the problems encountered previously in developing progressive psychologies, especially those that have attempted to establish a psychology to complement Marxist or Neo-Marxist political economic accounts. Any psychology must at some point address the question of "What is an individual?" Both politically progressive theorists as well as mainstream theorists have devised different responses to this question. Building on the work of Shames (1982), who outlined the first five categories; this can be summarized into six categories:

(1) The individual enters the world equipped with a set of biological predispositions, homologous to those that rule the animal world, which are then modified and transformed by "society" to produce a personality.
(2) The individual comes into the world equipped with a pre-existing set of potential faculties that is subsequently filled in through interaction with the "social environment."
(3) The individual has no real existence at all, but is a composite manifestation of: (a) internal biological processes, or (b) external behavioral contingencies.
(4) The individual has no real existence but is a subjective and objective illusion created by cultural conventions, or is simply a point of intersection of a nexus of relationships.
(5) An "ex-centered" view of individual in which the "essence" of human individuals, although manifesting itself within concrete persons, has its source outside the individual in the "ensemble of social relations." The origin of human capacities and attributes in general are the historical products of human activity. The singular individual develops his or her capacities and attributes through individual activity within this larger systems of social relations. The relationship between the general and the particular depend upon specific productive relationships of the social system, i.e., the concrete individual in each system is limited by the potentials of human beings in general.
(6) An expanded version of the excentered individual in which biological along with social processes comprise the individual in general as well as accounting for specific individuals.

Models 1 and 2 describe variants of the humanist perspective. Humanist models rely on some pre-existing human foundation or essence. Psychology, because of its focus on the individual, has a propensity to use fundamental individual qualities as the point of departure to explain psychological and social life. Even when socio-logical theories are incorporated into psychological theory, there is a tendency to use those theories that are individually focused, e.g., roles, norms. Humanist theories look outside of human history to explain human individuality. The individual is seen as prior to the relations into which he or she enters.

Max Horkheimer pointed out many years ago that humanist theories have a special difficulty in coming to grips with the fact that new individual and social qualities arise as a result of individual experiences and broader historical processes (Held, 1980). Rather, humanists' reaction to this fact takes one of two forms. One form is mechanical evolution: all human characteristics that arise at a later point were originally present in germ (presumably genetic). Alternatively, it takes the form of some variety of philosophical anthropology: these characteristics emerge from a metaphysical "ground" of being. "These mutually opposed theories fail to do justice to the methodological principle that human processes are marked by structural change no less than by continuous development" (Horkheimer cited in Held, 1980, p. 118). Althusser's (1977) view of ideology is also relevant here. Starting with an established *a priori* view of humans will ultimately lead back to the original assumption. This is essentially a closed (ideological) system. Moreover, such spec-ulations of human nature are rarely posed in any testable form, and certainly none have ever been empirically verified.

Let me provide a few illustrations of how this perspective pervades much of the conceptual thinking in psychology and social psychology. In non-Marxist theories, these models have used what Seve terms "abstract generalities" (Seve, 1978; Shames, 1981). Abstract generalities are based on taking differences (and correlatively similarities) between individual objects in order to create a "general object." For example, in the social science literature, observations are made on a particular population and then a "modal individual" is conceived (e.g., "The Bowery Man," "The Mexican Peasant"). This approach poses several problems. One of the fundamental deficiencies of the abstract generality is its inability to explain the concrete singular case. By abstracting out commonalities, the "general" is made to appear real and essential, and the singular becomes unreal and inessen-tial. Hence, there is no way to account for the development of the singular, concrete individual. One of the reasons is that it views individuals as separate entities, ignoring the real ties that unite individuals. Thus, the "abstract generality" model is paradoxical in that it begins with the singular concrete person, but is unable to return to it. If our task is to develop a psychology of the individual, this is a substantial obstacle.

Marxist humanists (e.g., Fromm, 1961; Ollman, 1976) have placed a heavy reliance on the early works of Marx, especially the 1844 Manuscripts that were re-discovered many years after Marx's death. For instance, Ollman (1976) divided the Marxist versions of models 1 and 2 into "natural man" and "species man," respectively. Bertell Ollman argues that Marx has "a conception of man outside of history" (Ollman, 1976, p. 74). He suggests that "power" and "need" are keys to understanding Marx's concept of human nature in general. Olllman describes human's "natural powers and needs" as those that are shared with every living entity. They are impulses toward objects outside the body, e.g., the drive to eat. However, natural powers are processes of life devoid of human attributes. On the other hand, "species powers and needs" are those that humans alone possess. They are what set humans apart as a "species being," from the rest of the animal world. Ollman lists the following as examples of species powers: seeing, hearing, smelling, tasting, feeling, thinking, being aware, sensing, wanting, acting, loving, willing, procreating, sex, knowing, and judging. However, here again, a variety of human characteristics are abstracted out and made into general essences of the human beings. The potpourri of attributes that Ollman lists as characteristics of "species being" contains all sorts of behaviors that have been divested of their historical and social contexts.

Similar speculative properties pervade the psychoanalytic literature and have influenced a number of structuralists, existentialists, and postmodernist thinkers. Because the proponents claim to be materialists and even scientific, they suggest that their concepts have a biological basis. Reich (1972) describes the libido "as a borderline concept between the psychic and the somatic" (p. 15). Lacan's notion of desire is seen as having a biological support, but the latter does not constitute or determine it (Althusser, 1971). Lacan had several views concerning "desire" (Deleuze & Guattari, 1972). One view conceptualizes desire as a type of production going beyond any idea of need, lack, or idea of fantasy. The second view is based on his concept of "the Other," which reintroduces the idea of lack, e.g., the desire for the mother. Deleuze and Guattari took up the notion of the former and characterized persons as desiring machines, and they saw the economy itself as rooted in the materiality of desire and it physical forces (Best & Kellner, 1991). Lyotard celebrates "desire" for providing intensities of experience, liberation from repressive conditions, and creativity (Best & Kellner, 1991). Sartre likewise talks about "desire" that propels persons into various relationships with things, e.g., doing and making, having, and being (Poster, 1975). The early Frankfurt School argued that "reason" and "freedom" are immanent to human beings. Later, Marcuse shifted the focus from Reason to Eros (Held, 1980).

For radicals, the attraction of humanist psychologies is that they begin with a fundamental (ideal) concept of humans (e.g., desire, Eros, freedom, reason) that has become distorted by the existing sociopolitical system and, by overthrowing this system, our true natures can flourish. The problem with these concepts is that, if desire, libido, or Eros are tied to a biological base, what constitutes this base? Moreover, what are the mechanisms that transform the biological base into psychological phenomena? It is difficult to address any of these questions because of the way these concepts are defined. Hence, these fundamental properties are not testable, and therefore not verifiable.

Model 3 describes "reductionism," which means that the all levels of phenomena are explained in terms of a single level. Reductionist thinking owes much of its difficulties to the choice of a point of departure. Theorists who begin at the individual level are more predisposed to reduce phenomena to a biological level, whereas those who begin with society are more likely to view phenomena at a social level. As a caveat, although our current state of affairs views the biological, psychological, and social as separate emergent levels of analysis (i.e., different organization of matter with properties not possessed by the other levels), it is at least theoretically conceivable that various aspects of psychology such as consciousness could eventually be understood on a physiological level, much as chemistry and physics began to merge over the centuries. However, for the present, we will assume that they are discrete levels of organization.

With respect to a theory of human psychology, sociobiology and its successor, evolutionary psychology (Gander, 2003), represent good illustrations of reductionistic thinking. For example, Wilson (1975) suggests that "altruism," "selfishness," and "slavery" have their parallels in the animal kingdom, thereby promising that genetics will ultimately account for these phenomena. Evolutionary theorists contend that various human behaviors exist because they have evolutionary survival value. Thus, they must be heritable or biologically based. However, this approach creates several problems: (a) It treats terms such as "altruism" or "selfishness" as unitary, concrete concepts and ignores their many different forms and how they may vary based on context; (b) Many of these concepts have irreducible social elements (e.g., suicide as a type of "altruism" varies based on cultural context); (c) Many of these concepts are not framed in testable form.

Behaviorism, is based on a social reductionism, in which the individual is reduced to external behavioral contingencies. For behaviorists, "all organisms are the same; all are empty, manipulable things without an organizing principle, without substance and solidity" (Ratner, 1971). There are various critiques of this model (Mishler, 1976; Ratner, 1971). Among the most important is the absence of social context and meaning. For example, there is no context for why certain causal agents exist. "Behavior" is reduced to discrete acts devoid of meaning, context, or embedded social relationships, and there is no sense of power relationships since the reinforcement model views society as an interdependent, symmetrical and reciprocal controlling mechanism.

With respect to Model 4, which proposes that the individual has no real existence but is a subjective and objective illusion, the structuralists anticipated the postmodernists by declaring that "there is no such things as individuals as such" (Callinicos, 1976). Whereas for the postmodernists, persons are products of language, for structuralists individuals are embodiments of processes. Persons are viewed as the agents of the mode of production – in the role of capitalists, workers, and so forth – according to the positions to which they are assigned through the mechanisms reproducing the social formation. Louis Althusser (1977), one of the leading structuralists, made an assault on humanism, especially on the notion that history can be explained as a predetermined drama in which the human essence is alienated and then reconciled. As noted previously, Althusser argued that any predetermined (teleological) process closes history to science and replaces it with ideology. Thus, to counter the a priori subject of history, Althusser eliminated the subject (i.e., "process without subject"). This opens up scientific analysis. History and individuals are then conceived as developing in accordance with particular overdetermined configurations (structures). Contradictions or conflicts in these structures produce movement in a particular direction. Consequently, individuals are nodal points (i.e., bearers) of these structures. Moreover, our sense of individuality (subjectivity) is produced by ideology; that is, the illusion that history was made for us.

One of the strengths of the postmodernist critique in psychology has been its emphasis on the social construction of the self and the various categories that figure prominently in modern psychology such as "emotions," "attitudes," "intelligence," "personality," and "motivation" (Danziger, 1997; Pfister & Schnog, 1997). With its move away from the modernist themes of universal truths and "objectivity," postmodernism focuses on local interactions and communal networks, and how persons are a "but a network of relations" (Kvale, 1992, p. 36). The individual becomes a medium for the culture and language. Kvale (1992) writes "that in contrast to the individualist and intra-psychic terminology of modern psychology, there is a deindividualization and externalization of the person in a postmodern discourse. There is a move from inside to outside, from knower to known" (p. 15). Foucault and his followers have figured prominently in this theoretical movement. They have addressed these issues on a micro-level (Best & Kellner, 1991). Rather than focus on broader structural arrangements, they have concentrated on how certain versions of self are created by power relations that control the language that defines individuals. Here again, we are dealing with decentered selves that depend on institutional and disciplinary forces to create individual identities.

These approaches put us on the path to a more scientific psychology, by eliminating the speculative foundationalism of the humanists. However, we pay a hefty price by sacrificing the concrete, biological individual. Humans are more than the repository of structures or language. Although these writers recognize the physical being, it is seems to be conveniently forgotten or obscured. For Althusser (1971), it is relegated to a footnote and considered in the shadowy background of "support." Foucault (1980) refers to "bodies and pleasures" in developing a bio-struggle against oppressive ways of defining the body. However, it is not clear as to what realm of the body he is referring, and he seems to be lapsing into an essentialist anthropology that he typically has attacked as humanism (Best & Kellner, 1991).

A second problem with the structuralists and Foucauldians are their inability to account for the singular individual. Structures and language create individuals in general, but can these structures and the forms of power and knowledge account for the real individual? Both Althusser and Foucault generally avoid pre-given human essences, but substitute pre-given relations. Thus, relations or knowledge/language are real and external with respect to unreal, nodal individuals. As Best and Kellner (1991) contend, "On Foucault's account, power is mostly treated as an impersonal and anonymous force which is exercised apart from the actions and intentions of human subjects. Foucault methodologically brackets the question of who controls and uses power for which interests to focus on the means by which it operates . . . it occludes the extent to which power is still controlled and administered by specific and identifiable agents in positions of economic and political power" (p. 70).

From a structural perspective, individuals can be viewed as having no independent ontological status except as nodes of relations or moments of relationship. An unsatisfactory alternative would be to believe that only individuals are real, and that relations are not real but derivative ways of describing how such individuals stand to each other. However, I am arguing for an ontology that maintains that there are *real* individuals in *real* relations. In other words, individuals and relations are inseparable concepts, and that such one-sided interpretations are conceptual abstractions from concrete reality.

This perspective means that neither the individual nor the social structure should be used as abstract points of departure. Bhaskar (1979) makes the point that we should not forget that individuals do not create society, they transform it. People are born into an active, social world from which he/she learns values, faces demands, and the like. Given this material world into which the person enters, the individual then acts into the world. The interaction of these individuals, their activities, their relations, and the material product of their activities comprise the higher level of complexity that we call society. Moreover, Reed (1996) observes that, while situations of embodied agents may constrain their actions, at the same time these constraints may suggest possibilities for action.

The fifth model has been espoused by the French Marxist Lucien Seve (1978), the Russian psychologist A. N. Leontyev (1978), and the German critical psychologists (Tolman & Maiers, 1991). They promote an "ex-centered" view of the individual in which a person's capacities and attributes, although manifesting within concrete individuals, have their source outside the individual – in the ensemble of social relations. Human capacities and attributes *in general* are the historical products of human activity. The singular individual develops his or her capacities and personal attributes through activity within the larger system of social relations. The relationship between the general and the particular depend upon specific productive relationships of the social system, i.e., the concrete individual is limited by the potential of human beings in general. Thus, as Seve (1978) proposed, if personality can be characterized as "an enormous accumulation of varied acts over time," then the type of activities an individual engages in is crucial for the development of the personality. Workers who sell their labor are involved in a whole set of relations to capital, to money, and to machinery. The social system also creates new needs such as consumer goods, leisure activities, and services. Moreover, through growth and technology, an expansion of human capacities in general occurs. Thus, social activities, need creation, and technological growth form the individual in general as well as shaping the specific activities, needs, and capacities of the singular individual.

The limitation of this approach is that it fails to address adequately the role that biology plays in psychological development of persons in general as well as in the singular individual. Seve (1978) believes that human psychological processes have become functionally independent of biological organization. Thus, the body provides the initial support for the appearance of human life in psychological forms. Leontyev (1978), allows a greater role for biological processes but describes the latter's role in a non-specific metaphysical way: there is a two-sided movement with a spiral form resulting in the formation of higher levels and the leaving or alteration of lower levels (e.g., such as biological adaptations), which in turn serves the possibility of further development of the system as a whole. What does this mean concretely? What precisely is the role of physiological processes in psychological development and functioning? Finally, these theorists are especially weak with respect to unconscious cognitive processes and the role of emotion in psychological functioning. Both view the unconscious as different layers of awareness, and they neglect the role that unconscious emotions play in psychological functioning.

In summary, there are two critical questions that must be addressed if we are to develop a liberatory psychology:

(1) How does the social and biological world mediate its effect on the psychology of each individual?

(2) What is the "motor" of individual development? That is, what factors move persons to develop in a certain direction?

In this section, I have shown that most progressive theorists have more systematically explored the mediations of the social world, and that the role of the biological realm has been minimized or ignored. Paradoxically, many of the theories ultimately depend on a biological underpinning, but this underpinning is poorly conceived and lacks any scientific credibility. For example, the humanists typically use a model in which begins with some pre-existing human foundation (e.g., species being, desire, libido) that interacts with social forces. Such foundations are attributed to biological processes, but are imprecisely defined. Consequently, it is impossible to systematically test these foundational elements.

How the social world mediates its effect on human development has been addressed in several ways. One approach is to use language as the mediator between culture and person, e.g., culture through language imposes constraints on desire/libido, and desire/libido finds symbolic expression in the social world. However, others believe that language does not exhaust all the ways society mediates its effects on people. Real activities and relationships, and the attendant constraints they place on individuals are also theorized as important.

Finally, based on my critique of existing models 1 to 5, I believe that Model 6 may be the most fruitful pathway towards a progressive psychology. It expands on the ex-centered individual so that biological along with social processes determine the individual in general as well as accounting for specific concrete individuals. However, everything remains speculative until we pose testable questions such as how social mediators are actually processed by physiological processes, and how they interact to create psychological processes? These are scientific questions and underscore the importance of examining the biological realm and the value of the scientific endeavor. As I have shown, progressive psychological theory has not only neglected the biological realm, but has often substituted metaphysical concepts for real biological processes. What should be clear from this discussion is the important role for biology in human psychology. Such an endeavor does not mean that we have to lapse until biological reductionism. We will address these issues in the next section.

Resurrecting the biological realm

There are several reasons to examine the biological sphere more systematically. First, as I noted, we need to be able to examine how the social world comes to affect psychology as well as the impact that physiological processes directly have on human psychology. Second, if one of our aims is to examine why persons don't act in their best interests, at least part of this explanation may lie in unconscious cognitive processes. Progressives have typically had difficulty addressing the role of the unconscious. For the most part, they have followed the Enlightenment views of consciousness and rationalism. For example, Marxism, typically uses "consciousness" as a type of awareness. Thus, capitalism creates illusions of independence and obscures the real underlying relations that serve to exploit workers. The aim of revolutionary activity is to make persons more conscious with respect to the impact of capitalist relations on their lives. Moreover, the future communist society will be guided by consciously rational principles that will eliminate the vagaries and inequities of capitalist economies.

Even when persons have some insight into their objective conditions, they often do not act rationally in their best interests. Theorists turned to psychoanalysis for the answer. Psychoanalysis proposes that, beneath the surface world of conscious intentions and meanings, there is a world of unconscious wishes and motives that affects these surface appearances. Both Wilhelm Reich (1972) and early Frankfurt School theorists relied heavily on Freud's instinct theory (Fromm, 1970; Held, 1980; Wolfenstein, 1993). The patriarchal family repressed legitimate individual desires and rational thinking. Reich proposed that character formation occurs during the Oedipal period when the patriarchal family suppresses sexual impulses. This suppression of sexual impulses has two effects: sexual energy is channeled into character structures that simultaneously ward-off sex impulses and provide partial gratification. Every society creates those character forms that it needs for its preservation. Character structure deadens people so that they do much of the repetitive, mind-numbing, non-fulfilling work of capitalist societies. Moreover, Reich contends that sexual repression paralyzes rebellious forces because any rebellion is laden with anxiety and produces, by inhibiting sexual curiosity and thinking in the child, a general inhibition of critical facilities. Hence, character structure concomitantly tends to make full sexual experience and rational social consciousness extremely difficult, if not impossible (Ollman, 1979).

The later Frankfurt School theorists, particularly Herbert Marcuse, maintained that in late capitalism the family was no longer used to impose moral directives and restrain gratification. Rather, the new society controlled individuals directly from above: "[The individual] is rendered one dimensional through the infusion of the content of her/his ego from the outside by the apparatus of social domination" (Brown, p. 158). Marcuse (1962) refers to a "repressive desublimation" that occurs to ensure that individuals consume whatever the needs of the economic system require. Thus, the classical anal character is relaxed in favour of a "loose structure characterized by desire for instant gratification, by the predominance of emotions over consciousness and conscience." This theme is similarly invoked by Deleuze and Guattari (1972) with to respect to "deterritorialization" in which unchaining of material production and repressive social codes allows desire to move outside of restrictive psychic and special boundaries. But capitalism also re-channels (reterritorializes) desire and needs into inhibiting psychic and social spaces that control persons within the state, family, consumerism, and other institutions. Much of this occurs through language and symbolism.

Both Habermas and Lacan, without denying Freud's instinctual theory, comprehend much of Freud's historical instinctual concepts (e.g., Oedipal relations) as forms of symbolic communication. For Habermas, institutions and technology "suppress the ability of the people to interpret their need dispositions as well as to sanction various needs so as to create a symbolic system of enforced substitute gratifications whose character becomes fixed and opaque. In this way, the institutional framework of class society comes to constitute a self-reproducing system of power which is imposed on all its members and serves to censor and channel . . . energies toward ends which are predefined as 'legitimate'" (Brown, 1973, p. 84).

Thus, the attraction of psychoanalysis for radicals has been its ability to provide a psychological component as to why persons do not rebel against seemingly oppressive and non-fulfilling life circumstances. The fact that the processes occur unconsciously contributes to their effectiveness. Numerous criticisms have been lodged against psychoanalysis such as its metaphysical concepts, particularly Eros, libido, and Thanatos, its cultural, class, and gender biases, and the lack of correspondence between infantile fantasies and scientific evidence about cognitive development (Lichtman, 1982; Wolfenstein, 1993; Kagan, 1998; Stern, 1985). However, its recognition of the unconscious and the role that symbolism plays in the substitution gratification of unconscious desires seems worth retaining. Nevertheless, for our present discussion, a key question is what we make of the underlying basis of the unconscious – is it biological or not?

Richard Lichtman (1982) insists that the unconscious must be viewed as thoroughly social. The unconscious is "that portion of ourselves which we alienate from conscious awareness under pressure of intolerable social forces: it is the region of our being in which we flee from those aspects of ourselves which threaten us with dissolution" (Lichtman, 1982, p. 178). The social structure creates a double-bind for individuals. It creates desires and emotions that it requires of individuals but that cannot be acknowledged such as hostility or envy. These emotions and desires are forced into the unconscious where of variety of mechanisms are employed to deal with them. Lichtman contends that psychological defense mechanisms are historically conditioned, and are shaped by what they defend, by whom, for what purpose, against which authority, in what particular manner. He cites the observations by psychoanalyst Otto Fenichel in the 1940s that sexual impulses were often repressed whereas aggressive impulses were handled through other defense mechanisms. This is because, at that time, education handled the subject of sex by not mentioning it, whereas aggressiveness is mentioned but is designated as bad.

Although Lichtman's formulation undermines the ahistorical quality of the psychoanalytic unconscious, it does not eliminate the biological underpinnings that must exist to some extent with respect to the processing and expression of desires and emotions. In fact, Lichtman's hypothesis combined with recent cognitive neuroscientific findings, allows for transforming some of the metaphysical concepts into measurable variables. Moreover, the "psychoanalytic unconscious" may be best viewed as part of a larger cognitive unconscious.

This leads to the crux of this last section of the chapter, which is a call to radicalize biology. For a liberatory psychiatry to emerge we must make biological findings our own. I will show that neurophysiological and neurocognitive findings can be used for liberatory purposes. That we can push biological research in ways to promote emancipation. It has become clear that Descartes was wrong on two points. (1) The mind and body are not separate. We now recognize that "the body plays an active role in mental life" (Pally, 2000, p. 80). (2) Consciousness and mind are not the same thing (Wilson, 2002); rather, many mental processes occur below our awareness. Although much further elaboration is needed, it is evident that consciousness involves linking widely distributed areas of the brain into complicated patterns, rather than feeding all the information into a central coordinating region. This is probably why consciousness takes time (Pally, 2000), and why most mental activity is conducted below conscious awareness.

Neuroscientists have found that the most interesting processes about the human mind – judgments, feelings, motives – typically occur outside of awareness for reasons of efficiency. Timothy Wilson (2002) points out that unconscious mental activities involve not only low-level processes such as perceptual processes but also higher-order psychological processes and states. The adaptive unconscious differs considerably from the Freudian unconscious that was based on repressed unconscious urges and desires, and held the possibility of accessing these unconscious thoughts if repression was overcome. The adaptive unconscious always remains out of awareness. Bargh and Chartrand (1999) have described it as "the unbearable automaticity of being." There are marked differences between conscious and unconscious processes. Some of these differences are outlined below in Table 1.1, which is adapted from Wilson (2002).

The characteristics of the adaptive unconscious have implications with respect to understanding human behavior and, consequently, it may help us better apprehend receptiveness to social and political change. Below, I provide a few illustrations of how the adaptive unconscious works with respect to making judgments, emotionality, and dealing with stress.

The social interactionist approach theorizes that people think about the consequences of their action, whereas the "social intuitionist" approach believes in the social part but questions the causal role of reflective conscious thinking (Haidt,

Table 1.1. Comparison of conscious and unconscious processes

Conscious	Adaptive unconscious
Slow	Fast
Limited data	Almost unlimited data
Voluntary/intentional	Involuntary/unintentional
Demands attention/resources	No demand on attention
Flexible	Rote-rigid
Controlled (slow, effortful)	Automatic (fast, unintentional)
Serial processing	Parallel distributed processing
Symbolic manipulation/analytic	Pattern matching; metaphorical/holistic
Context independent	Context dependent
Fine-tuned details	Rough details
Fine motor control	Rough motor control
Platform independent	Platform dependent (brain/body dependent)
Unique to humans over age 2	Common to all animals
Sensitive to positive information	Sensitive to negative information

2001). The social intuitionist model states that reasoning is rarely the direct cause of judgments. Freud viewed people's judgments as driven by sexually determined unconscious motives and feelings, which was then rationalized with publicly acceptable reasons. The social intuitionist model expands the Freudian framework.

The case for the social intuitionist model is as follows (Haidt, 2001).

(1) Automatic evaluation: emotional evaluations typically occur so quickly and follow a principle of least effort.

(2) Motivating problem: reasoning is more like a lawyer defending a client than a judge or scientist seeking the truth. It is usually sufficient to attain social harmony, coherency, and some supporting evidence. The mind needs to make fairly quick but accurate perceptions and predictions.

(3) The reasoning process readily constructs justifications of intuitive judgments creating the illusion of objective reasoning.

(4) Moral action correlates with moral emotion more than with moral reasoning: emotional and self-regulatory factors affect moral action. For example, persons with brain damage to the orbitofrontal cortex, which assesses emotions, can solve problems but show poor judgment and indecisiveness. Emotions (e.g., empathy, reflexive distress, sadness, guilt, shame) primarily lead to altruism.

Several writers have referred to these findings regarding rationality as a "bounded rationality" instead of classic rationality (Gigerenzer & Goldstein, 1996). That is, information processing needs to "satisfice" rather than optimize.

"Satisfice" is a blend of satisfying and sufficing. People neither look up nor integrate all information but they *take their best bet*. People under limited time can't carry out an unlimited rational analysis. They must make fast inferences or predictions. Such approaches typically outperform other methods for speed and accuracy. Most predictions are rough guesses. They are good enough matching most of the time. People use consciousness for the new, unpredictable, and the ambiguous; primarily as a correcting device. People are primed to predict based on past experiences. What a person expects to happen will affect perception. Predictions are also made regarding interpersonal activities. Empathy and imitation occur unconsciously. People react to what they expect in others. People anticipate disappointments, hurts, rejection, and humiliation. They repetitively experience the past.

The role of emotion is to coordinate the body and mind (Pally, 2000). Antonio Demasio (2003) argues that every experience is accompanied by some degree of emotion and this is obviously important with respect to social and personal problems. Emotion organizes physiology, memory, perception, motivation, thought, behavior, and social interaction so as to enhance coping with the particular situation that is generating the emotion. For example, fear and anxiety increase the tendency to interpret the stimuli as dangerous, have frightening thoughts and memories, and to prime the person for a particular action. The amygdala, located in the forebrain, is thought to be one of the primary centers of emotional control, especially of fear, although no one brain region operates in isolation (LeDoux, 2000). Other brain areas that influence and assess emotion include the orbitofrontal cortex and the cingulate (Pally, 2000).

There is an interaction between emotional systems (mostly amygdala-based) and non-emotional memory related systems (mostly hippocampus-based). Thus, emotions affect memory and memory can affect emotions (Richter-Levin, 2004). We can also begin to see how language/symbols become embedded with emotional content. Emotions can be conscious as well as independent of consciousness. Thus, we are in the position to integrate emotional theory into the mechanisms of judgments and decision-making that were elaborated above. Emotions are not a substitute for proper reasoning, but it increases the efficiency of reasoning and makes it speedier (Damasio, 2003). As previously noted, there seem to be two paths involved in decision-making. One path – the fast, automatic one – involves the prompt activation of prior emotional experiences in comparable situations, and decisions can be made immediately ("gut" response). Demasio (2003) believes that emotions reflect body states (e.g., viscera, musculoskeletal system, and various organ systems) mapped out in the brain. The second path involves cortical involvement and more conscious reasoning strategies. However, even in this instance, prior emotional experiences may act *consciously or unconsciously* to influence working memory, attention, and reasoning so as to bias the decision based on prior emotional experiences.

Wilson (2002) believes that we essentially live with two selves, one residing in the adaptive unconscious that interprets the environment and establishes motives that guide people's behavior. The conscious self has no access to the unconscious self and if must construct stories to account for one's feelings and behaviors. The adaptive unconscious largely affects people's uncontrolled, more spontaneous responses whereas the conscious self tends to more important with respect to people's deliberative explicit responses. "Because people do not have access to all determinants of their beliefs and feelings, their reasons for doing things are often a function of cultural or personal theories that can be wrong or at best, incomplete" (Wilson, 2002, p. 168). Daniel Gilbert (2006) has found that people are poor predictors of future mood. For example, contrary to what most healthy people would anticipate, persons experiencing major trauma (e.g., accidents, rapes, war) often return to their pre-trauma emotional state. People are likewise poor predictors of what things would make them happy. Many beliefs about happiness are socially generated needs (e.g., wealth, having children) that often do not yield the anticipated pleasures.

Research has also found that the right brain is better able to detect anomalies and to make decisions to revise belief systems. The left brain interprets multiple inputs and tries to not be overwhelmed by all possible explanations in order to maintain a coherent belief system, even at the cost of denial or generating false reports (Gazzaniga, 1998). Thus, not only do people resist unconscious mental contents, but they also resist knowledge of conscious material if it does not fit well with their consciously held interpretations of reality. When no salient or meaningful changes occur in the environment, people do not have to attend consciously (Pally, 2000). Consciousness is needed when we notice changes and need to flexibly choose the most adaptive response to that change. As a result of the flexibility of consciousness, it is prone to forgetting and distortion as well as learning, growth, and change.

Finally, over the past decade many studies on stress have focused primarily on the hippocampus and amygdala (Sapolsky, 1996; Shors, 2006; Tsigos & Chrousos, 2002; Vyas *et al.*, 2002). In normal stress situations, the hippocampus provides feedback to break the stress response mediated by the hypothalamic–pituitary–adrenal (HPA) axis. The amygdala, on the other hand, tends to increase the stress response of the HPA axis. Research has shown that with chronic stress, or perhaps as a sequelae of traumatic stress, these feedback mechanisms begin to fail. Consequently, the hippocampus begins to lose cells and density, and the amygdala may increase in density. Although the impact of these changes is far from certain, in light of the hippocampus' and amygdala's role in memory, motivation, and emotion, it is likely that the effect of chronic stress on these brain regions will influence emotions and thinking. Will it make those who have experienced higher levels of stress more fearful or anxious? Or through its impact on the hippocampus (because of its memory and contextualization functions) will it make it difficult for persons to appropriately recognize and effectively channel emotions such as rage, frustration, or anger? Will this make persons less likely to act to change their circumstances?

Thus, to fully understand the individual, we must return to biology to appreciate the implication of cognitive processes on unconscious and automatic social behaviors. Indeed, it is likely that the information overload in modern society induces greater use of automatic behaviors, thereby increasing conformity and resistance to change – what we might call "surplus automaticity." Moreover, if the mental structures for maintaining belief systems are hard-wired into the nervous system, they will be more resistant to change. And for those individuals experiencing greater levels of stress, the normal relationship between the emotion and cognition may be disrupted, and affect persons' ability to act in their best interests.

Conclusions

To summarize the key points of this chapter:

(1) Progressives can embrace science if we do not restrict ourselves to a limited view of the enterprise. That is, it does not have to be based solely on positivism (atomistic elements) and predictions, but can also include relations/interactions as well as tendencies with explanations.

(2) Scientists and scientific theories are separate from real objects and forces. The validity of a theory depends on it being tested against the latter.

(3) All scientific theories contain social elements, but it is possible to critique them and take them into account as theory is developed and tested.

(4) In developing a progressive psychology we must account for real people within real relations.

(5) Failures to develop a progressive psychology have occurred because conceptual models have relied on speculative, untestable theories, or have ignored or minimized the concrete, biological individual, or real social relationships.

(6) In developing a progressive psychology we must recognize conscious and unconscious cognitive and emotional forces that act on the individual. This entails recognition of biological as well as social elements. An appreciation of neuroscience will be needed to understand how these elements become integrated.

(7) Progressives need to embrace science and biology, to radicalize it, and direct it towards the goal of promoting and sustaining human liberation.

REFERENCES

Althusser, L. (1971). *Lenin and Philosophy*. New York: Monthly Review Press.

Althusser, L. (1977). *For Marx*. London: New Left Books.

Bargh, J. A. & Chartrand, T. L. (1999). The unbearable automaticity of being. *American Psychologist*, **54**, 462–479.

Best, S. & Kellner, D. (1991). *Postmodern Theory. Critical Interrogations*. New York: Guilford Press.

Bhaskar, R. (1978). *A Realist Theory of Science*. Sussex: Harvester Press.

Bhaskar, R. (1979). *The Possibility of Naturalism*. Atlantic Highlands: Humanities Press.

Brown, B. (1973). *Marx, Freud, and the Critique of Everyday Life. Toward Permanent Cultural Revolution*. New York: Monthly Review Press.

Brown, N. O. (1959). *Life Against Death*. Middletown, CT: Wesleyan University Press.

Brown, S. D., Pujol, J., & Curt, B. C. (1998). As one in a web? Discourse, materiality, and the place of ethics. In *Social Constructionism, Discourse and Realism*, ed. I. Parker. London: Sage Publications.

Callinicos, A. (1976). *Althusser's Marxism*. London: Pluto Press.

Collier, A. (1979). In defence of epistemology. In *Issues in Marxist Philosophy. Volume 3.* ed. J. Mepham & D.-H. Rubin. Atlantic Highlands: Humanities Press.

Collier, A. (1994). *Critical Realism*. London: Verso.

Damasio, A. (2003). *Looking for Spinoza. Joy, Sorrow, and the Feeling Brain*. Orlando: Harcourt.

Danziger, K. (1997). *Naming the Mind. How Psychology Found Its Language*. London: Sage Publications.

Deleuze, G. & Guaattari, F. (1972). *Anti-Oedipus*. New York: Viking Press.

Dyson F. (2007). *The Scientist as Rebel*. New York: New York Review of Books.

Feyerabend, P. (1975). *Against Method*. London: New Left Books.

Foucault, M. (1980). *The History of Sexuality*. New York: Vintage.

Fromm, E. (1970). *The Crisis of Psychoanalysis. Essays on Freud, Marx, and Social Psychology*. Greenwich, CO: Fawcett Publications.

Fromm, E. (1961). *Marx's Concept of Man*. New York: Frederick Ungar Publishing.

Gander, E. M. (2003). *On Our Minds. How Evolutionary Psychology is Reshaping the Nature-Versus-Nurture Debate*. Baltimore: Johns Hopkins University Press.

Gazzaniga, M. S. (1998). The split brain revisited. *Scientific American,* July issue, 50–53.

Gigerenzer, G. & Goldstein, D. G. (1996). Reasoning the fast and frugal way: Models of bounded rationality. *Psychological Review*, **103**, 650–669.

Gilbert, D. (2006). *Stumbling on Happiness*. New York: Alfred A. Knopf.

Haidt, J. (2001). The emotional dog and its rational tail: a social intuitionist approach to moral judgment. *Psychological Review*, **108**, 814–834.

Harding, S. (1991). *Whose Science? Whose Knowledge? Thinking For Women's Lives*. Ithaca: Cornell University Press.

Held, D. (1980). *Introduction to Critical Theory. Horkheimer to Habermas*. Berkeley: University of California.

Jacoby, R. (1975). *Social Amnesia*. Boston: Beacon Press.

Kagan, J. (1998). *Three Seductive Ideas*. Cambridge, MA: Harvard University Press.

Kuhn, T. (1962). *Structure of Scientific Revolutions*. Chicago: University of Chicago Press.

Kvale, S. (ed.) (1992). *Psychology and Postmodernism*. London: Sage Publications.

Latour, B. (1993). *We Have Never Been Modern*. Cambridge, MA: Harvard University Press.

LeDoux, J.E. (2000). Emotional circuits in the brain. *Annual Review of Neuroscience*, **23**, 155–184.

Leontiev, A.N. (1978). *Activity, Consciousnes, and Personality*. New York: Prentice Hall.

Lewis B. (2006). *Moving Beyond Prozac, DSM, and the New Psychiatry. The Birth of Postpsychiatry*. Ann Arbor: University of Michigan.

Lichtman, R. (1982). *The Production of Desire*. New York: The Free Press.

Lodge, D. (1984). *Small World*. London: Penguin Books.

Marcuse, H. (1962). *Eros and Civilization*. New York: Vintage Books.

Mishler, E.G. (1976). Skinnerism: materialism minus the dialectic. *Journal of Theory and Social Behavior*, **6**, 21–46.

Ollman, B. (1976). *Alienation. 2nd edn*. Cambridge: Cambridge University Press.

Ollman, B. (1979). *Social and Sexual Revolution*. Boston: South End Press.

Pally, R. (2000). *The Mind-Brain Relationship*. London: Karnac Books.

Parker, I. (ed.) (1998). *Social Constructionism, Discourse and Realism*. London: Sage Publications.

Parker, I. (2000). Story-theories about and against postmodernism in psychology. In *Postmodern Psychologies, Societal Practice, and Political Life*, ed. Holzman, L. & Morss, J. New York: Routledge.

Popper, K. (1963). *Conjectures and Refutations*. New York: Harper Torchbooks.

Poster, M. (1975). *Existential Marxism in Postwar France*. Princeton: Princeton University Press.

Pfister, J. & Schnog, N. (eds.) (1997). *Inventing the Psychological*. New Haven: Yale University Press.

Ratner, C. (1971). Principles of dialectical psychology. *Telos*, Fall, no. 9, 83–109.

Reed, E.S. (1996). The challenge of historical materialist epistemology. In *Psychology and Society. Radical Theory and Practice*, ed. I. Parker & R. Spears. London: Pluto Press.

Reich, W. (1972). *Sex-Pol*. New York: Vintage Books.

Richter-Levin, G. (2004). The amygdala, the hippocampus, and emotional modulation of memory. *The Neuroscientist*, **10**, 31–39.

Robinson, P. (1969). *The Freudian Left (Wilhelm Reich, Geza Roheim, Herbert Marcuse)*. New York: Harper and Row.

Rossi, P. (2003). Magic, science, and the equality of human wits. In *Nature and Narrative. An Introduction to the New Philosophy of Psychiatry*, ed. B. Fulford, K. Morris, J. Sadler, & G. Stanghellini. Oxford: Oxford University Press.

Sampson, E.E. (1998). Life as an embodied art: the second stage beyond constructionism. In *Reconstructing the Psychological Subject. Bodies, Practices and Technologies*, ed. B.M. Bayer & J. Shotter, London: Sage Publications.

Sapolsky, R.M. (1996). Why stress is bad for your brain. *Science*, **273**, 749–750.

Seve, L. (1978). *Man in Marxist Theory and the Psychology of Personality*. Sussex: Harvester Press.

Shames, C. (1981). The scientific humanism of Lucien Seve. *Science and Society*, **45**, 1–23.

Shames, C. (1982). Dialectics and the theory of individuality. Unpublished manuscript.

Shors, T. J. (2006). Stressful life experiences and learning across the lifespan. *Annual Review of Psychology*, **57**, 55–85.

Spears, R. & Parker, I. (1996). Marxist theses and psychological themes. In *Psychology and Society. Radical Theory and Practice*, ed. I. Parker & R. Spears. London: Pluto Press.

Stern, D. N. (1985). *The Interpersonal World of the Infant. A View from Psychoanalysis and Developmental Psychology*. New York: Basic Books.

Tolman C. W. & Maiers, W. (eds.) (1991). *Critical Psychology. Contributions to an Historical Science of the Subject*. Cambridge: Cambridge University Press.

Tsigos, C. & Chrousos, G. P. (2002). Hypothalamic–pituitary–adrenal axis, neuroendocrine factors and stress. *Journal of Psychosomatic Research*, **53**, 865–871.

Vyas, A., Mitra, R., Shankaranarayana Rao, B. S., & Chattarji, S. (2002). Chronic stress induces contrasting patterns of dendritic remodeling in the hippocampal and amygdaloid neurons. *Journal of Neuroscience*, **22**, 6810–6818.

Wilson, E. O. (1975). *Sociobiology: A New Synthesis*. Cambridge, MA: Harvard University Press.

Wilson, T. D. (2002). *Strangers to Ourselves. Discovering the Adaptive Unconscious*. Cambridge, MA: Belnap Press of Harvard University Press.

Wolfenstein, E. V. (1993). *Psychoanalytic Marxism*. New York: Guilford Press.

Young, R. M. (1996). Evolution, biology and psychology from a Marxist point of view. In *Psychology and Society. Radical Theory and Practice*, ed. I. Parker & R. Spears. London: Pluto Press.

2

Power, freedom, and mental health: a postpsychiatry perspective

Philip Thomas and Pat Bracken

Through these different practices – psychological, medical, penitential, educational – a certain idea or model of humanity was developed, and now this idea of man has become normative, self-evident, and is supposed to be universal. Humanism may not be universal but may be quite relative to a certain situation … This does not mean that we have to get rid of what we call human rights or freedom, but that we can't say that freedom or human rights has to be limited at certain frontiers. For instance, if you asked 80 years ago if feminine virtue was part of universal humanism, everyone would have answered, yes. What I am afraid of about humanism is that it presents a certain form of our ethics as a universal model for any kind of freedom. I think that there are more secrets, more possible freedoms, and more inventions in our future than we can imagine in humanism as it is dogmatically represented on every side of the political rainbow: the Left, the Centre, the Right. (Foucault, 1988)

Some time ago, we were trying to help a young woman who heard voices. She had always found it impossible to talk about her experiences. People were unaware that she had the experience. She kept it hidden, a secret. And when the psychiatrists did find out, her worst fears were realized. She was told that she had schizophrenia (she knew that this was not so). She rejected their opinion.

On one occasion she was asked how long she had heard voices. Since I was seven, she replied. She then went on to tell *her* story. At that age, a neighbor had started to abuse her sexually. She was threatened not to tell anyone under pain of death. Shortly after this, she started to hear the voice of her abuser, threatening her with death. But she was (and remains) a courageous person. Even at the age of seven she wanted to talk with others about what was happening to her. One day she plucked up courage and asked her best friend at school. "Do you ever hear voices?" she asked, tentatively. "What do you mean?" her friend replied. "You know, like hearing someone when there's no one there." "No," her friend replied with a mixture of horror and derision, "that only happens to 'loonies'. You are going to be locked up in the loony bin."

Much later, she was detained in hospital for over 2 years. Large doses of neuroleptic drugs were injected forcibly into her body. She detested this. It was

Liberatory Psychiatry: Philosophy, Politics, and Mental Health, ed. Carl I. Cohen and Sami Timimi.
Published by Cambridge University Press. © Cambridge University Press.

humiliating, and besides, the medication caused her to put on weight. It also numbed her mind, making it impossible for her to use her own coping mechanisms, evolved over 20 long years of having to survive with the voices. However, her courage created a plane of resistance to her psychiatrist's attempts to purge her soul of her voices. She was determined that she would resist, that she would oppose their interpretations and actions upon her. She demanded a second opinion. She was refused. She repeated her demand, and continued to insist until her wishes were met.

This anecdote serves as an introduction to the issues we want to deal with in this chapter. It illustrates the ways in which constraints operate in our social lives. We do not control the ideas, constructions, words, and priorities of the worlds in which we live and grow. Instead, these representations present us with a picture of what it is to be human, to be normal, to be free. Wittingly or unwittingly, we are all bound by them. They hold our conduct within certain limits, but also incite us in certain directions and ultimately present us with a vision of what liberation and freedom are all about.

The years after the World War II witnessed an explosion in new ideas that challenged orthodox and established systems of belief. In the 1960s talk of liberation and freedom filled the air. The old colonial powers were relinquishing their grip on their former colonies. Black Power, the Women's Movement and Gay Liberation were flexing their muscles. In the midst of this, psychiatry added its voice. Well, to be precise, the anti-psychiatry movement did. For many, anti-psychiatry epitomized this spirit of rebellion. In 1967, four anti-psychiatrists (Joseph Berke, David Cooper, R. D. Laing and Leon Redler) organized the *Dialectics of Liberation Congress* at the Roundhouse in North London. The event drew together leading international figures, advocates of revolution and social change in the service of liberation. Stokely Carmichael spoke about Black Power; Herbert Marcuse a leading figure from the Frankfurt School of critical theorists, spoke about liberation from the affluent society (Cooper, 1968). Two intellectual traditions underscored this event: Marxism and psychoanalysis. For many of the participants the hope was that, by applying insights from these discourses to the ills of society, the world would be changed for the better. The congress was confident: revolution and real freedom were just around the corner. From where we are now, 40 years later, this appears hopelessly naïve. Our generation has witnessed terrible acts under the banners of revolution and liberation. In our postmodern times, progress is something full of contradictions; even freedom itself is no longer straightforward. And yet we know that things could be better, should be better, and we want to move forward. Progress, for all its difficulties, is something we aspire to. This book is called *Liberatory Psychiatry*. While this incorporates a noble aspiration, in our opinion this term is an oxymoron: psychiatry cannot be liberatory. In this chapter, we shall explore the complexities and paradoxes that arise when the words liberation and psychiatry are brought into conjunction.[1] We begin by examining some of the assumptions implicit in the ideas of the critical theorists and anti-psychiatrists of the 1960s and 1970s. We are particularly concerned with the role of psychoanalysis in these ideas, and that of the experts who use this knowledge. In our view, the work of Michel Foucault yields penetrating insights into the nature of power, and the relationship between power and subjectivity. We examine this work in some detail, and that of his followers, especially Gordon and Rose. We end by considering the implications of this Foucauldian analysis of power for our task today, as critical psychiatrists, and the future of the relationship between medicine and madness.

Our argument essentially is that the process of liberation and the state of freedom are simply more complex than allowed for in the thought of the 1960s radicals. As we enter the twenty-first century, we believe that there is a need to debate what these terms mean, particularly in regard to our thoughts, feelings, relationships, and behaviors. Furthermore, we argue that, whatever it is, liberation is not something that is in the gift of one professional group or another, or something to be defined by one professional discourse or another. Psychiatry *can* offer more real help and support to experts by experience;[2] it *can* be less controlling and more transparent, but it *cannot* offer liberation. The most that we can do as critical psychiatrists is to work towards more openness and honesty and through this to show how a great deal of psychiatric discourse is nothing more than mythology. In doing this, we hope to open spaces where other voices can be heard, particularly the voices of experts by experience. Maybe it is more appropriate to think of a critical psychiatry that works towards the facilitation of different liberations.

Liberation, anti-psychiatry and critical theory[3]

Both the anti-psychiatry movement and the Frankfurt school shared a common desire to move away from the influence of positivism, which they considered to have an oppressive influence on the human sciences. Both agreed on the importance of interpretation (as opposed to the causal explanation of science and positivism) in human affairs, and both settled on psychoanalysis as an appropriate hermeneutic tool[4] to understand human actions. In Chapter 2 of *The Divided Self*, Laing (1965) sets out the importance of understanding and hermeneutics, drawing on Dilthey's analogy concerning the interpretation of human action with the interpretation of hieroglyphics and other ancient texts. He makes a direct comparison between the interpretation of ancient hieroglyphs and the interpretation of "... psychotic 'hieroglyphic speech and actions.'" (Laing, 1965, p. 31). He also attacks positivism, pointing out that science can lead us to detailed knowledge about the genetics of manic depression or schizophrenia without us being able to understand a single schizophrenic person. In a similar manner, members of the Frankfurt School rejected the influence of positivism in the social sciences. David Ingleby (1981) is probably one of the best-known advocates of critical theory in relation to psychiatry, and psychoanalysis figures prominently in his ideas about hermeneutics. In an earlier paper, one of us (Bracken, 1995) has examined these earlier liberatory discourses in the light of Foucault's work. They share three features; self-reflection, repression, and liberation. Habermas (1971) argues that, just as psychoanalysis could liberate the patient from neurosis, when used in the service of critical social theory it could contribute to the liberation of society from ideology and cultural oppression. Habermas argued that, for this to happen, there had to be a universal standard of reason, or rationality. Without this there could be no rational criticism of social institutions. In addition, the "critical intellectual" whose expertise, understanding and insights could liberate society played a significant role in both critical theory and anti-psychiatry. In Marxist–Leninist terms the critical intellectual was to be in the "vanguard." Through the rational scientific analysis of our current situation, he/she was able to map the future. Ultimately, these ideas stem from the Enlightenment preoccu-pation with reason and progress, the belief that the nature of society could be improved progressively through the application of human reason to human problems. A good example of this is Marcuse's (1966) use of psychoanalytic theory to examine the problems of contemporary culture. He argued that modern society is dehumanized by what he called "repressive desublimation" in which sexual urges were channelled in socially acceptable ways. This meant that our need for love and intimacy were "desublimated" and directed away from family and loved ones to consumerism, serving the interests of consumer capitalism. In other words, capitalist culture is repressive of human instincts.

Foucault challenged this. He attacked the idea that society is repressive of sexuality (Foucault, 1978). Human nature and sexuality are not so much repressed by power as created by it. Repressive theories of sexuality are unable to account for the proliferation of different forms of sexuality during the twentieth century, as well as the impetus to categorize them. He also rejects the notion of a universal rationality through which we may judge whether we are making progress, arguing that it is not possible to separate reason from ideology (Foucault, 1977a). This is because his analysis of power and knowledge challenges the Marxist distinction between ideology and truth. For Foucault there is no such thing as a universal rationality that speaks the truth. Truth is contingent, tied to local practices and power relations. This means that there are many different rationalities. He argued that we must stop thinking of power simply in negative terms:

. . . power produces knowledge (and not simply by encouraging it, because it serves power or by applying it because it is useful). . . power and knowledge directly imply one another . . . there is no power relation without the correlative constitution of the field of knowledge, nor any knowledge that does not presuppose and constitute at the same time power relations. (Foucault, 1977a, p. 27)

This presents a challenge to the role of the critical intellectual who, through promoting social reflexivity based on a universal rationality, progresses society towards liberation and freedom. We can compare the actions of such an intellectual to the role of a psychoanalyst. In making interpretations, the analyst reinforces a particular view of the mind and subjectivity. Likewise, the critical intellectual analyses and interprets society's ills according to the principles of universal reason. However, if there is no such thing as universal reason, and truth is locally contingent, there can be no fixed meanings to a text. All that the act of interpretation achieves is to reveal earlier layers of interpretation. In other words our understanding of the world is not dependent upon some ultimate objective truth based in reason, but has been created by our predecessors and ourselves. This challenges the role of the critical intellectual as the "helmsman of progress." It means that society can no longer rely on the privileged position of the intellectual. Ordinary people:

. . . know perfectly well, without illusions; they know far better than he and they are certainly capable of expressing themselves. (Foucault, 1977b, p. 207)

Beyond anti-psychiatry

The years that followed the demise of anti-psychiatry saw three significant developments. First, there was a regrouping of biomedical psychiatrists. Stung by the attacks of those like Szasz, who argued that mental illness did not exist, and enraged by the anti-psychiatrists' accusations that the practice of psychiatry was oppressive, orthodox psychiatry rekindled the spirit of Kraepelin. DSM-III, published in 1980, represents the start of a process that continues today. Neo-Kraepelinism expunged psychoanalytic concepts and theories because they were unscientific. The salvation of psychiatry was to be achieved through the alliance of nosology with neuroscience. Second, psychiatric care moved into the community. This was seen by many as offering a less oppressive, more humane form of psychiatric care. Finally, new voices were being raised in question of psychiatry, particularly its claim to speak the truth about madness. These, of course, were the voices of those who had used mental health services.

Gordon (1986) points out that the origins of psychiatry are not only bound up with the Enlightenment, but also with modern conceptions of democracy and liberalism. Psychiatry is enmeshed with judgments, values and practices (or sanctions) that help to maintain an "appropriate" public consciousness. In order to be full citizens, we have to be rational autonomous beings. Psychiatry works to police the boundaries of what is deemed rational and claims expertise in judgments about capacity. But words like community care and citizen are problematic. Their meanings are many-hued, and thus subject to broad and imprecise definition. For example, "community care" may appeal as an ill-defined positive value in which the negative connotations of asylum and the identity of mental patient are replaced by something new, progressive, and better. However the expression can also be used to obscure undemocratic and oppressive practices such as the forced administration of medication in the community. It can thus be seen as a rhetorical device that casts those who use it in the light of liberatory practice, whilst continuing to practice oppressively in the shadows. This is not to deny that there have been genuinely liberatory achievements by psychiatrists and others working in the community,[5] but, as Gordon points out, such achievements were not possible through psychiatry alone. To a large extent, these more positive developments depended on legislative changes such as Law 180 in Italy and, as we shall see, direct action by those who had experienced madness.

Community care has been accused of creating a new class of non-citizen, the so-called revolving door patient, whose life is lived in a variety of disciplinary spaces, hospitals, prisons, and bail hostels. This group is more reviled and oppressed than the former asylum inmates largely because the policies of community care mean that they have much higher public visibility. It is not surprising that community psychiatry today has for some, especially members of Britain's Black and Minority Ethnic communities, become little more than a form of community policing. Gordon sees similar problems with citizenship. The prominent role played by psychiatry in diagnosing society's ills in part relates to its role in the restitution of the individual's citizenship. He suggests that this is a cover for the imposition of political order. Thus the position of psychiatry in advanced liberal democracies is deeply ambiguous. Unless we are able to examine critically these contradictory aspects of psychiatry, we will make no progress in answering questions about liberation and mental health. This is where Foucault's ideas concerning power and subjectivity are helpful.

Foucault: power and subjectivity

Foucault's later ideas make it possible for us to explore the connection between power and freedom in a way that reflects the complexity of the relationship. He argues that power and liberty are closely intertwined, and directly related to human subjectivity. In a late interview with Dreyfus and Rabinow, in 1982 (Foucault died in 1984), he looked specifically at the idea of liberation. He says that liberation involves engaging not just with the state and its rulers but also with how we are brought into being as subjects in a particular society:

> I would like to say, first of all, what has been the goal of my work during the last twenty years. It has not been to analyse the phenomena of power, nor to elaborate the foundations of such an analysis. My objective, instead, has been to create a history of the different modes by which, in our culture, human beings are made subjects. (Foucault, 1982, p. 208)

He points out that the word subject has two meanings. It can refer to a person who is subject to the control of another person. This is the sense in which some people in England speak of themselves as subjects of the monarch. But it can also refer to my awareness of my own identity as a person through self-knowledge. Both senses "... suggest a form of power which subjugates and makes subject to" (Foucault, 1982, p. 212). Foucault does not disavow earlier interpretations of power, like Marxist analyses couched in terms of the forces of production or class struggle (although as we saw earlier, he denies the claim of many Marxists that such analyses are foundationalist). He argues that the mechanisms of subjection are more complex than allowed for in foundationalist discourses such as traditional Marxism. He concludes:

> ... that the political, ethical, social, philosophical problem of our days is not to try to liberate the individual from the state, and the state's institutions, but to liberate us both from the state and from the type of individualization which is linked to the state. We have to promote new forms of subjectivity through the refusal of this kind of individuality which has been imposed on us for several centuries. (Foucault, 1982, p. 216)

He describes what it is that a number of contemporary social movements (or "oppositions" to use his expression) have in common, for example, feminist opposition to the power of men, those who were formerly colonial subjects to their colonizers, or the voices of mental health service survivors and consumers to psychiatry. It is difficult to dismiss these movements simply as anti-authoritarian struggles. They have a deeper significance because they have features in common. They extend beyond national boundaries, and are unrelated to specific political systems or economies. In addition, the aim of these struggles is primarily directed at power as it is manifested in our domestic lives and with regard to our bodies. This is liberation as a process, not a single and singular act of revolution. They are also "immediate" in the sense that those involved are those who are most closely affected by those who are the source of their oppression:

In such struggles people criticize instances of power which are the closest to them, those which exercise their action on individuals. They do not look for the "chief enemy," but for the immediate enemy. Nor do they expect to find a solution to their problem at a future date (that is, liberations, revolutions, end of class struggle). In comparison with a theoretical scale of explanations or a revolutionary order which polarizes the historian, they are anarchistic struggles. (Foucault, 1982, p. 211)

This point about the immediacy of the struggle is, in our view, particularly significant. It represents a point of departure from earlier liberatory discourses. To our knowledge, no experts by experience or survivors of psychiatry spoke at or were involved in the *Dialectics of Liberation* conference.

Another important feature of these struggles is that they are primarily concerned to assert the right of those involved to be different, by emphasizing the *value* of their individuality and difference. They resist attempts to separate and detach the individual from his or her community of difference, and to tie him or her to his or her own identity. They also stand in opposition to power linked to professional expertise (or "knowledge, competence and qualification" – Foucault, 1982, p. 212), such as psychiatry. They represent a struggle against mystification and the imposition of secretive representations on people. Such struggles, argues Foucault, are concerned most fundamentally with the question of human subjectivity:

Finally, all these present struggles revolve around the question: Who are we? They are a refusal of these abstractions, of economic and ideological state violence which ignore who we are individually, and also a refusal of a scientific or administrative inquisition which determines who one is. (Foucault, 1982, p. 212)

In his earlier lectures on psychiatry given at the *Collège de France* in 1973–1974, Foucault's genealogy[6] of French psychiatry draws him to the conclusion that, from the nineteenth century to the present day, one of the main features of psychiatric power has been its attempts to classify madness, and the futile invocation to clinical science to establish a medical truth about madness (Foucault, 2006). In addition, we can now begin to see that the knowledge and practices of psychiatry, its diagnostic categories, theories and therapies, play a particular role in the affairs of the State. It polices the boundaries of rationality, and does so by setting out clear criteria for normal subjectivity. It is not "normal" to hear voices. Furthermore, it dictates how such experiences are to be understood. People who hear voices must be suffering from schizophrenia. Voice hearing becomes a symptom of mental illness, not a gift, or a message from a divine presence. Ivan Leudar and one of the current writers (PT) have described the profound cultural shift in the meaning of the experience of voice hearing since the time of Socrates (Leudar & Thomas, 2000).

Foucault's analysis of the different modes of subjectivity suggests that there are other ways of challenging power, and thus thinking about how psychiatry might possibly be liberatory:

> I would like to suggest another way to go further towards a new economy of power relations, a way which is more empirical, more directly related to our present situation, and which implies more relations between theory and practice. It consists of taking the forms of resistance against different forms of power as a starting point. To use another metaphor, it consists of using this resistance as a chemical catalyst so as to bring to light power relations, locate their position, find out their point of applications and the methods used. Rather than analyzing power from the point of view of its internal rationality, it consists of analyzing power relations through the antagonism of strategies. (Foucault, 1982, pp. 210–211)

This can be seen in action in a wide variety of social movements over the last 30 years. Following the success of the Gay Pride movement, which from the 1970s on has celebrated and asserted gay identity and difference, Mad Pride and Mad Chicks are now doing the same for madness. These groups emphasize the value of the difference of madness. They see this difference in positive terms, and refuse to see it cast in terms of fear and horror. Since the 1980s the survivor movement has raised its voice with increasing effectiveness in opposition to psychiatry. This opposition takes many forms. It challenges the right of psychiatry to lock up and incarcerate; it opposes the use of psychiatric languages to interpret subjective experience in terms of mental disorder. Lisa Blackman (2001) has described the Hearing Voices Network as an "ethical space" in which people who hear voices can come together to explore different meanings and understandings of their experiences. In general, professionals are excluded from these groups, of which there are now in excess of 150 throughout Britain. The meanings and interpretations of experience is self-directed by those who attend these groups. They demonstrate Foucault's assertion that, in general, ordinary people know best how to interpret their worlds.

Power, conduct and government

In the fourth lecture at the *Collège de France*, Foucault (2006) uses Bentham's Panopticon to symbolize a new form of power, one that is aimed at regulating the conduct of the individual not the group. This is achieved through mental, not physical, power. Because those under surveillance have no idea when they are being observed, they must conduct themselves on the assumption that they could be observed at any moment. In other words, disciplinary power is internalized by each individual who then self-regulates his or her behavior. This is an important moment in the economy of power systems. It results ultimately in new forms of governmentality (Foucault, 1982, p. 224). But in his later works, Foucault is less interested in how power is exercised than he is in the effects of power. Power is ubiquitous. We are all affected by it in one way or another, but for Foucault, "Power exists only when it is put into action ..." (Foucault, 1982, p. 219), so a defining feature of power is that it is a mode of action on others that does not necessarily act immediately. It acts across time and space, and in doing so acts on human actions, present and future. In terms of the effects that power has, there are two components to consider. First, the "other" over whom power is exercised must be recognized as a person who has choices and is free to act, and second, that within a power relationship a wide range of possible responses and consequences of actions are revealed and made possible. Exercising power cannot simply be accounted for in terms of violence:

It is a total structure of actions brought to bear upon possible actions: it incites, it induces, it seduces, it makes it easier or more difficult: in the extreme it constrains or forbids absolutely; it is nevertheless always a way of acting upon an acting subject or acting subjects by virtue of their acting or being capable of action. A set of actions upon other actions. (Foucault, 1982, p. 220)

Foucault's concept of power moves us substantially away from Marxist and liberal accounts, which usually speak of power controlling, constricting, dominating, curtailing, and obscuring. Foucault's point is that power has polarity; it can be negative, but it can also be positive and productive, and in our historical period this is its most characteristic mode. Power in this sense is not opposed to freedom or liberation. Rather, it incites us to feel free and to express ourselves in terms of choices. In addition, power relations are woven inevitably into the fabric of society. Power is no longer something that is simply imposed on us from above, "A society without power relations can only be an abstraction." (Foucault, 1982, pp. 222–223). The ambiguous meaning of the word "conduct" can help us to understand the complexity of power. Conduct can mean how we behave and regulate our actions, but it can also refer to "leading" others, like the conductor of an orchestra. This suggests that the exercise of power involves guiding and leading the possibilities for the conduct of others, as well as specifying possible outcomes of conduct, such as rewards or sanctions. This is how government exercises power. Foucault argues that it is only possible to exercise power over subjects who themselves are free, that is to say individuals or groups who face choices as to how they might conduct themselves. He takes the example of slavery. Slaves are enchained. They have no choices and thus no possibilities for action. Slaves are not free, and so the relationship between the slave and slave-master cannot be a governmental power relationship in the way in which Foucault is using these terms. For him, government implies a more complex relationship in which freedom is a precondition for the exercise of power. In democracies, freedom and power are bound together in a reciprocal struggle.

If this is so, and the essence of power relationships involves a conflict between power and freedom, then there is no relationship of power without the possibility of escape. Power relationships cannot exist without points of insubordination and subversion that are axiomatically points of escape. This gives rise to what he calls confrontation strategies:

Accordingly, every intensification, every extension of power relations to make the insubordinate submit can only result in the limits of power. The latter reaches its final term either in a type of action which reduces the other to total impotence (in which case victory over the adversary replaces the exercise of power) or by a confrontation with those whom one governs and their transformation into adversaries. Which is to say that every strategy of confrontation dreams of becoming a relationship of power and every relationship of power leans toward the idea that, if it follows its own line of development and comes up against direct confrontation, it may become the winning strategy. (Foucault, 1982, pp. 225–226)

Rose takes these ideas about the nature of power further. He regards the rise of the "psy" complex (or psychology, psychiatry, and psychoanalysis) (Rose, 1985) as being closely related to changes in the way that advanced liberal democracies exercise power. He (Rose, 1986) has traced the genealogy of psychiatry, showing that the origins of nineteenth-century asylums were an essential feature of the governmental processes that were responsible for instilling the idea of discipline as a pre-requisite for liberty. Thus the "psy" complex is linked intrinsically not only to political power, but to government, a word that Foucault uses (as we have seen) in a broader sense than the activities of politicians and the political structures of state, and which is directed at the "conduct of conduct" (Rose, 1998, p. 12). According to Rose, these developments have important implications for freedom:

What is at stake in these analyses at their most general, therefore, is nothing less than freedom itself; freedom as it has been articulated into norms and principles for organizing our experience of our world and ourselves; freedom as it is realised in certain ways of exercising power over others; freedom as it has been articulated into certain rationales for practicing in relation to ourselves. (Rose, 1998, p. 16)

However, freedom in the governmental sense is conditional; in advanced liberal democracies we are *obliged* to be free but only in terms that are set out for us. These terms are normative and relate to different areas of our lives, for example, how we choose to dress and present ourselves to the world, our consumption of goods, how we express our sexuality, how we conduct ourselves when we are ill, sad or angry. But at the same time they constrain the possibilities that we have for action. Although we have choice, the choices that are on offer are normative choices with certain values attached. The rise of psychological and psychiatric expertise in the twentieth century is to be understood in terms of this normative function. It provides the expertise through which almost all areas of our lives are normatively interpreted and conducted for self-fulfilment – "Freedom, that is to say, is enabled only at the price of relying upon the experts of the soul." (Rose, 1998, p. 17).

Rose follows Foucault in considering the ambiguity of power. Freedom and power are not polar opposites; freedom is bound power. This is why it is necessary that we re-think the relationship between knowledge and subjectivity. If we are to use power in the service of freedom, we must move away from hegemonic notions of knowledge and expertise, of knowledge as a privileged, objective universal, and the expert as the privileged bearer of the light of truth.

The future of psychiatry?

In practical terms, this means that, if psychiatry is to realize what liberatory potential it has, then it must first relinquish any claim to have a foundational account of human subjectivity, or for that matter the social and political contexts in which individual subjectivity is embedded. Barker and Buchanan-Barker (2006) argue that postpsychiatry has failed to engage with the problem of the future of psychiatry. They propose that medicine has little or nothing to offer those who experience madness or distress. Other professionals can offer such things as psychological help, practical inputs, and human supports. Nurses are now trained to diagnose and prescribe. There is no *raison d'être* for a "medicine of the mental," for a psychiatry. We are broadly sympathetic to this position and the very concept of "postpsychiatry" implies some sort of endgame for the discourse and practice we now call psychiatry. We also share their sensibility to the oppressive history of psychiatry and have attempted in our writings to expose the limitations of psychiatric theory and the hurt caused by many psychiatric interventions. However, there are two issues that are neglected by Barker and Buchanan-Barker. First, they have little to say about the processes whereby psychiatry can be changed or even demolished. The issue here is that short of a revolution, there is no realistic prospect of simply dismantling the edifice of psychiatry overnight. In reality, psychiatry will, for the time being, continue to be the main response for a great many people when they experience distress. As long as this situation continues, for as long as the main statutory interventions for people who experience psychosis and distress are dominated by biomedical "truths," then postpsychiatry and critical psychiatry have a key role to play in challenging and questioning these "truths." This may not in itself be liberatory, but what it does achieve is to engage with and legitimate the voices of those people who are involved in the immediate struggle, as Foucault puts it. In other words, such critiques create spaces in which other voices may emerge, and in which they may speak for themselves of liberation. We cannot speak for those voices.

The second point that Barker and Buchanan-Barker fail to consider is the embodied nature of human existence. Like Thomas Szasz, they argue for a sort of dualistic world where there is real (i.e., physical) illness on one side and un-real (mythological or metaphorical) illness on the other. Indeed, like Szasz, they almost seek to demarcate a territory of human reality into which it is simply illegitimate for medicine to enter. Experience has taught us that any attempt to apply such binary thinking is doomed to failure and in the end can become a new source of oppression. Such a view polarizes the debate about how society should respond to madness in ways that are unhelpful, and is redolent of 1960s anti-psychiatry; "bad" somatic interventions, "good" psychotherapeutic, or narrative interventions. In our view, it is simply not possible to write the body out of madness, and this is where medicine has a role. Our point is that psychiatry represents a failed attempt to bring the world of medicine to bear on states of madness, distress and alienation. The answer is to re-think this relationship, not to demand a divorce.

This echoes a growing body of work from the field of medical anthropology. While anthropologists work with the idea that cultural systems shape illness experience to a greater degree than we sometimes realize, most are careful not to neglect the reality of our embodied nature and have sought to theorize this in different ways. For example, Csordas (1994) describes how attempts to reduce experience (in this case "organic" voices following on from brain surgery for epilepsy) to the level of biology, psychology, or culture do not do justice to the complexity of subjective experience. He argues that we need to approach subjectivity in a way that recognizes that we are embodied beings, and that the physical body takes us into the world of culture. Attempts to write culture *or* biology out of human experience simply serve to deny one or other aspect of human reality. Healing that reality when it is hurt and suffering also needs an approach that respects this complexity.

This view is supported by historical perspectives on healing. For thousands of years the physician and the priest have had a joint role in healing. Rynearson (2003) points out that, alongside the revolutionary theories about the body and illness that were developed by Hippocratic medicine in Greece in the late fifth century BCE, an ancient alternative to Hippocratic medicine, the cult of the healing god Asklepios, was highly popular throughout the Greek world. In this medical movement, which existed alongside Hippocratic medicine, suppliants slept in the temples of Asklepios, where the god visited them in their dreams and cured their illnesses. The interventions used by the God included surgical procedures (cutting an eye, for example) and the use of medicines (pouring in *pharmakion*). In other words healing from illness has always involved both rational and material (Hippocratic) interpretations, as well as the magical and spiritual (Asklepios). Cultural and bodily processes are at the heart of healing. Rivers

(1924) draws attention to the links between medicine, magic and ritual, particularly the use of religious and magical ritual in prognosticating and curing in Melanesian culture. He points out that, for physicians to function as healers, they must be aware that they are emulating priestly activities, especially in regard the moral aspects of healing. They must be engaged with their cultures. This holds an important truth about the future of our role as doctors both in medicine and for the way in which we work with people who experience distress. It implies that we must reach out and engage with culture in its widest sense, in recognition of the complex relationship between suffering, human life and culture. No matter how much we are opposed to the oppressive and barbaric practices of psychiatry, the problem of the future of psychiatry will not be answered simply by wishing psychiatry out of existence. We cannot un-invent the technologies that are associated with the practices of psychiatry. We must learn to control them, rather than let them control us.

Conclusion – beyond psychiatry

We argue that the question of the future of psychiatry should be reformulated in terms of the question of the relationship between medicine and madness. Postpsychiatry argues that we need to move beyond the idea that any professional discourse (be it psychiatry, anti-psychiatry, or psychotherapy) can lead to liberation. Postpsychiatry proposes that liberation in the area of mental health can only be achieved by experts by experience themselves. As we have seen above, this is happening already. Groups like Mad Pride, Mad Women and The Hearing Voices Network in the UK, and the Icarus Project in New York or the Freedom Centre in Northampton, Massachusetts, are creating new ways of thinking about their experiences, ways that refuse the narrow perspectives of traditional psychiatry and its allies. What is most exciting about these groups is that they are not only reshaping the contours of mental health discourse but they are also reshaping our views of what it is to be normal, to be human and to be free. When Foucault says that "that there are more secrets, more possible freedoms, and more inventions in our future than we can imagine in humanism," we believe that this is exactly what he had in mind. This is also becoming a vitally important matter internationally, as Western values, beliefs and patterns of consumption spread across the globe, a development that well fits the interests of the global pharmaceutical industry, and elites like the World Health Organization and World Psychiatric Association (Thomas *et al.*, 2005).

Neither critical psychiatry nor postpsychiatry can lead liberatory processes, and neither should attempt to do so. They can, however, provide a critique and rationale of existing practice, and help to open up new spaces for the voices of those who are usually excluded (Bracken & Thomas, 2001, 2005). But we also need to start rethinking how medicine should engage with the "mental."

Engaging with suffering

The single most harmful aspect of modern psychiatry is its failure to face up to and engage with personal suffering, stories of tragedy, loss, abuse, and oppression. The biological reductionism that now dominates has served to marginalize approaches that foreground these issues. This in our view is a deep moral and spiritual failing that can only be rectified by a major overhaul of the epistemology of psychiatry, and the way that doctors are trained. This reductionism lies behind current practices of psychiatric assessment and diagnosis. These and the interventions that are subsequently prescribed are very often experienced as limiting and oppressive and have been described in detail by first person narratives of experts by experience (see, for example, the anthology of narratives edited by Read and Reynolds, 1996). The historian Kathleen Jones describes how, as psychiatrists turned to biological models, they:

... could carry out [their] work as other doctors did – relieved of the burdens of attempting to follow the processes of disturbed minds, the strains and complexities of unfamiliar lifestyles, the pressures of unemployment, squalid housing conditions and poor nutrition. There was no need to enter the jungle of human emotions – love, hatred, pain, grief. (Jones, 1988, p. 83)

This is what we referred to earlier as the "moral aspects of healing." Physicians, if they are to heal, must find ways of bearing witness to suffering and not work to obscure the causes of this suffering. While doctors who work in the field of mental health will still need to study the biology of the human body, we believe that there is a need for a much greater emphasis on the humanities and the social sciences as well as forms of education that involve learning from service users in different ways.

Bearing witness to suffering is an important moral process both within the life of the individual who suffers, and the lives of those who suffer in broadly similar ways, as can be seen, for example, in the collective oppression and suffering of Black people in predominantly white societies, of women by male power, or of those who are oppressed by the mental health system. There is a wider political dimension to the role of the doctor who is thus aware of the extent and impact of suffering that arises from oppression on individual well-being, and an obligation to stand in solidarity with those who experience such oppression.

Challenging psychiatry from within and without

Critical psychiatry has a crucially important role to play in terms of challenging those aspects of clinical practice that are abusive, as well as challenging those features of the culture of psychiatry that contribute to the domination of the profession by neuroscience, particularly the influence of the pharmaceutical industry. One of the most important insights gleaned from critical analyses of the epistemology of psychiatry has been the uncovering of hidden agendas and interests paraded in the guise of science that result in disease mongering, the creation of "cosmetic psychopharmacology" and the existence of close financial ties between the industry and those responsible for developing diagnostic criteria such as the *Diagnostic and Statistical Manual* of the American Psychiatric Association (see, for example, Moynihan & Henry, 2003; Rose, 2003). In England, the Critical Psychiatry Network is making its own modest challenge by raising the matter in medical journals (Moncrieff *et al.*, 2002), as well as opposing government attempts to introduce coercive legislation aimed at introducing compulsory treatment in the community (Moncrieff *et al.*, 1999; Crawford *et al.*, 2001), and the general trend to extend the boundaries of psychiatry into all aspects of our lives (Timimi *et al.*, 2004). These actions, though small in themselves, contribute to a broader debate about the future of psychiatry that engages with the voices of service users and survivors, and adds legitimacy to their views.

NOTES

(1) It is important that we acknowledge in passing the work of two other thinkers, Frantz Fanon and Paulo Freire, both of whom have given us important insights into the processes of liberation. Fanon's powerful accounts of his personal experiences of racism when he left Martinique after World War II to study medicine and psychiatry in France, resulted in a social phenomenology of racism in *Black Skin, White Masks* (Fanon, 1986). His last work, *The Wretched of the Earth* (Fanon, 1967) became a liberatory handbook for anti-colonial revolutionary movements. Freire was an educationalist whose work with the oppressed and socially excluded in the Brazilian city of São Paulo threw new light on the social processes that can lead to liberation (Freire, 1996). There is, perhaps, a resonance between Freire's idea that the oppressor cannot hand over liberation to the oppressed, and some aspects of Foucault's later ideas about power and resistance, which we will explore towards the end of this chapter. Here, for reasons of conciseness, we have to limit the scope of our contribution to the ideas of critical theory and anti-psychiatry. This is not meant to deny or underplay the importance of the ideas of these two thinkers.

(2) We are well aware of the difficulties in terminology that plague discussions between the USA and Britain. From this point on we shall use the expression "expert by experience" because this challenges the idea that there is a single, privileged way of interpreting the experiences of madness, and foregrounds the importance of the voices of those who have direct personal experience of madness.

(3) Critical theory here is synonymous with the ideas of what has come to be known as the Frankfurt School. This was founded in 1923 by Max Horkheimer in the University of Frankfurt. The school closed in 1934 when its leading members, Horkheimer, Adorno, and Marcuse, emigrated to America, where they opened the New School of Social Research in New York. After the War Horkheimer and Adorno returned to Frankfurt, leaving Marcuse in New York. Jurgen Habermas has become one of the leading contemporary advocates of critical theory within this school of thought.

(4) The word hermeneutics derives from the Greek messenger of the Gods, Hermes, and refers to the processes of interpretation. Originally used in Christian theology, where it was used to describe efforts to access the true meaning of biblical texts, it was introduced into philosophy in the nineteenth century by Dilthey, who argued that the interpretation of the meaning of human actions could be understood through a manner similar to that used to interpret sacred texts.

(5) Most notably here we think of the work of Loren Mosher in the USA, Franco Bassaglia in Trieste, and Marius Romme and Sandra Escher in Holland.

(6) Genealogy is a term that has risen to prominence following the work of Foucault, although it was first used by Nietzsche. It is a method of historical critique, the purpose of which is to challenge established norms and ways of seeing the world. Foucault achieved this through historical-sociological analyses.

REFERENCES

Barker, P. & Buchanan-Barker, P. (2006). Post-psychiatry: good ideas, bad language and getting out of the box. *Journal of Psychiatric and Mental Health Nursing*, **13**, 619–625.

Blackman, L. (2001). *Hearing Voices: Embodiment and Experience*. London: Free Association Books.

Bracken, P. (1995). Beyond liberation: Michel Foucault and the notion of a critical psychiatry. *Philosophy, Psychiatry and Psychology*, **2**, 1–13.

Bracken, P. & Thomas, P. (2001). Postpsychiatry: a new direction for mental health. *British Medical Journal*, **322**, 724–727.

Bracken, P. & Thomas, P. (2005). *Postpsychiatry: Mental Health in a Postmodern World*. Oxford: Oxford University Press.

Cooper, D. (1968). *Introduction*. In *The Dialectics of Liberation*, ed. D. Cooper. Harmondsworth: Penguin, pp. 7–11.

Crawford, M. J., Hopkins, W., Thomas, P., Moncrieff, J., Bindman, J., & Gray, A. J. (2001). Most psychiatrists oppose plans for new mental health act. *British Medical Journal*, **322**, 866.

Csordas, T. (1994). Words from the Holy People: a case study in cultural phenomenology. In *Embodiment and Experience: The Existential Ground of Culture and Self*, ed. T. Csordas. Cambridge: Cambridge University Press.

Fanon, F. (1967). *The Wretched of the Earth*. (Trans. C. Farrington.) Harmondsworth: Penguin.

Fanon, F. (1986). *Black Skin, White Masks*. (Trans. C. Markmann.) London: Pluto.

Foucault, M. (1977a). *Discipline and Punish, The Birth of the Prison*. (Trans. A. Sheridan.) Harmondsworth: Penguin.

Foucault, M. (1977b). In *Michel Foucault, Language, Counter-Memory, Practice*, ed. D. F. Bouchard. Ithaca: Cornell University Press.

Foucault, M. (1978). *The History of Sexuality. An Introduction*. (Trans. R. Hurly.) Harmondsworth: Penguin.

Foucault, M. (1982). Afterword. In *Michel Foucault: Beyond Structuralism and Hermeneutics*, ed. H. Dreyfus & P. Rabinow. New York: Harvester Wheatsheaf, pp. 208–226.

Foucault M. (1988). Truth, power, self: an interview with Michel Foucault – October 25th, 1982. In *Technologies of the Self: A Seminar with Michel Foucault*, ed. L. H. Martin *et al*. London: Tavistock, pp. 9–15.

Foucault, M. (2006). *Psychiatric Power: Lectures at the Collège de France 1973–1974*, ed. J. Lagrange; trans. G. Burchell. Basingstoke: Palgrave Macmillan.

Freire, P. (1996). *Pedagogy of the Oppressed*. (Trans. M. Ramos.) Harmondsworth: Penguin.

Gordon, C. (1986). Psychiatry and the problem of democracy. In *The Power of Psychiatry*, ed. P. Miller & N. Rose. Cambridge: Polity Press, pp. 267–280.

Habernas, J. (1971). *Knowledge and Human Interests*. Boston: Beacon Press.

Ingleby, D. (1981). Understanding mental illness. In *Critical Psychiatry: The Politics of Mental Health*, ed. D. Ingleby. Harmondsworth: Penguin.

Jones, K. (1988). *Experience in Mental Health*. London: Sage.

Laing, R. D. (1965). *The Divided Self: An Existential Study in Sanity and Madness*. Harmondsworth: Penguin.

Leudar, I. & Thomas, P. (2000). *Voices of Reason, Voices of Insanity*. London: Routledge.

Marcuse, H. (1966). *Eros and Civilization*. Boston: Beacon Press.

Moncrieff, J., Thomas, P., Crawford, M., & Henderson, C. (1999). Psychiatrists should oppose community treatment orders. *British Medical Journal*, **318**, 806.

Moncrieff, J. & Thomas, P. (2002). The pharmaceutical industry and disease mongering. *British Medical Journal*, **325**, 216.

Moynihan, R. & Henry, D. (2003). The fight against disease mongering: Generating knowledge for action. *Public Library of Science (Medicine)*, **3**(4), e191.

Read, J. & Reynolds, J. (eds.) (1996). *Speaking Our Minds: An Anthology*. London: Macmillan, Open University.

Rivers, W. H. R. (1924). *Medicine, Magic and Religion*. London: Kegan Paul, Trench and Trübner. (Reprinted by Routledge Classics, 2001.)

Rose, N. (1985). *The Psychological Complex: Psychology, Politics and Society in England 1869–1939*. London: Routledge and Kegan Paul.

Rose, N. (1986). Psychiatry: the discipline of mental health. In *The Power of Psychiatry*, ed. P. Miller & N. Rose. Cambridge: Polity Press pp. 43–84.

Rose, N. (1998). *Inventing Ourselves: Psychology, Power and Personhood*. Cambridge: Cambridge University Press.

Rose, N. (2003). Neurochemical Selves. *Society*, Nov./Dec., 40–59.

Rynearson, N. (2003). Constructing and deconstructing the body in the cult of Asklepios. *Stanford Journal of Archaeology*, **2**, available on http://archaeology.stanford.edu/journal/new-draft/2003_Journal/rynearson/ accessed 7th October 2004.

Thomas, P, Bracken, P., Cutler, P., Hayward, R., May, R., & Yasmeen, S. (2005). Challenging the globalisation of biomedical psychiatry. *Journal of Public Mental Health*, **4**, 23–32.

Timimi, S., Moncrieff, J., Jureidini, J. *et al.* (2004). A critique of the international consensus statement on ADHD. *Clinical Child and Family Psychology Review*, **7**, 59– 63; discussion 65–9.

3

Challenging risk: a critique of defensive practice

Duncan Double

Perhaps one of the most obvious manifestations of liberatory psychiatry was the Congress on the Dialectics of Liberation held in London at the Roundhouse in Chalk Farm in July 1967. David Cooper (1968) designated the four organizers of the Congress as anti-psychiatrists. Besides himself, these were R. D. Laing, Joseph Berke, and Leon Redler. Both Laing and Cooper gave papers at the conference, as did celebrated social theorists such as Herbert Marcuse and political activists such as Stokely Carmichael.

To Free a Generation was the alternative title of the book of the conference *The Dialectics of Liberation* (Cooper, 1968). This description makes clear that the book was concerned with how liberation may be achieved. The strands of anti-psychiatry were interwoven with the 1960s counterculture, whose aim was to free the spirit of the age from the nightmare of the world (Nuttall, 1970). The writings of R. D. Laing, perhaps especially *The Politics of Experience and The Bird of Paradise*, helped to articulate this perspective. Laing (1967) was explicit that civilization represses transcendence and so-called "normality" too often abdicates our true potentialities.

Psychedelic drugs seemed to expand the limits of imminent experience (Wolfe, 1989). One of the originators of hippie culture, Ken Kesey who, with his Merry Pranksters drove across America in a brightly painted bus, wrote *One Flew Over the Cuckoo's Nest* (Kesey, 1963). This successful novel depicts Randle McMurphy's attempt, possibly on behalf of the counterculture, to overthrow the bureaucratic control of Nurse Ratched in the psychiatric institution.

David Cooper was the most radical of the anti-psychiatrists in his quest for freedom. He wanted liberation from the family, which he saw as an ideological conditioning device that reinforces the power of the ruling class in an exploitative society (Cooper, 1971). Besides being Marxist in his political refusal to submit to bourgeois society, he thought that spontaneous self-assertion of full personal autonomy should be a decisive act of counter-violence against the system. He argued for sexual liberation of an orgasmic ecstasy (Cooper, 1974). He even

Liberatory Psychiatry: Philosophy, Politics, and Mental Health, ed. Carl I. Cohen and Sami Timimi.
Published by Cambridge University Press. © Cambridge University Press.

believed that initiation of young children into orgasmic experiences should become part of a full education.

What is not always clear is that R. D. Laing distanced himself from Cooper's excesses. Where they were agreed was that the social practice of psychiatry needed to change. They both wanted to give people freedom from the social control of psychiatry. I want to explore further what this means in this chapter, and relate it to the current psychiatric scene. I describe the therapeutic alternatives of anti-psychiatry and, in particular, note the motivation for reform because of the institutional effects of the asylum. Psychiatry does have a social role and this cannot be avoided, however much the anti-psychiatrists may have wished they could. Mental health services manage the risk of mental illness on behalf of society and how they do this determines how liberated people will be. We have moved on from the time of anti-psychiatry as the traditional psychiatric hospital has continued to be run down. Where anti-psychiatry railed against the excesses of the institution, the development of community care has created a different environment. I discuss the effect of inquiries in the UK: first of all, in relation to mistreatment in hospital; and then in criticisms of community care because of homicides by psychiatric patients. I conclude that the over-bureaucratic way in which modern psychiatric services tend to respond to the management of risk in the community has many of the features of the worst excesses of the asylums.

Anti-psychiatry and liberation

David Cooper (1967) set up Villa 21 in Shenley Hospital between 1962 and 1966. He tried to create a community in which patients would have the chance to discover and explore an authentic relatedness to each other. To do this required "an effort to cease interference, to 'lay off' other people and give them and oneself a chance" (Cooper, 1967, p. 89). Being allowed to "go to pieces" was necessary before one could be helped to come back together again. When staff controls had to be re-introduced to gain some semblance of order on the ward, Cooper concluded that a successful unit could only be developed in the community rather than in hospital.

Both Laing and Cooper were part of the Philadelphia Association that established Kingsley Hall in 1965, although Cooper had nothing more to do with this project after it started (Mullan, 1995). Laing lived at Kingsley Hall for 18 months in 1965/6. Kingsley Hall was an experiment in unstructured living. It sought to allow psychotic people the space to explore their madness and internal chaos. It did not attempt to "cure" but provided a place where "some may encounter selves long forgotten or distorted" (Schatzman, 1972). The local community was mostly hostile to the project. After 5 years Kingsley Hall was largely trashed and uninhabitable. Laing's dream of a place "without those features of psychiatric practice that seemed to belong to the sphere of social power and structure rather than to medical therapeutics" was only partially successful, even from his own perspective (Laing, 1985).

The association of anti-psychiatry with the counterculture of the 1960s and 1970s may have helped to propel anti-psychiatry into the limelight. It may also have contributed to its demise. Without this cultural support, anti-psychiatry seemed to lose its popular appeal. Also, some of its major proponents, such as Laing, were more obviously interested in personal authenticity than changing psychiatry practically. After Kingsley Hall, Laing went on retreat to Ceylon and India to pursue his interests in meditation, Buddhism and Hinduism. Later in life, Laing (1987) regarded his main achievement as being in the area of social phenomenology in philosophy, not psychiatry. Generally, anti-psychiatry is seen as having had no lasting influence on psychiatry and its practice (Tantam, 1991). For all its calls for liberation, these aspirations were sidelined largely into promoting personal and spiritual freedom with little interest in redeeming psychiatry itself. This diversion helped to allow mainstream psychiatry to marginalize anti-psychiatry's influence.

One exception to this evaluation of the significance of anti-psychiatry would be the achievement of Franco Basaglia in changing mental health law in Italy. Basaglia's awareness of the effects of institutionalization led to his struggle to abolish the asylum. He recognized the necessary political, class-related character of this fight. From his point of view, the asylum contained poverty and misery not madness. As expressed by his wife, with whom he worked closely, the asylum was "a dumping ground for the under privileged, a place of segregation and destruc tion where the real nature of social problems was concealed behind the alibi of psychiatric treatment and custody" (Basaglia, 1989). Politically Basaglia was influenced by the writings of Antonio Gramsci, a cofounder of the Italian communist party (Mollica, 1985). Health care workers, such as doctors, nurses, and students, regarded as "technicians of practical knowledge," were encouraged to contest their roles and recognize the social and political context of psychiatric problems. This attitude led to the mass resignation of the doctors at Gorizia in protest at the failure to invest in community services. In terms of liberatory psychiatry, this could be seen as a pre-eminent refusal to be accomplices of the system.

Psichiatria Democratica was founded in 1973 and acted as a pressure group leading to the passing of Law 180 by the Italian parliament in May 1978. The new law prevented new admissions to existing mental hospitals and decreed a shift of perspective from segregation and control in the asylum to treatment and rehabilitation in society. The mental health services in Trieste, where Basaglia worked, became seen as the most important representation of the success of democratic psychiatry.

The negative effects of institutionalization

The example of Basaglia confirms that liberatory psychiatry is closely entwined with the social aspects of psychiatric practice. Initially, Basaglia was struck by the effects of institutionalization, which Russell Barton (1959) called a disease, for which he coined the term "institutional neurosis." This syndrome was characterized by symptoms such as apathy, lack of initiative, loss of interest, and submissiveness. The cause was said to be factors such as loss of contact with the outside world, enforced idleness, brutality and bossiness of staff, loss of friends and personal possessions, poor ward atmosphere, and loss of prospects outside the institution.

The negative effects of the process of institutionalization were Basaglia's motivation for change. This notion fits with the interests of the anti-psychiatrists, in general, in the negative effects of institutionalization in the asylums (Goffman, 1961). For example, both Joseph Berke and Leon Redler came from the USA to work with Maxwell Jones at Dingleton before moving to collaborate with Laing. The therapeutic community movement, based on ideas of equality, informality, and frank and open discussion, was pioneered in psychiatry by Jones (1952). It challenged traditional asylum assumptions. One of the constructive and lasting outcomes of anti-psychiatry could be seen as the therapeutic communities established by the Philadelphia Association, founded by Laing and others, and the Arbours Association, set up by Berke and Morton Schatzmann.

Although debates about community care are no longer as polarized as they were in the past, many psychiatrists felt threatened by their perceived loss of power due to the rundown of the traditional psychiatric hospital. Anti-psychiatry reinforced this challenge to psychiatric power and became identified with the closure of the traditional asylum, even though there is not necessarily a logical link. For example, in a brief appendix to the third edition of *Being Mentally Ill*, Thomas Scheff (1999) notes that the first edition of his book was regarded as the "Bible" of the group that wrote a bill that became the new mental health law for California, and later for the rest of the United States. The new law made it more difficult for people to be kept in hospital indefinitely, which, in turn, is likely to have contributed to the subsequent closure of mental hospitals.

The motivation to create a therapeutic milieu from the traditional psychiatric hospital has a long history and is much wider than anti-psychiatry. For example, Harry Stack Sullivan established a small ward for schizophrenic men that was staffed with hand-picked attendants, set apart from the rest of the Sheppard Pratt Hospital in the 1920s (Barton Evans III, 1996). He gave his staff autonomy to operate on their own with patients. He found unexpected genuine relationships flourished between patients and staff leading to an improvement in institutional recovery (Sullivan, 1962). Another example is from Laing again, before Kingsley Hall, when he was involved in an experimental therapeutic venture within the health service as a psychiatric trainee at Gartnavel hospital in Scotland (Andrews, 1998). The nurses called the project the "Rumpus Room." It recognized the role that the hospital environment had in "enforced inactivity" of patients, and encouraged patients and nurses to develop personal relationships of a reasonably enduring nature.

Although anti-psychiatry was explicit in its wish to overthrow psychiatric control, there were more general moves to open up psychiatric practice through recognition of human relations and group dynamics. For example, the World Health Organization (1953) promoted the creation of an atmosphere of a therapeutic community as an important element in treatment, heralding the opening of the locked doors in mental hospitals and the rundown of the traditional asylum. Elements of this therapeutic atmosphere included encouraging patients' self-respect and sense of identity; and the general assumption that patients are trustworthy and retain capacity for a considerable degree of responsibility and initiative. Purposeful, planned activity was promoted in a patient's day.

I want to explore further the social nature of psychiatry by studying its political context over recent years in the development of community care. Questions about how to care for the mentally ill and whether this should take place in hospital or in the community make apparent the propensity for abuse and neglect of these people. Evident failures in care highlight the tension between controlling patients on behalf of society and helping them to find individual and personal fulfilment and liberation.

The development of community care and the role of inquiries

Psychiatry's social role is reinforced through mental health legislation. Using the UK as an example, the Lunatic Asylums Act 1845 made it mandatory for each borough and county to provide adequate asylum accommodation at public expense for its pauper lunatic population. This led to an asylum building programme, but the asylums quickly became overcrowded institutions.

In the 1950s, the locked doors of the psychiatric hospitals started to be opened. The peak of the mental health population in the UK and USA was the mid-1950s and later in other Western countries (Goodwin, 1997). The traditional asylums became increasingly irrelevant to the bulk of mental health problems and began their decline as alternative services were developed, including psychiatric units in general hospitals, residential homes and day centres. Many old long-stay patients grew old and died in hospital, and the number of new long-stay patients to replace them has been much lower. Despite the massive reduction in bed space and the closure of most of the traditional asylums, there has, in fact, been an increase in the admission rates to psychiatric hospitals. What has happened is that the average length of stay has been considerably reduced, although a small minority of people still experience protracted hospital admissions (Goodwin, 1993).

Abuses and over-restrictive practices within institutions

One of the features that encouraged the rundown of the psychiatric hospital was the recognition of the potential harm caused by psychiatric hospitalization. In the UK, for example, there were a number of scandals that uncovered mistreatment of patients in hospital (Martin, 1984), with detaining the mentally ill under the Mental Health Act appearing to exacerbate the potential for abuse. A phase of public concern and debate was launched by the Ely Hospital inquiry (see Martin, 1984, for further details). In 1967 a nursing assistant at Ely Hospital in Cardiff made a series of allegations about the treatment of patients and the pilfering of property by staff. These allegations were published in the Sunday newspaper *News of the World*. The inquiry found examples of callous, "old fashioned and unsophisticated" techniques of nursing control. Although in most instances this practice was not "wilful or malicious," nursing standards were low, supervision weak, reporting of incidents inadequate, and training of nursing assistants virtually nonexistent. Staff were also found to have pilfered supplies of food. There were determined and vindictive attempts to silence complainants. In addition, it transpired that members of the Nursing Division of the Ministry had visited Ely some years before and had reported "scandalous conditions, bad nursing," and yet nothing had been done about it. In essence, the inquiry report confirmed the basis of all the *News of the World* revelations.

Another example of an influential inquiry was the Whittingham Hospital inquiry (again, see Martin, 1984, for further details). In 1969 two senior members of the staff at Whittingham Hospital near Preston, Lancashire, made allegations of ill-treatment of patients, fraud and maladministration, including suppression of complaints from student nurses. Two male nurses were convicted of theft. Shortly after the police investigation, a male nurse assaulted two male patients, one of whom died. The nurse was convicted of manslaughter and imprisoned. An inquiry was set up after the trial was over. What was significant about the report was that it placed the responsibility on the management for the institutional conditions that led to callous and incompetent nursing and some deliberate cruelty. The inquiry also uncovered suppression and denial of student nurses' complaints about ill-treatment.

The political response in the UK to this series of inquiries was to set up the Hospital Advisory Service, which, independent of the normal departmental machinery, provided visiting teams for inspecting hospitals. The other main consequence was the government's renewal of its promotion of the policy of community care. The view was strengthened that society should not reject its mentally ill and handicapped people. No longer was it appropriate to consign these people to distant institutions where they lived their lives out of sight and mind of the rest of society, with the potential for them being abused (Martin, 1984). The white papers *Better Services for the Mentally Handicapped* (Department of Health and Social Security & Welsh Office, 1971) and *Better Services for the Mentally Ill* (Department of Health and Social Security, 1975) were published. Psychiatric hospitals were to be replaced by more local and wider-ranging facilities.

These inquiries generally had a positive effect and aimed to encourage ethically acceptable professional behavior in the institution. However, inquiries may not always be as perspicacious as they seem (Walshe & Higgins, 2002). They can have a serious effect on staff morale if they reach incorrect conclusions because of, for example, poor methodology or their inquisitorial nature. Although we live in a "risk society" (Beck, 1992), there is a responsibility to avoid "scapegoating" and a culture of blame. The accountability of clinical governance should be sound, open, and fair, but in practice this is not always the case. The notion that errors, particularly those that have bad outcomes, are manifestations of incompetence, carelessness or recklessness in the individual has consequences on broader practice. After all, fallibility is an inherent part of being human; fear of being found to be "fallible" will have an impact on professionals' willingness to take potentially therapeutic risks.

Flaws with inquiries have perhaps become particularly manifest with inquiries into failure of community care over recent years. In the UK, since 1994 health authorities have been obliged to hold an independent inquiry in cases of homicide committed by those who have been in contact with the psychiatric services (Buchanan, 1999). These inquiries reflect a shift from focusing on abuses and over-restrictive practices within institutions towards anxiety about the lack of control in the community (Crichton & Sheppard, 1996). The presence of asylums may have sustained a belief that it is part of the role of psychiatric services to shield society from its madness (Salter, 2003). Without these structures for confinement, society may feel more at risk.

Problems with these inquiries have been highlighted by a number of commentators. There is a danger as a result, for potentially destructive outcomes with negative rather than positive effects on practice, leading some to argue that reform of the current system of such investigations is necessary (King *et al.*, 2006). I want to look at the context in which these inquiries developed.

Anxiety about lack of control in the community

Community care has been a controversial policy. Campaigners against the rundown of the traditional psychiatric hospitals opposed the policy in various ways.

Initially, they focused on the apparent risk of homelessness after discharge from hospital (Weller, 1989). Because of the evident relatively high level of mental illness amongst the homeless population, it was concluded that patients were being discharged irresponsibly from the traditional asylums "onto the street." However, follow-up studies of discharged patients showed that the rundown of the psychiatric hospital, at least in the UK, was not the main factor contributing to the increase in the numbers of homeless mentally ill (Leff, 1993). The number of homeless people seems to have been affected more by housing policy than by psychiatric deinstitutionalization. The reason in particular may have been the reduction in direct access hostels, which had, since the mid-1950s, seemed to serve as unacknowledged refuges for some mentally ill people (Craig & Timms, 1992).

When evidence accumulated against the view that psychiatric dehospitalization was increasing homelessness and criminal imprisonment, the tack of campaigning by organizations such as SANE (http://www.sane.org.uk/) changed to concern about public safety due to homicides by psychiatric patients. The tragic killing of Jonathan Zito on the London Underground led to the formation of the Zito Trust. The victim's widow, Jayne Zito, was understandably motivated to improve mental health services. She was prevented from pursuing a negligence claim in relation to her husband's death because UK courts are loath to rule that public bodies, such as mental health services, owe a duty of care to third parties.

Campaigners such as these led the newly elected Labour government to conclude that community care had failed (Department of Health, 1998a). The government strategy document *Modernising Mental Health Services* (Department of Health, 1998b) stated that the policy of community care had brought many benefits. It also suggested that underfunding, inadequate care, and poor management had caused the failures in policy.

The public cannot be totally safeguarded against homicides by mentally ill people. As homicide is rare, attempts to prevent such tragedies risk high false negative prediction. Assuming it were possible to recognize patients at high risk of committing homicide with sufficient sensitivity and specificity, it has been estimated that, for every one person detected correctly, 5000 people will be identified as being at high risk of committing homicide but will not do so (Crawford, 2000). Despite the hype in the media, single cases do not constitute evidence of the failure of the system of community care. UK national homicide figures in fact show a 3% annual decline in the proportion of mentally disordered people contributing to homicide figures (Taylor & Gunn, 1999). Such findings by themselves give no basis to the argument for change in community care policy.

The results of this public outcry about mental health services may have been counter-productive, as it encourages defensive rather than therapeutic practice. Over recent years, more people have been locked up in secure beds in the UK as numbers of other adult mental health beds have reduced. Numbers of people detained under the Mental Health Act have increased (Wall *et al.*, 1999).

Moreover, homicide inquiries can have devastating consequences for mental health services (Szmukler, 2000). They are not always based on rational foundations. The stereotype of the "dangerous lunatic" is reinforced and public fears of the mentally ill are fuelled. To quote from Szmukler:

An assumption reigns, among the media and politicians at least, that all such homicides are preventable, despite the fact that every country has, and has always had them. For some reason, ours has become terrorised by them. (Szmukler, 2000, p. 6)

Many reports are long and have been very expensive to complete. For example, there are two volumes of the report of the Luke Warm Luke mental health inquiry (Scotland *et al.*, 1998), which cost £750 000. Luke Warm Luke (formerly Michael Folkes) stabbed to death Susan Milner, aged 33, in 1994. Michael Folkes had changed his name by deed poll to Luke Warm Luke, apparently taking the name from a character in the *Porridge* (a popular British sit-com set in a prison) series on television. He was convicted of manslaughter and made the subject of a hospital order with restrictions and sent to Broadmoor Hospital, a high-security special hospital. The murder he committed was known in the press as the "scissors death," as he stabbed his girlfriend to death 70 times with scissors at his London flat.

Luke Warm Luke had been diagnosed as suffering from paranoid schizophrenia and had been in and out of mental health facilities since 1983. He was released by a Mental Health Review Tribunal against Home Office and expert advice on the condition that he continued to take his medication. However, he later refused to take his depot injection and was allowed to take his medication orally. Tests after the attack demonstrated no traces of medication in his body. The day before the attack he had gone to the Maudsley hospital (a psychiatric hospital in London) in a distressed state. He was put on an emergency list for a community psychiatric nurse to visit.

The inquiry team criticized the lack of communication in the community care team dealing with the case. The three members of the aftercare team did not meet together in the 25 months leading up to the killing. They also criticized the decision to allow Luke Warm Luke to discontinue his depot medication. The report also said he should have been discharged into a staffed hostel so that he was not forced to look after himself and noted that the killing bore a striking similarity to an attack committed the year before. They concluded that both attacks could have been prevented if Luke Warm Luke had been admitted to hospital.

Despite the length of the report, it is unclear why Luke Warm Luke killed Susan Milner. The only explanation offered is that he was schizophrenic. This is regarded as a sufficient and complete explanation. There is no questioning of this connection. The simple, almost naïve view is that schizophrenia is a biological illness that determines how a person behaves, especially if they are violent. Any court exercising its proper role would never let a forensic psychiatrist get away with such an over-simplification. Yet inquiries can produce authoritative reports based on this kind of assumption.

As Szmukler (2000) points out, Luke Warm Luke's history of serious violence, which antedated the illness, was passed over without comment by the inquiry panel. Furthermore, the focus on mental health services tends to exclude the role of other actors in the drama. For example, Luke Warm Luke's victim visited the patient at 3 a.m. despite advice from friends not to do so. Earlier that night, he had threatened (with scissors) another young woman he had known. This woman called the police at about 10 p.m., but the police did not follow up on the incident because she did not want to press charges.

Szmukler (2000) goes on to discuss whether it is reasonable to be held responsible for the action of another and suggests it is unprecedented in medicine. It occurs in social work where child protection teams may be held responsible for the behavior of an abusing parent. However, at least in social work, the child protection team can focus on preventing harm to children. Moreover, the overall evaluation of child abuse inquiries has been that the preoccupation of many inquiry panels with apportioning blame has limited the lessons that could be learnt (Reder *et al.*, 1993). Understanding complex cases requires an approach that goes beyond blaming.

To reinforce this message, I give another example of a homicide inquiry from my own UK National Health Service (NHS) provider organization (Norfolk & Waveney Mental Health Partnership NHS Trust, 2005). Richard King was convicted of the manslaughter of his mother-in-law's partner on August 6 2004 and made the subject of a hospital order with restrictions. He had been in receipt of adult mental health services since 1989. The panel concluded the homicide occurred because of his mental illness and that, although it was not predictable, it was preventable because he should have been detained under the Mental Health Act.

It is clear that the Trust panel was motivated by what it saw as the public expectation that mental health services should exert some influence over the behavior of individuals in their care. The report was written to maintain this public confidence in mental health services by identifying mistakes and errors of judgment. However, it is not necessarily the role of an inquiry report to meet these stated public expectations. If that were the case, it would mean that homicide inquiries were being used to achieve political aims.

The report did not demonstrate that staff acted in bad faith, nor without reasonable care. These are the criteria that should first of all be used to assess their actions rather than mistakes and errors of judgment. No professional system ever works perfectly. There will always be weaknesses. The panel report, like other homicide inquiries, was also written with the benefit of hindsight, which often leads to a biased perspective on clinical judgments that have to be made in the course of everyday clinical work. Nor is it as clear as the panel make out that detention under the Mental Health Act was indicated. Compulsory treatment is only necessary if treatment cannot be provided unless the person is detained. Informal admission without use of the Mental Health Act seems to have been a viable alternative to detention in this case.

My comments on the panel's report should not be seen as encouraging complacency. They are intended to improve the quality of care for patients. The problem with such reports is that they are likely to encourage defensive practice and thus may lead to a worsening of care. After all, inquiries are as likely to make as many mistakes as the services they criticize, particularly if undertaken by the organization itself. It seems unfortunate that homicides by psychiatric patients have become the vehicle with which to attack mental health services.

Risk and mental health

I want to move on to discuss the role of "risk" more generally. Over-defensiveness because of "risk" can be alienating and counter-productive. For example, one of the common outcomes of homicide inquires has been to encourage an ever more rigid and bureaucratic interpretation of the "Care Programme Approach" (CPA) (CPA is the UK's attempt to systematize the approach to care of the mentally ill). This is despite the difficulties of showing that deficiencies in this regard are, in fact, related to outcome (Szmukler, 2000).

Anthony Giddens (1991) sees Britain as living in a post-traditional society in which the "Risk Society" is the context of politics. Over recent years, risk has become an academic growth area. Some of the stimulus for this increase has been the work of Mary Douglas (1992), in particular, her book *Risk and Blame*. The subtitle of her book, *Essays in Cultural Theory*, indicates that her work is at least partly about method. What I want to look at, like Mary Douglas, is how we view risk, in particular in relation to mental health.

People have certain ways of living in relation to institutions. There is always a political question about what is acceptable risk. In particular, there is a debate about the balance between risk taking and risk avoidance. What appears to be happening in the "Risk Society" is a shift towards the risk aversive end of this relationship. The word "risk" has been pre-empted to mean bad risks. The promise of a good political outcome is couched in other terms. Yet any society which did not take risks would not be making the most of its opportunities. Over-cautious behavior can be counter-productive and crippling. The debate also relates to authority, and oscillates between the pressures to move on from the old institutional constraints and the pressures to sustain the institutions in which authority and solidarity are seen to reside.

We need to be aware that debates about "risk" in mental health are political debates. As mentioned above, when New Labour came to power there was an increased emphasis on public safety in mental health in the context of suggesting that community care had failed. Even though this rhetoric may be used less commonly now by a more experienced administration, government concern about public safety remains a priority in their mental health policies. Any history of the opening of the traditional asylum doors, such as that by David Clark (1996) of Fulbourn Hospital, highlights the risks that were taken at the time, and the emotional turmoil that ensued from taking such decisions. Nonetheless, overall the changes were therapeutic for patients and could be seen as the most progressive advance in psychiatric treatment over recent years. What was needed was to move on from the state of affairs which involved "issuing memoranda, forbidding activities, putting up warning notices, setting up disciplinary enquiries and penalising staff who take risks or show initiative. Staff have learned to be cautious, to get everything in writing, to avoid initiative" (Clark, 1996).

We seem to have gone full circle and, at times, our systems in community care are as bureaucratic as those in the traditional asylums. We need to be bold enough to point out that regarding risk assessment in mental health as a purely clinical activity is not sensible. It has become very common following inquiries into homicides by psychiatric patients to hear the recommendation that risk assessment needs to be improved and that staff should receive further training in risk assessment. But will this really lead to any improvement? Does merely knowing about risks improve practice? Is risk assessment really such a separate part of the overall evaluation of a patient? We actually have very little reliable knowledge about the accurate clinical quantification of risk (Geddes, 1999).

A guiding influence in UK government mental health policy over recent years has been the National Confidential Inquiry (NCI) into Suicide and Homicide by People with Mental Illness. The NCI collects data on deaths by suicide and homicide by psychiatric patients. It makes recommendations on clinical practice with the aim of reducing the risk of suicide and homicide. Its Director, Professor Louis Appleby, is also the National Director of Mental Health, commonly known as the mental health "tsar," and an important advisor to government. The work of the NCI has been said to provide evidence that amending the Mental Health Act to extend powers for compulsory treatment in the community will help save lives.

The simplistic argument is made that treated, even forcibly treated, mentally ill people are less likely to commit suicide and murder than mentally ill people who are untreated. Services can make improvements in mental health, but they can also make matters worse. Having control and influence means that there is the potential for doing harm. Psychiatric interventions aim to be effective, but a good outcome does not necessarily follow. Inappropriate psychiatric treatment could potentially increase the risk of deaths by suicide or homicide. However inconceivable this may be for politicians and mental health services, it does need to be considered. As it is so difficult to think about it, only the advantages of the introduction of enforced community treatment are proclaimed officially, rarely the disadvantages. But overactive intervention may be counter-productive. Inappropriate imposition of compulsory community treatment may precipitate the acting out of more risky behavior, rather than contain the risk.

The UK has been slower than some other countries in introducing enforced community treatment. Outpatient commitment is permitted in virtually all US states (e.g., New York's "Kendra's Law"). The operation and use of outpatient commitment varies dramatically between states. Undesirable effects are acknowledged, particularly the creation of barriers to care. For example, treatment adherence and therapeutic alliance can be adversely affected (van Dorn et al., 2006). The evidence for effectiveness in, for example, reducing either admissions or bed-days is very limited and other effects are uncertain (Kisely et al., 2006).

Despite the passing of the Mental Health Act in the UK, debate will continue, driven by the notion that deaths by homicide and suicide are avoidable by increased coercion. The NCI even went as far in one of its reports, *Safer Services*, to estimate the potential number of deaths that would be prevented by the introduction of community treatment orders (Appleby et al., 1999). This relied on making various assumptions. It could have produced a higher or lower figure dependent on different assumptions. The fact is that whatever figure was produced is not evidence of the value of compulsory community treatment, as it is only an estimate calculated *if* this intervention is effective. Unthinking implementation of enforced community treatment risks undermining patients' rights. This momentum could be seen as reflecting a lack of tolerance for mental illness in society. Unrealistic efforts to control risk may inappropriately restrict freedom of thought and action. A government which promulgates the aim of social inclusion should be judged by its policies towards the mentally ill.

Defensive practice and critical psychiatry

I have discussed the recent history of psychiatry in the context of the development of community care. Psychiatry does have a social role. It is the sign of a humane society that it has high quality mental health services. When disturbed, mentally ill people may need to be protected from the harm they may cause to themselves and others. Assessment of risk needs to be realistic and not exaggerated for fear of exacerbating stigma. Prediction of future behavior is very difficult and society will never prevent all tragedies such as suicide and homicide. How society reacts to irrationality, disturbance, and madness does matter.

As well as this social aspect, individuals seek personal fulfilment and liberation. The danger is that the fear that things may go wrong in mental health services is distracting us from the task of how to make things better for people (Cooper, 2001). We may follow procedures that are more for the purpose of protecting staff than helping patients. Examples of such defensive practice in psychiatry would be admitting patients over-cautiously and placing patients on higher levels of observation than necessary (Passmore & Leung, 2002). "Specialing" of patients on acute psychiatric wards highlights the impersonal nature of such bureaucratic practice (Buchanan-Barker & Barker, 2005). As I have tried to illustrate above in the discussion of inquiries into psychiatric hospitals, the extreme end of this trend is that patients are abused and neglected.

Certain aspects of defensive practice hinge on the role of professional knowledge and clinical judgment. Health managers can influence direct clinical care through imposing regulations. Over recent years attempts have been made to make professionals more accountable and this has led to a crisis of trust (O'Neill, 2002). Such "proceduralism" emphasizes external criteria for assessing and evaluating our work, rather than internal factors (Cooper, 2001). The danger is that concern for improvement is not authentic and merely a facade to placate society's fears. Managerial guidelines can never be a complete substitute for clinical judgment.

I am not saying there are no potential advantages of an audit culture. Increasing understanding, learning from practice, and a desire to improve performance should be encouraged. However, fear of being criticized and unfairly judged does not lead to creative thinking about the quality of services. What is needed is a learning culture with excellent leadership that provides an ethos where staff are valued and supported as they form partnerships with patients (Halligan & Donaldson, 2001). Few mental health services have the courage to provide such an environment when they are overly concerned to protect themselves against criticism.

Health care systems are complex, which means there is much uncertainty in clinical practice. Gaps in care, such as losses of information or interruptions of delivery of care, are commonplace (Cook *et al.*, 2000). Fortunately, these gaps rarely produce too many difficulties. Usually they are anticipated, detected, or bridged in some way. What may lead to adverse clinical incidents are gaps which practitioners are unsuccessful in bridging. Conditions to improve patient safety are, therefore, those that facilitate practitioners in bridging gaps, not the reverse. Focusing too much on failures to adhere to narrow procedural guidelines misses the point about how health care systems produce good results.

Helping ill people is not an easy task. A focus on risk avoidance may unconsciously distract us from this aim. In particular in psychiatry, there is a need to sustain personal relationships with patients to understand their difficulties. The temptation may be to retreat from the anxiety this engagement creates by insisting on the biological nature of their illness. An advantage of this strategy is that it protects those trying to provide care from the pain experienced by those needing support.

"Critical psychiatry" wishes to avoid this objectification of the mentally ill (Double, 2006). The biomedical model of mental illness currently dominates psychiatric practice. Critical psychiatry proposes that psychiatry does not need to postulate that abnormalities of brain functioning are the cause of mental illness. Critical psychiatry may not intrinsically be opposed to a "blame culture" in mental health practice. However, it is likely to avoid defensive practice because it explicitly encourages a focus on the psychosocial contexts of mental health difficulties and their ethical implications. It also recognizes the expertise of users of the service and works towards a combination of this expertise by experience with professional expertise to create a partnership in treatment. Critical psychiatry also argues for a new relationship between coercion and care that recognizes the way values inform clinical decisions.

Critical psychiatry may therefore provide a framework that avoids the worst extremes of defensiveness because it explicitly promotes reflection on practice. Through attempting to counter the reductionism of "biologism" it focuses on the person in assessment and treatment. This approach has the advantage of recognizing the potential for human growth and authenticity. I do not want to make too much of the difference from mainstream psychiatry. Of course, we can all be panicked by our fears of risk and being blamed. But a deliberate focus on the patient perspective is more likely to make transparent their needs, rather than distort the primary aim of mental health services into the protection of the organization.

CONCLUSION

In this chapter I have tried to update the focus of liberatory psychiatry in the modern context of "risk" – not in an exhaustive way, but to appreciate that issues of liberation are still relevant in the modern context of community care. The point of the chapter has been to indicate that critical psychiatry may provide a new synthesis through its analysis of defensive practice. Anti-psychiatry flourished in the counter-culture of the 1960s and reinforced the critique of the oppressive nature of the traditional psychiatric hospital. Psychiatry still needs to be vigilant if it is to be successful in helping to create an environment that promotes the independence of people.

REFERENCES

Andrews, J. (1998). R. D. Laing in Scotland: facts and fictions of the 'Rumpus Room' and interpersonal psychiatry. In *Cultures of Psychiatry and Mental Health Care in Postwar Britain and the Netherlands*, ed. M. Gijswijt-Hofstra & R. Porter. Amsterdam: Editions Rodopi.

Appleby, L., Shaw, J., Amos, T. *et al.* (1999). *Safer services: Report of the National Confidential Inquiry into suicide and homicide by people with mental illness.* London: Stationery Office.

Barton, R. (1959). *Institutional Neurosis.* Bristol: Wright.

Barton Evans III, F. (1996). *Harry Stack Sullivan. Interpersonal Theory and Psychotherapy.* London: Routledge.

Basaglia, F. O. (1989). The psychiatric reform in Italy: Summing up and looking ahead. *International Journal of Social Psychiatry*, **35**, 90–97.

Beck, U. (1992). *The Risk Society.* London: Sage.

Buchanan, A. (1999). Independent inquiries into homicide. *British Medical Journal*, **318**, 1089–1090.

Buchanan-Barker, P. & Barker, P. (2005). Observation: the original sin of mental health nursing? *Journal of Psychiatric and Mental Health Nursing*, **12**, 550–555.

Clark, D. H. (1996). *The Story of a Mental Hospital: Fulbourn 1858–1993.* London: Process Press.

Cook, R. I., Render, M., & Woods, D. D. (2000). Gaps in the continuity of care and progress on patient safety. *British Medical Journal*, **320**, 791–794.

Cooper, A (2001). The state of mind we're in: social anxiety, governance and the audit society. *Psychoanalytic Studies*, **3**, 349– 362.

Cooper, D. (1967). *Psychiatry and Anti-psychiatry.* London: Tavistock.

Cooper, D. (ed.) (1968). *The Dialectics of Liberation.* Harmondsworth: Penguin.

Cooper, D. (1971). *The Death of the Family.* Harmondsworth: Penguin.

Cooper, D. (1974). *The Grammar of Living.* London: Allen Lane.

Craig, T. & Timms, P. W. (1992). Out of the wards and onto the streets? Deinstitutionalisation and homelessness in Britain. *Journal of Mental Health*, **1**, 265–275.

Crawford, M. (2000). Homicide is impossible to predict. *Psychiatric Bulletin*, **24**, 152.

Crichton, J. & Sheppard, D. (1996). Psychiatric inquiries: learning the lessons. In *Inquiries after Homicide*, ed. J. Peay. London: Duckworth.

Department of Health (1998a). Frank Dobson outlines third way for mental health. Press release reference 98/311. (Available at http://www.dh.gov.uk/PublicationsAndStatistics/PressReleases/ PressReleasesNotices/fs/en?CONTENT_ID=4024509&chk=G4JMRG).

Department of Health (1998b). *Modernising Mental Health Services: Safe, Sound and Supportive.* London: Department of Health.

Department of Health and Social Security (1975). *Better Services for the Mentally Ill.* London: HMSO.

Department of Health and Social Security and Welsh Office (1971). *Better Services for the Mentally Handicapped.* London: HMSO.

Double, D. B. (ed.) (2006). *Critical Psychiatry: The Limits of Madness.* Basingstoke: Palgrave Macmillan.

Douglas, M. (1992). *Risk and Blame: Essays in Cultural Theory*. London: Routledge.

Geddes, J. (1999). Suicide and homicide by people with mental illness. *British Medical Journal*, **318**, 1225–1226.

Giddens, A. (1991). *Modernity and Self-identity*. Cambridge: Polity Press.

Goffman, E. (1961). *Asylums. Essays on the Social Situation of Mental Patients and Other Inmates*. Harmondsworth: Penguin.

Goodwin, S. (1993). *Community Care and the Future of Mental Health Service Provision*. Aldershot: Avebury.

Goodwin, S. (1997). *Comparative Mental Health Policy: From Institutional to Community Care*. London: Sage.

Halligan, A. & Donaldson, L. (2001). Implementing clinical governance: turning vision into reality. *British Medical Journal*, **322**, 1415–1417.

Jones, M. (1952). *Social Psychiatry*. London: Tavistock.

Kesey, K. (1963). *One Flew Over the Cuckoo's Nest*. London: Methuen.

King, M. & 59 other signatories (2006). Community psychiatry inquiries must be fair, open and transparent [Letter]. *The Times*, Dec 4.

Kisely, S., Campbell, L. A., Scott, A., Preston, N. J., & Xiao, J. (2006). Randomized and non-randomized evidence for the effect of compulsory community and involuntary out-patient treatment on health service use: systematic review and meta-analysis. *Psychological Medicine*, doi:10.1017/S0033291706008592 (published online 21 Aug).

Laing, R. D. (1967). *The Politics of Experience and The Bird of Paradise*. Harmondsworth: Penguin.

Laing, R. D. (1985). *Wisdom, Madness and Folly*. London: Macmillan.

Laing, R. D. (1987). Laing's understanding of interpersonal experience. In *The Oxford Companion to the Mind*, ed. R. L. Gregory (assisted by O. L. Zangwill) Oxford: Oxford University Press.

Leff, J. (1993). All the homeless people – where do they all come from? *British Medical Journal*, **306**, 669–670.

Martin, J. P. (1984). *Hospitals in Trouble*. Oxford: Blackwell.

Mollica, R. F. (1985). From Antonio Gramsci to Franco Basaglia: the theory and practice of the Italian psychiatric reform. *International Journal of Mental Health*, **14**, 22–41.

Mullan, B. (1995). *Mad to be Normal. Conversations with R. D. Laing*. London: Free Association.

Nuttall, J. (1970). *Bomb Culture*. London: Paladin.

Norfolk & Waveney Mental Health Partnership NHS Trust (2005). *Panel report from the inquiry into the care and treatment of Richard King*. (Available at http://www.nmhct.nhs.uk/FOI/Class%207/inquiry%20doc.pdf).

O'Neill, O. (2002). *A Question of Trust*. Cambridge: Cambridge University Press.

Passmore, K. & Leung, W-C. (2002). Defensive practice among psychiatrists: a questionnaire survey. *Postgraduate Medicine*, **78**, 671–673.

Reder, P., Duncan, S., & Gray, M. (1993). *Beyond Blame: Child Abuse Tragedies Revisited*. London: Routledge.

Salter, M. (2003). Serious incident inquiries: a survival kit for psychiatrists. *Psychiatric Bulletin*, **27**, 245–247.

Schatzman, M. (1972). Madness and morals. In *Laing and Anti-psychiatry*, ed. R. Boyers & R. Orrill. Harmondsworth: Penguin.

Scheff, T. J. (1999). *Being Mentally Ill: A Sociological Theory*, 3rd edn. New York: Aldine de Gruyter.

Scotland, Baroness, Kelly, H., & Devaux, M. (1998) *The report of the Luke Warm Luke mental health inquiry* (Vols I & II). London: Lambeth and Lewisham Health Authority.

Sullivan, H. S. (1962). *Schizophrenia as a Human Process*. New York: W. W. Norton & Co.

Szmukler, G. (2000). Homicide inquiries: What sense do they make? *Psychiatric Bulletin*, **24**, 6–10.

Tantam, D. (1991). The anti-psychiatry movement. In *150 Years of British Psychiatry, 1841–1991*, ed. G. E. Berrios & H. Freeman. London: Gaskell.

Taylor, F. J. & Gunn, I. (1999). Homicides by people with mental illness: Myth and reality. *British Journal of Psychiatry*, **174**, 9–14.

Van Dorn, R. A., Elbogen, E. B., Redlich, A. D., Swanson, J. W., Swartz, M. S., & Mustillo, S. (2006). The relationship between mandated community treatment and perceived barriers to care in persons with severe mental illness. *International Journal of Law and Psychiatry*, **29**, 495–506.

Wall, S., Hotopf, M., Wessely, S., & Churchill, R. (1999). Trends in the use of the Mental Health Act: England, 1984–96. *British Medical Journal*, **318**, 1520–1521.

Walshe, K. & Higgin, J. (2002). The use and impact of inquiries in the NHS. *British Medical Journal*, **325**, 895–900.

Weller, M. P. I. (1989). Mental illness – who cares? *Nature*, **339**, 249–252.

Wolfe, T. (1989). *The Electric Kool-aid Acid Test*. London: Black Swan.

World Health Organization (1953). *Expert Committee on Mental Health: Third Report*. Geneva: WHO.

4

Democracy in psychiatry: or why psychiatry needs a new constitution

Bradley Lewis

Nothing about us without us!!

(protest poster at a rally against American Psychiatric Association)

Psychiatry's contemporary efforts to increase its liberatory potential are heir to a range of historically similar efforts. Carl Cohen and Sami Tamimi point out in their introduction to this book that the founding images of psychiatry start with Philip Pinel's liberatory gesture of unchaining the eighteenth-century Parisian insane. We can add to this liberatory gesture William Tuke's efforts to create a moral treatment, Sigmund Freud's efforts to discover and interpret unconscious conflicts, Jacques Lacan's efforts to keep Freud's work true to its potential, community psychiatry's efforts to spread psychiatric treatment to a broader public, Thomas Szasz's efforts to rid psychiatry of philosophical category mistakes, R. D. Laing's efforts to make space for the existential value of psychic suffering, and, even Robert Spitzer's efforts to make psychiatry more scientifically consistent. Throughout the history of psychiatry, in other words, we see a range of liberatory efforts. Each of these efforts has been designed to benefit the psychically different and those who suffer from psychic pain.

Despite the tremendous diversity of these liberatory efforts, they all have at least one thing in common. They all were created and designed by experts through a similar process. In each case, an expert, or small band of experts, undertook a critique of current psychiatric paradigms and institutions. After the critique, the expert imagined alternative psychiatric systems – which offered different and sometimes radically different approaches to psychiatry. The expert then joined with others to spread the new system out into the field. The net result in each case was that new ideas for psychiatry came from a small handful of relevant stake-holders. And, more striking, the most important stakeholders, the service users, were excluded from the process. Even in the most radical of these liberatory examples, service users themselves did not articulate the critique or design the improved system. In each of these historical efforts the process moved from expert analysis to expert solution.

Liberatory Psychiatry: Philosophy, Politics, and Mental Health, ed. Carl I. Cohen and Sami Timimi.
Published by Cambridge University Press. © Cambridge University Press.

None of these liberatory efforts imagined an alternative infrastructure of inquiry that would be more inclusive of psychiatric stakeholders. None found a way to analyze problems and discover solutions that included the people who would use and be most affected by the outcome of that inquiry. It is true that some of these liberatory efforts did attempt to increase service user's role and contribution at the point of service. That can certainly be said for Laing and Szasz, and in many ways it can also be said for Freud and Lacan. But even in these reform efforts – the inaugurating ideas, the rules, norms and expectations of practice, the material infrastructure, and the groundwork of legitimate inquiry – were all set up by expert stakeholders.

I argue in this chapter that we can draw a clear lesson from this history. Reforming psychiatry's clinical practice at the point of service must also include a larger reform of its research and decision making infrastructure. No matter how well meaning one's reform intentions, when a clinical system of knowledge and practice is set up without input from the main stakeholders, the system ends up skewed and biased away from stakeholders needs. In all probability, the system ends up skewed in rough proportion to the relative input and power of those involved.

Future liberatory reforms efforts in psychiatry must not fall in this "expert trap." Rather, future liberatory efforts must be developed through a process of inclusiveness. Key stakeholders must be involved in all levels of the reform – not just at the point of service, but also in the process of considering system wide problems and weighing possible alternatives. As a result, the next wave of liberatory reform in psychiatry should not be expert driven, it should be democracy driven. Indeed, the call for progressive liberatory reform in psychiatry should be a call for democracy in psychiatry.[1]

The power of democracy

Democratic theorists Ernesto Laclau and Chantal Mouffe argue that the language and goals of democracy have been key "fermenting agents" behind a variety of progressive politics. Citing from recent history, they give examples of the women's movement, African-American civil rights, gay and lesbian liberation, and environmental activism (Laclau & Mouffe, 1985, p. 155). Going back further, this same democratic imaginary has also been used by abolitionists to combat slavery, suffragettes in their struggles for the vote, and anti-imperialist in their resistance against colonial rulers (Smith, 1998, p. 9).

These examples show the power of democratic aims not only for specific liberatory goals, but also as a catalyst for generalizing and spreading liberatory goals. Once democratic discourse gets started, the call for "democracy" functions as a rallying cry for collective action in ever new domains. Even domains previously removed from democratic language are effected. Laclau and Mouffe point out that egalitarian discourses have played an increasing role throughout history in the construction of collective identifications: "At the beginning of this process in the French Revolution, the public space of citizenship was the exclusive domain of equality, while in the private sphere no questioning took place of existing social inequalities. However, as de Tocqueville clearly understood, once human beings accept the legitimacy of the principle of equality in one sphere they will attempt to extend it to every other sphere" (Laclau & Mouffe, 1990, p. 128). In short, once democracy gets started, it tends to spread into ever new domains.

The question arises: is it possible that psychiatry could be the next sphere to embrace democracy? The expert trap in the history of psychiatric reform certainly suggests the need for a democratic process, but the leap to democracy in psychiatry will not be easy. The difficulty comes partly from current experts who benefit from the current arrangement. But, even more so, the difficulty comes from the wide-spread idealization of "science" in psychiatry, which leaves psychiatric stake-holders extremely passive about their own contributions to knowledge.

The currently dominant view of science in Western influenced societies goes back to the Enlightenment. Key features of this view include a cluster of strongly held beliefs that science is objective, value-free, and that its method systematically corrects for human prejudice and bias. Most people understand the knowledge produced by science to be the closest thing humans have to the truth – to an understanding of the way the world actually works independent of human interests and desires. This ideal of ever-increasing approximation of the truth connects directly with an ideal of progress. Since science supposedly brings humans pro gressively true understanding of the world, science is deeply connected with a sense of human progress and civilization.

The power of these ideas runs deep in modern cultures, and science holds a uniquely privileged position in contemporary thought. Few people would grant other domains of inquiry and knowledge production such a privileged position. Science is, as a result, the last domain of the culture wars. In most other domains, people largely agree that producers of human statements contain within them the producers' frames of reference, their values, and their interests. In other words, knowledge claims about domains outside science – such as art, fashion, politics, popular culture – are thought to be connected to the local practices and the world views of their origins. For these domains, most people would agree with cultural studies scholar Stuart Hall that, if the producers are part of a "dominant cultural order," they will encode into their statements the larger "maps of social reality" which simultaneously impose specific classifications of the social and political world (Hall, 1980, p. 134). They would also agree that these social maps have a "whole range of social meanings, practices, and usages, power and interest 'written in' to them"

(p. 134). Though these dominant social maps are neither univocal nor uncontested, they tend toward creating a pattern of "preferred" meanings, which have the producers' "institutional/political/ideological order imprinted in them" (p. 134).

When it comes to science, however, people have trouble making the connections between facts and values, between scientific knowledge and social contexts. Bruno Latour argues in his book *We Have Never Been Modern* that this should not be surprising (Latour, 1993). The difficulty moderns have in making connections between human culture and non-human nature is in many ways the foundational divide of modernism. To be modern is, in short, to separate the two. Latour considers this divide to be such a core feature of modernism that he makes an analogy with other separations of modernism. The separation between the human and non-human "could be compared to the division that distinguishes the judiciary from the executive branch of a government" (Latour, 1993, p. 13). It is a constitutional separation, and it is a foundational feature of modernism. To be modern is to adopt the constitution. And to make the constitution work, modernists must adopt a deeply held sense that science and scientific method are independent of the human aspects of inquiry.

But are science and scientific method really so "neutral" toward the "values" of researchers? Most science studies scholars would say no. Scientific inquiry, like other forms of inquiry, is a human practice. In a review of science studies, Sharon Traweek argues that over the past 30 years science studies have produced "a near avalanche of research on the way communities of scientists, engineers, and physicians [produce] knowledge" (Traweek, 1993, p. 4). Often this literature consists of detailed ethnographic studies of the social interactions involved in the creation of supposedly neutral, or objective, science. Over and over again, this literature documents that *people make science*, not some abstract scientific method, and these people have a variety of interests, blind spots, and unequal power relations that dramatically affects the products of science. Scientific method, as a set of procedures, guidelines, rules, norms, institutional structures, etc., is slippery enough to allow considerable variability of choice in the selection of problems, paradigms, perceptions, evidential priorities, methodological adjustments, and interpretive possibilities. The result of these many human choices within science is that the human factor in scientific outcome remains high. Trying to tighten scientific method (through more science and more rigorous scientific method) does not change this situation.

Even in the most rigorous of science, to use Latour's terms: "the status of a statement [made by some people] depends on later statements [made by other people]" (Latour, 1987, p. 27). Without people there would be no science. And, in the last instance (and increasingly in the bottom line of economic rationality), it is *people* who verify truth statements with statements about statements. Certainly not anything can be said and science studies scholars are not "anything goes" relativists.

The world is real. It resists some interpretations and supports others. Statements about the world cannot be complete social constructions because they must accommodate the world, but the world itself does not make statements and the statements it accommodates are multiple. There are, in other words, many ways for people to carve up nature, and this inevitable human participation makes science anything but an objective reflection of the world. Rather than seeing science as objective reflection, science studies understand science-as-culture. Science studies, Latour explains, retie "the Gordian knot ... that separates exact knowledge and the exercise of power" (Latour, 1993, p. 3). As such, science studies understand all products of science as "nature–culture" hybrids.

These insights from science studies effectively demote scientific inquiry from its hierarchical status as unconditionally more worthy and more valuable than other forms of knowledge and other forms of inquiry. The science-as-culture perspective does not make science less worthy than other forms of inquiry, but it does (at least theoretically) level the playing field between forms of inquiry. As a result, scientific representational practices must prove their worth by virtue of their effects, uses, and the life-worlds they foster – they are not automatically more worthy by virtue of being "scientific." For Traweek, "most [science studies] researchers take these statements to be a sort of boring baseline of shared knowledge in the field" (Traweek, 1996, p. 145).

Recent work in science studies has accordingly moved beyond descriptive ethnographies, which detail science's all too human sources, and has turned toward the question of democracy. If science is not exceptional or independent of humans anymore than other forms of inquiry, then we must ask how are the human relations of science organized? What kinds of social institutions and protocols are set up to negotiate potential controversies like: What kinds of research are good to pursue and for whom are they good to pursue? Which of the available methods of inquiry are best? On what ethical or political grounds do we include or exclude possible knowledge contributors?

Philosopher of science Philip Kitcher argues that currently most science answers these questions through a political system he calls "internal elitism" (Kitcher, 2001, p.133). In "internal elitism"

the channeling of research effort is subject to pressures from a largely uninformed public, from a competitive interaction among technological enterprises that may represent only a tiny fraction of the population, and from scientists who are concerned to study problems of very particular kinds or to use the instruments and forms of expertise that are at hand. (p. 126)

Internal elitism means that scientific experts, coming from a narrow stratum of society, make all of these key value decisions among themselves and effectively decide the knowledge agenda for everyone else.

The problem of this kind of elitism in science is the same as the problem of elitism in other domains. It tends toward a pattern of preferred meanings, which as Hall explained, have the "institutional/political/ideological order" of their producers imprinted in them (Hall, 1980, p. 134). This problem leads to the next question. If current science set up through internal elitism is unacceptable, what alternative approaches should be considered? Or as philosopher of science Sandra Harding puts it, "What can be done to enhance the democratic tendencies within the sciences and to inhibit their elitist, authoritarian, and distinctively androcentric, bourgeois, Eurocentric agenda?" (Harding, 1991, p. 217). Harding's answer, similar to most people who have looked seriously at this issue, is some form of democratic representation in science. In democratic societies, in other words, there need to be formations of scientific practice which support democratic values, not the values of an elite minority.

Theorizing a democratic psychiatry

What does all this mean for psychiatry? At its most basic, it means that, before psychiatry can meaningfully reform itself, it must let go of its modernist illusions. The science studies work I reviewed along with a range of work in contemporary philosophy (loosely aggregated under the rubric of "postmodern theory") makes it clear that psychiatry must embrace an understanding of itself outside a modernist world view. Like Thomas and Bracken (see Chapter 2), I recommend that we call this alternative worldview "postpsychiatry" (Lewis, 2006). For those who do not like the concept of postmodernism, Bruno Latour would suggest adopting the notion of "amodernism" or "non-modernism" instead. Latour uses these terms rather than "postmodern" because he argues Western science never achieved the fabled modernist separation between facts and values in the first place. Western science, like other forms of knowledge-making, has always created complicated imbroglios of nature and culture, facts, and values. As such, Latour would argue that there's no need to make a "postmodern turn" since we never really took a "modern turn" to begin with.

Either way, the point for psychiatry remains the same. Psychiatry must let go of a modernist constitution that draws a sharp line between nature and culture, facts and values. It must rework its basic infrastructure so that it moves beyond idealized notions of this binary. Once psychiatry accepts the human and political dimensions of inquiry, it will be able to accept the need for setting up fair and just human relations of inquiry. It will be able to move beyond internal elitism to a more democratic structure of inquiry.

Unfortunately, most psychiatrists are deeply entrenched in the modern constitution, and they do not see the current structure of internal elitism in psychiatric inquiry as a problem. Using the modernist constitution as their guide, most psychiatrists would argue that that despite the fact that psychiatric experts, coming from a narrow stratum of society, make all of these key research and treatment protocol decisions among themselves, the interest of patients are still fairly represented without any need for democracy. Consider, for example, the lead motto of the American Psychiatric Association: *Member Driven. Science based. Patient Focused.*[2] This motto provides a good representation of the modernist constitution at work in psychiatry. The motto implies that the interests of the most relevant group – patients – are already the focus of the field because, through a "science base," psychiatry develops its knowledge and interventions for the sole purpose of benefiting patients.

But since science cannot completely factor out the interests of its producers, then the APA motto is problematic. The current APA membership consists of "36 000 physician leaders in mental health"(http://www.psych.org/). There are no patient leaders, or family leaders, or civic leaders, etc. So, one can fairly ask, how can an association that represents 36 000 physicians *and no patients* actually be "patient focused?" This is where the supposed magic of the middle part of the motto, "science based," comes in. Science magically allows the organization to be simultaneously patient focused and exclusively driven by physician leaders. But, as I have been arguing, not even science can work this much purifying magic.

Indeed, no matter what method experts use to assess, understand, and intervene into problems, they cannot completely leave their own interests out of the process. This would be no less true if we replaced "science based" with another expert driven slogan. If we switched psychiatry from "science based" to "phenomenology based," or "philosophy based," or "experience based," or "ethics based," the same problem would arise. When the balance of expertise is 36 000 to 0, no logic of expertise can magically correct for a very serious, and very problematic, skewing effect toward the interests of the 36 000. The only way to truly achieve "patient focus" in psychiatry is to move from "science based" to "democracy based."

Three concrete steps toward a democratic psychiatry

But, even if increasing numbers of psychiatrist let go of their modernist obsession with science, how can the world of psychiatry actually move from being expert based to democracy based? How can psychiatry make concrete steps that shift the field from a domain where experts are the principal architects of inquiry to a domain where non-expert stakeholders have a significant input? In this section, I offer up three ways in which psychiatry can start moving toward this goal: (1) reform the APA; (2) create a critical psychiatry network; and (3) shift clinical care to a narrative frame.

The first and most obvious step toward creating a more democratic psychiatry is to reform the membership and organizational structure of the APA.[3] At the moment, only professional psychiatrists are members of the APA. In order to work toward a more democratic psychiatry, the APA would have to open up its doors to other groups who are involved with, interested in, or effected by psychiatric practice and procedures, e.g., patients, family members, interested citizens, clinicians, administrators, researchers, legal personnel, government officials, police, and interested scholars.

However, simply allowing a few token members from each of these groups to join the APA is not enough. The APA membership must be structured in relation to the size of the stakeholder group and the degree to which psychiatry affects a particular group. This means that the primary group represented in the APA community would be patients or "c/s/x" (to use the more progressive term which is now being used instead of the more problematic, "patient").[4] After c/s/x, family members would be the next biggest group, followed by clinicians, administrators, scholars (from all sides of campus), clinical researchers, and relevant persons from the legal community. Coupled with this new *weighted* membership structure, the APA would also have to diversify along the lines of race, ethnicity, ability, gender, sexual preference, class, and age. Although, of course, such identity labels would not be seen as fixed or essential and members could be acknowledged as having multiple and hybrid identifications.

In terms of organization, the members of this more diverse APA would be elected and would function for psychiatry, as members of congress function for the United States. At annual APA conventions, these members would participate in, what I have called elsewhere, "psychiatric community tribunals" (Lewis, 2006, p. 158). In these tribunals, APA members would be given background information (via hearings) on particular topics of psychiatric research, education, and treatment protocols. These information sessions would be followed by opportunities to cross-examine presenters. These tribunals would vote on key issues and have the power to make decisions about, for example, psychiatric guidelines, services, training requirements, journals, research, infrastructure, and financial issues.

Altering the membership and organization of the APA in this way would no doubt lead to the dilemma of consensus. What happens, in other words, when this new group of diverse APA members cannot agree on research, practice, or treatment proposals? I argue that a reformed APA could overcome this dilemma by rejecting the need for unanimous consensus or even a majority vote. Instead, the APA would allow proposals which achieve, for example, 20% (or more) of the vote to be considered "legitimate" knowledge. Such "legitimate" knowledge would be written up in teaching materials, offered as a real possibility in practice situations, granted funded for further research, etc.; albeit with a caveat that the knowledge is controversial, that there are doubts involved, and that the APA community differs on how to deal with it.

Although completely democratic institutions of psychiatric governance may never be possible, it is very possible to make progressive movement from today's structure of internal elitism and exclusive professional membership toward more democratic participation in psychiatry. The main impediment to making this kind of progress is not feasibility, but contemporary attitudes and the strength of the modernist constitution. Current modernist mindsets are so strong that psychiatric governing bodies are very unlikely to invite democracy into their organizations. They are unlikely to move from "science based" to "democracy based" on their own initiative. Therefore, in the next section, I recommend a second set of strategies that work toward increasingly democratic participation in psychiatry – regardless of whether psychiatry recognizes the need for this participation. If the main psychiatric institutions, like the APA, are not willing to consciously reorganize themselves along democratic lines, other strategies can be set in motion which could affect today's psychiatry and also lay the foundations for a truly democratic psychiatry in the future.[5]

The second step toward democratizing psychiatry is to create critical psychiatry networks and grassroots coalitions to foster alternative possibilities to the mainstream. This step can begin even without organized psychiatry's stamp of approval. No vote or agreement to reorganize the APA membership is required. All that is required is the grassroots coalition building. In the last several years there has spontaneously emerged a range of interdisciplinary scholars and activists who expand common assumptions about psychiatry and mental illness. These include: (1) consumer activists who have developed alternative approaches to psychic pain and psychic difference; (2) interdisciplinary humanities and social science scholars working at the interface of psychiatry, mind, and culture; and (3) critical psychiatrists and other mental health professionals working toward progressive change in psychiatry. Although there is considerable overlap in these domains, they often work in relative isolation from each other. A critical psychiatry network would bring these voices together to showcase this important work and to help create a more connected research community.

But what would such a network really look like? To answer this, I suggest that inspiration be drawn from the arena of disability studies. Disability studies serve as a useful model in the way it has built and supports new disability scholarships and also the way it has forged a coalition between scholars and activists. Similar to scholars who are looking at the political, social, economic and cultural dimensions of psychiatry, disability scholars have been looking at these social, political, economic and cultural dimensions of disability. In particular, they have studied the way various cultural and political forces have led to the labeling, normalizing, and medicalizing of "disabled" bodies.[6]

These disability scholars, as well as building a substantial body of scholarly disability studies, have also built healthy alliances with disability activists. Together, these scholars and activists have fought to challenge the medicalization and normalization of mainstream approaches to disability. They have done this through community interventions that focus on consciousness raising and collective action. Similar to other new social movements (such as feminism or gay and lesbian movements), consciousness raising helps create new disability identifications. These identifications allow disability activists to form political connections with people who have been similarly treated. As disability scholar Michael Oliver points out, "by reconceptualising disability as a social restriction or oppression, [disability identifications] open up possibilities of collaborating or cooperating with other socially restricted or oppressed groups" (Oliver, 1996, p. 129). These collaborating groups become a powerful coalition toward collective action and social change.

The disability studies example shows that a "critical psychiatry network" between scholars, activists, and "c/s/x" is possible and could have very fruitful and potentially powerful results. Indeed, such a network may not be far off. As Duncan Double, a UK psychiatrist, outlines in his chapter in this book, early work has already begun put together a "critical psychiatry network." This network not only draws together scholarship from around the world which looks critically at psychiatry, it also encourages and supports activist efforts which challenge the most problematic aspects of modern psychiatry. The website's political statement reads:

> We believe that there is a need to resist attempts to make psychiatry *more* coercive. In its attempts to take forward this agenda, the Network has:
> - Made clear its opposition to compulsory treatment in evidence submitted to the Government's Scoping Group set up to review the Mental Health Act.
> - Submitted evidence to the Government, arguing against the idea of preventive detention.
> - Carried out a survey of senior English psychiatrists to seek their views about preventive detention.
> - Worked closely with other groups, coordinated by MIND, in trying to influence government policy (http://www.critpsynet.freeuk.com/position.htm).

This kind of "critical psychiatry network" is an important start. With the right funding and support, the network could grow into a powerful global forum from which today's psychiatry could be increasingly rethought and, if necessary, challenged. The network begins the process of bringing new voices to psychiatry even without psychiatry's willingness to change. As such, the network offers a vital foundation from which a more democratic psychiatry might blossom.

That said, even with the real potential of critical psychiatry networks, reforming the APA into a more democratic institution remains a major task. While those interested in a more democratic psychiatry must push in this direction, it is going to take a lot of work to change the institution and knowledge base of contemporary psychiatry. In the mean time, what about today's clinical encounters? Even while democratic reform efforts organize, people will still be in the clinics seeing psychiatrists. This concern for today's clinical encounters brings me to my third strategy for a more democratic psychiatry. How can psychiatrists operate more democratically in the clinical encounter while the psychiatric institutions and knowledge base remain the same (or while the work to change the institutions and knowledge base is being done)? The answer, in brief, is *narrative psychiatry*.[7]

Although there have been relatively limited applications in contemporary psychiatry, a growing number of people in medicine use narrative approaches in their clinical work. Rita Charon coins the phrase "narrative medicine" to describe this emerging field that employs literary and narrative studies to augment the scientific understandings of illness (Charon, 2005, p. 261). According to Charon, when clinician's possess "narrative competency," they can enter the clinical setting with a nuanced capacity for "attentive listening . . ., adopting alien perspectives, following the narrative thread of the story of another, being curious about other people's motives and experiences, and tolerating the uncertainty of stories" (p. 262).

Advocates of narrative medicine believe that doctors "*need* rigorous and disciplined training" in narrative reading and writing not just for their own sake (helping deal with the strains and traumas of clinical work); but also "*for the sake of their practice*" (p. 262). Without such "narrative competency," clinicians lack the ability to fully understand their client's experience of illness. For Charon and others in narrative medicine, narrative studies are not a mere adornment to a doctor's medical training; they are a crucial and "basic science" that must be mastered for medical practice (Charon, 2004, p. 863).

Narrative competency allows doctors to understand that the scientific models of illness (in which clinicians are predominantly trained) are also narratives. Along these lines, Kathryn Montgomery Hunter points out that narrative medicine allows a movement away from the illusion "of objectivist, scientific reportage" and toward an acknowledgement that medical case histories are "humanly constructed" accounts: "Two things are essential: first, both tellers and listeners must recognize the narrator of the case history as contextually conditioned, and, second, the lived experience of the patient must be experienced" (Hunter, 1991, p. 166).

Contemporary physician-writer Abraham Verghese, in a speech to fellow physicians at the American Society of Internal Medicine, explained why narrative competency is vital: "As physicians, most of us become involved in the stories of our patient's lives . . . we become players in these stories. Our actions change the narrative trajectory . . . and our patient's stories come to depend heavily on repetition of what we say" (Verghese, 2001, p. 1012). He then went on to point out that the inescapable thesis for medicine is three fold: "(1) *story* helps us link and make sense of events in our lives; (2) we as physicians *create* stories as often as we record them . . .; and (3) we are characters in [these] various stories, walking on and off the stage in tales that take place in our hospitals and clinics" (p. 1012).

Insights like these from narrative medicine are directly applicable to psychiatry. Not only do narrative approaches allow psychiatric practitioners to more fully understand their clients' experiences of illness, but they also allow practitioners to see through the illusion that their understandings of patients are objective, scientific, value-free, and thus the one "right" interpretation. With narrative competency, clinicians understand the contextually conditioned nature of their own psychiatric knowledge, and they understand that their knowledge is just one narrative among many. This is particularly prescient in the current climate when biopsychiatry prevails so powerfully, and other interpretations of mental distress are progressively marginalized as biopsychiatry becomes seen as the one "correct" interpretation of mental distress.

As with narrative medicine, narrative psychiatry does not seek to reject these prevalent biological understandings of illness. Unlike anti-psychiatry critics who reject biopsychiatry because of its reductionism and oversimplifications, narrative psychiatry helps clinicians see a world where alternative interpretations of mental illness, including biopsychiatric ones, are not so much wrong or bad, but different. Narrative psychiatry, in other words, encourages clinicians to see multiple interpretations of illness and not just stick doggedly, and even dogmatically, to one single interpretation.[8] Encouraging this kind of narrative competency among psychiatric practitioners allows much more freedom, flexibility, and democracy in the clinical setting. In this way, narrative psychiatry may be understood as similar to democratic psychiatry only on a much smaller scale. Narrative practitioners and their clients are not confined to single approaches and are free to explore the many, rich and varied, approaches available. This openness to alternative approaches allows a much more democratic clinical setting than authoritarian "doctor knows best" of most expert-driven treatment protocols.

Achieving this kind of narrative competency does not require a revolution in psychiatry or even the work of a critical psychiatry network. It can enter the clinics immediately. To achieve narrative competency, practitioners need only understand the basics of narrative theory and learn to read widely in a range of different contexts. Through this exploration, clinicians must learn to appreciate the many stories of biopsychiatry, psychoanalysis, cognitive therapy, interpersonal therapy, family therapy, humanistic approaches, cross-cultural approaches, feminist approaches, disability activist approaches, postmodern approaches, spiritual approaches, and ecopsychology, to name a few. Furthermore, they must come to understand the value of biography, autobiography, and literature for developing a narrative repertoire. In the end, narrative competency means familiarity with the many possible stories of psychic suffering and psychic difference. The more stories clinicians know, the more likely they are to help their clients find a narrative frame that works for them.

The narrative frame that is most helpful for a particular person may involve a story of psychiatric "disease" and "medical model" treatment, but it may well involve a variety of other narrative structures. The narrative psychiatrist, even when working in the limited role of "med checks" and "evals," can allow the process of clinical story making to remain open to stories beyond dominant disease models. If the disease model helps and fits with the person's preferences, then it can be used. If not, there's no reason to insist or to be dogmatic. Clearly, from a narrative perspective, there can be no gold standard or simple answers along the way. Clinicians and clients alike must work together, using judgment, wisdom, and experience as their guides.

Conclusion

The next round of liberatory reform in psychiatry must not fall into the modernist trap of expertise. It must recognize the intimate connections between knowledge and power and begin the process of setting up a new constitution that brings democracy to psychiatry. Like Bracken and Thomas, I recommend that we call this new approach to psychiatry "postpsychiatry." Some, like Bruno Latour, might prefer that we call the approach "non-modern" psychiatry. But whatever we call it, the steps toward a more democratic psychiatry are similar. They involve three basic tasks. First, the organizational structure of psychiatry must be opened to membership from a more representative stakeholder group. Second, while working toward that goal, critical psychiatric networks and coalitions must begin to organize and circulate additional, alternative, and critical perspectives and approaches to mainstream (undemocratic) psychiatry. And, finally, clinical practitioners must let go of their modernist dogmatism to adopt more flexible practice models. Narrative psychiatry is an excellent example of this more open and flexible approach.

NOTES

(1) The following sections contain material first explored in *Moving Beyond Prozac, DSM, and the New Psychiatry: Birth of Postpsychiatry* (Lewis, 2006). I am grateful to Michigan University Press for permission to publish some of it here.

(2) I take this motto from the top banner of the American Psychiatric Association web page (http://www.apa.org/).

(3) My use of the "APA" as the collective body for psychiatric governance and democratization in this section is only meant as a conceptual placeholder, a thought experiment. Reimagining the APA so that it is less of a guild or special interest group and more of a psychiatric governing body is just one option. Many alternative groupings for organizing the politics of psychiatry are possible.

(4) The term "patient" has been increasingly unsatisfactory within various critiques of psychiatry. Many are suggesting instead "c/s/x" which stands for "consumer/survivor/ex-patient." Putting these different identity positions (consumer/survivor/ex-patient) all together into a single neologism (c/s/x), rather than using only "ex-patient," allows a coalition among people with diverse identifications. It also implies that the relationship between these identity positions is not simply linear. People often shift from one identity position to another, and back again, or inhabit more than one at the same time. Thus, many folks involved with the mental health system, or attempting to avoid involvement with it, are often a hybrid mixture of these multiple identifications (Morrison, 2003). I use the term "c/s/x" rather than "patient" for the remainder of this discussion.

(5) I should add to this discussion that some object to the possibility of democratizing psychiatry (and other forms of "democracy and science" initiatives) not because they believe politics and science are separate, but because they have a basic skepticism with regard to democracy. These skeptical objections are often based on contemporary frustrations with what democratic theorists call "thin democracy," and they are based on the recent abuses of democracy as a legitimizing rhetoric for neo-imperialism. There is a far cry, however, from "getting to vote" in a thin democracy and the experience of significant stakeholder participation in a "thick democracy." How to move thin democracies toward meaningful stakeholder participation is a problem of democratic theory and a topic too large for this paper. Clearly, democracy as it is currently practiced is far from ideal. We may continue to argue, with Winston Churchill, that democracy is a more inclusive form of governance than other actual alternatives, but that hardly means that democracy is a panacea or that its practices are not loaded with mine fields. If psychiatry takes seriously the need to organize its knowledge politics around democratic values, it will also need to make democratic theory one of its core competencies. Knowledge of biological, psychological, and social domains of "patients" will not be enough. Psychiatry will also have to be smart about its own political organization.

(6) See "Mad Fight: Disability Activism and Psychiatry" (Lewis, 2006) for an extended discussion of disability and psychiatry. For basic background on disability studies see Michael Oliver, 1990, *The Politics of Disablement: A Sociological Approach*, Rosemarie Garland-Thomson, 1997, *Extraordinary Bodies: Figuring Physical Disability in American Culture and Literature*; James Charlton, 1998. *Nothing About Us Without Us: Disability, Oppression, and Empowerment*, and Lennard Davis, in press, *The Disability Studies Reader*.

(7) For an extended discussion of narrative psychiatry see Listening to Chekhov: Narrative Approaches to Depression" (Lewis, 2006). Also see Richard Martinez, "Narrative Understanding and Methods in Psychiatry and Behavioral Health" in *Stories Matter: The Role of Narrative in Medical Ethics*, ed. Rita Charon and Martha Montello (New York: Routledge, 2002) and Glen Roberts and Jeremy Holmes, *Healing Stories: Narrative*

Psychiatry and Psychotherapy (Oxford: Oxford University Press, 1999). For overviews of earlier uses of narrative theory in psychotherapy see Jill Freedman and Gene Combs, *Narrative Therapy: The Social Construction of Preferred Realities* (New York: W. W. Norton, 1996) and Michael White and David Epston, *Narrative Means to Therapeutic Ends* (New York: W. W. Norton, 1990).

(8) For a discussion of "dogmatism" in contemporary psychiatry, see Nassir Ghaemi, *The Concepts of Psychiatry: A Pluralistic Approach to the Mind and Mental Illness* (Baltimore, Johns Hopkins University Press, 2003). Ghaemi concludes, based on an analysis of psychiatric practice, that approximately "64% of psychiatrists are dogmatists" (p. 301).

REFERENCES

American Psychiatric Association. (accessed June 3, 2006), http://www.psych.org.

Charlton, J. (1998). *Nothing About Us Without Us: Disability, Oppression, and Empowerment.* Berkeley: University of California Press.

Charon, R. (2004). Narrative and Medicine. *New England Journal of Medicine*, **350**, 862–864.

Charon, R. (2005). Narrative medicine: attention, representation, affiliation. *Narrative*, **13**, 261–270.

Critical Psychiatry Network. (accessed June 3, 2006), http://www.critpsynet.freeuk.com.

Critical Psychiatry Network. Position Statement. (accessed June 3, 2006), http://www.critpsynet. freeuk.com/position.htm.

Davis, L. (ed.) (in press). *The Disability Studies Reader*. 2nd edn. New York: Routledge.

Freedman, J. & Combs, G. (1996) *Narrative Therapy: The Social Construction of Preferred Realities.* New York: W. W. Norton.

Garland-Thomson, R. (1997). *Extraordinary Bodies: Figuring Physical Disability in American Culture and Literature.* New York: Columbia University Press.

Ghaemi, N. (2003). *The Concepts of Psychiatry: A Pluralistic Approach to the Mind and Mental Illness*, Baltimore: Johns Hopkins University Press.

Hall, S. (1980). Encoding, decoding. In *Culture, Media, Language*, ed. Hall *et al*. London: Routledge. pp. 128–139.

Harding, S. (1991). *Whose Science? Whose Knowledge? Thinking from Women's Lives*. Ithaca, NY: Cornell University Press.

Hunter, K. M. (1991) *Doctors' Stories: The Narrative Structure of Medical Knowledge*, Princeton: Princeton University Press.

Kitcher, P. (2001). *Science, Truth and Democracy*. Oxford: Oxford University Press.

Laclau, E. & Mouffe, C. (1985). *Hegemony and Socialist strategy: Towards a Radical Democratic Politics*, London: Verso.

Laclau, E. & Mouffe, C. (1990). Post-Marxism without apologies. In *New Reflections of the Revolutions of Our Time*, ed. E. Laclau. London: Verso.

Latour, B. (1987). *Science in Action: How to Follow Scientists and Engineers through Society*. Cambridge, MA: Harvard University Press.

Latour, B. (1993). *We Have Never Been Modern*. Trans. Catherine Porter. Cambridge, MA: Harvard University Press.

Lewis, B. (2006). *Moving Beyond Prozac, DSM, and the New Psychiatry: Birth of Postpsychiatry*, Ann Arbor: University of Michigan Press.

Lewis, B. (in press). Listening to Chekhov: Narrative approaches to depression. *Literature and Medicine*.

Lewis, B. (in press). A mad fight: psychiatry and disability activism. In *The Disability Studies Reader*, 2nd edn. ed. L. Davis. New York: Routledge.

Martinez, R. (2002). Narrative understanding and methods in psychiatry and behavioral health. In *Stories Matter: The Role of Narrative in Medical Ethics*, ed. R. Charon & M. Montello. New York: Routledge.

Oliver, M. (1990). *The Politics of Disablement: A Sociological Approach*. New York: St. Martin's Press.

Oliver, M. (1996). *Understanding Disability: From Theory to Practice*. London: Macmillan.

Roberts, G. & Holmes, J. (1999). *Healing Stories: Narrative Psychiatry and Psychotherapy*, Oxford: Oxford University Press.

Smith, A. M. (1998). *Laclau and Mouffe: The Radical Democratic Imaginary*. London: Routledge.

Traweek, S. (1993). An introduction to the cultural and social studies of sciences and technologies. *Culture, Medicine, and Psychiatry*, **17**, 3–25.

Traweek, S. (1996). Unity, dyads, triads, quads, and complexity: cultural choreographies of science. In *Science Wars*, ed. A. Ross. Durham, NC: Duke University Press, pp. 139–150.

Verghese, A. (2001). The physician as storyteller. *Annals of Internal Medicine*, **135**, 1012–1017.

White, M. & Epston, D. (1990). *Narrative Means to Therapeutic Ends*, New York: W. W. Norton.

5

German critical psychology as emancipatory psychology

Charles W. Tolman

Introduction

The focus of this chapter is a psychology that had its origins in the student movements of the 1960s and 1970s. When it first acquired a name, it was called "critical-emancipatory psychology," but in time the label was shortened to "critical psychology," though it never lost its emancipatory intent. By way of introduction, I shall first say something about its history and the conceptual and ideological issues that motivated it. As we move on, we shall see how, crucial to its emancipatory goals, it formulated the subject matter of psychology as human subjectivity.[1] We shall then look at how psychology itself was reconstructed in order to reflect the nature of its subject matter.

There were many catalysts that precipitated the collective actions of a highly politicized postwar student generation in the Germany of the 1960s. These included restrictions by both governments and university officials on free speech. Many students and others complained of a lack of relevance of the material taught at universities. There was a general unrest stemming from the universities' authoritarian approach to the curriculum. In the end, however, the complaint that had by far the greatest impact on subsequent developments concerned the ideological nature of the subject matter being taught, particularly in philosophy and the social sciences.

Two debates were particularly crucial to the later development of Critical Psychology in Germany. The first took place in 1967 and had to do with the relevance of psychological or any other kind of scientific knowledge. The traditional view, one defended by the "liberal" wing of the Psychology Institute at the Free University of Berlin, was that knowledge was essentially neutral and that its relevance was created in the link between that knowledge and its application or use. That link was alleged to be the individual psychologist or scientist. It was, in short, a matter of individual conscience as to how knowledge was applied outside the academy.

Liberatory Psychiatry: Philosophy, Politics, and Mental Health, ed. Carl I. Cohen and Sami Timimi.
Published by Cambridge University Press. © Cambridge University Press.

The opposition to this view was strong and eloquent. All knowledge and practice, it was maintained, were necessarily generated and exercised in accordance with one interest or another. Moreover, there was a seamless web of relations in which philosophy, science, ideology, and society were necessarily interconnected. The universities, their priorities, and the knowledge they produced and propagated were all serving the interests of those who had the power to influence them. And that power was not in the hands of students or workers but in those of the state and the capitalists it served. One of the student participants put forward a list of psychology's involvement with ruling interests. There was, she maintained, research directed at improving the effectiveness of the military and psychological warfare, all in the service of imperialism; there was research in marketing and advertising, all in the service of the capitalist economy; work on communications and opinion sampling served bourgeois ideology; work on personnel selection, industrial psychology, and occupational counseling were concerned only with efficiency of capitalist production; and all sorts of counseling and psychotherapy were contributing to conformity. The list could easily be expanded (Staeuble, 1968). The well-known Hawthorne experiments,[2] for example, had not been intended to help the workers. Moreover, the reduction in behaviorist learning theory of learning and performance to deprivation states and reinforcement revealed little about the learners but did serve to justify wage slavery in the workplace. In short, psychology was necessarily partial and this partiality needed to be brought to the center of attention.

This debate was joined by Klaus Holzkamp, who published a paper expounding on the relevance of scientific knowledge for societal practice (1970, reprinted in 1972). Among other things, he distinguished between technical and emancipatory relevance. All knowledge was relevant; it was really a question of the parties to whom it is relevant. Behavioral psychology had proved very relevant to those who were interested in controlling others. It offered little, however, to those whom it controlled. It must be possible, he maintained, to develop knowledge that serves the interests of individuals in their efforts to improve the quality of their lives.

Holzkamp's points were among those taken up in the second crucial debate. The debate was initiated by a student intervention at a meeting of the German Society for Psychology in Tübingen in September 1968. It was effectively a challenge to the presumed political neutrality of the usual contributions to such meetings. How, for instance, the students asked, could psychologists sit around talking about the technical details of a personality inventory, while ignoring the political misuses to which such inventories were being put? According to the interveners, it was just these misuses that needed to be discussed. The result at this meeting was not to resolve any of the related issues but to organize a meeting for the following year, namely in May 1969, at which precisely these issues would be examined.

The two principal delegations at the meeting held in Hanover came from Berlin, one from the Free University and one from the Technical University. The thrust of the arguments put forward by the TU delegates was that psychology was inherently in the service of the ruling ideology, which, it was agreed, was oppressive. There could therefore, be no such thing as a critical or oppositional psychology. Psychology itself must be opposed, not only in the universities but in all areas of practice. It was suggested, for example, that copies of intelligence tests and other tests used for selection of people be given wide public distribution so as to undermine their use in schools and industry.

The FU delegates disagreed. The problem, they said, was not with psychology as science in principle, but with the powers that, as a discipline, it blindly served. They admitted that the prevailing psychology was shaped by, and in thrall to, an oppressive and exploitive ideology, but just as a psychology had been formed to serve those interests, a genuinely critical psychology could be developed to serve more broadly human, emancipatory interests. At the very least, it should be possible for such a psychology to clarify just what constitutes a liberated existence and to identify the psychological processes that mediate domination.

Over the next few years a group, mainly located at the FU Berlin and led by Klaus Holzkamp, a prominent senior member of the faculty at the Psychological Institute, undertook to lay the groundwork for a genuinely critical and emancipatory psychology. This involved a thorough critique of existing mainstream psychologies in order to identify their deficiencies from a liberatory standpoint. It was immediately clear that a psychology serving the interests of ordinary people would have to be based on a sound theoretical understanding of the relation of the individual to society. This was totally lacking in existing psychologies. Moreover, a critical psychology would have to be clear on what it meant to be a specifically human subject. The leading psychologies of the time had set generality as a goal and achieved it in the form of theories, such as the theory of reinforcement, that appeared to apply to all organisms, regardless of where they stood on the phylogenetic scale. They thus obscured the specifically human character of their subject matter. Generality would still have to be a goal, but a distinction would have to be made between the abstract kind that eliminated specifics and the concrete kind that preserved and explained them.

The shape of anti-emancipatory psychology

It is apparent that many psychologies that became current in the twentieth century did not promote emancipation. Behaviorism was most influential. Indeed, the extent of its influence is commonly underestimated. It is easy to identify this position with the psychology championed by John B. Watson or B. F. Skinner, but it must be remembered that virtually all the mainstream psychologies of the last century, though often less blatant, shared defining characteristics with these starker theories. Functionalism, for example, allowed talk about consciousness and purposes, but this was largely just that: talk. Even many of the protest psychologies, when they had to legitimate themselves academically by accommodating the prevailing criteria for acceptable (i.e., publishable) research, adopted key features of behaviourism.

It is therefore important to understand what these key features were. It will be recalled that John B. Watson gave twentieth-century psychology its direction by proclaiming it the science with the theoretical goal of predicting and controlling behavior. The formula that arose from this was S–R, the stimulus–response connection. Given the response, the goal was to identify the stimulus; given the stimulus, the goal was to predict the response. The psychologist, according to Watson, understands behavior "only as he can manipulate or control it" (1924, p. 7). The S–R model is of course a causal model that makes no concession to experimental or theoretical indeterminacy of its subject matter. The apparently "softer" functionalist S–O–R model introduced by R. S. Woodworth (1929) merely introduced another link in the chain; it did not change its causal nature.

The method that developed out of this kind of thinking was one that placed great store in the measurement of input and output, which became known as independent and dependent variables. To complete the picture, the "O" in Woodworth's model became known as an intervening variable. The idea of correlating independent and dependent variables was, of course, not new. Whether or not thus self-identified, it captures a defining feature of all scientific method, which, of course, is based on causal assumptions about nature. A significant move for scientific method in psychology came with the introduction of the statistical methods involving sampling and analysis of groups of data. This, in turn, introduced a further sophistication into the thinking behind psychological methods. This was the notion of "multiple causation." The S–R model had implied that once the stimulus was identified, the response would be absolutely predictable. But, of course, that seldom if ever happened. This showed up in the statistical methods as error variance. But this was not taken to mean that the researcher had made a mistake; it meant rather that only some of the independent variables had been identified and that there remained others yet to be discovered. The underlying idea was still one of complete predictability in principle.

The statistical method yielded still another benefit to causally driven psychology. This was that, when there was in fact a complete failure to predict the response of an experimental subject – that is, when a subject did not follow instructions or otherwise misbehaved – the event could be accounted for by the sampling theory upon which the statistical methods were based. The difficult subject became an "outlier" and non-representative of the population being sampled and could therefore be ignored. The statistical–causal model was thus completely self-confirming; all exceptions to the rule could be accounted for on good theoretical grounds without threatening the model's integrity. Psychologists might not be able to sell to industry and other interested parties the promise of absolute control of individuals, but they could sell the promise of control "on average," which, of course, made sense to the book-keepers who kept an eye on costs and benefits.

The behavioral–functional mode of psychology became all but universal in the twentieth-century. It formed (and still forms) the mainstream, with protests and exceptions clearly lying on the periphery. An interesting challenge from the inside, however, came from B. F. Skinner, an utterly unashamed behaviorist. His complaint was that the original aim of prediction and control was compromised by the statistical method. While multiple causation and sampling error might account for failures to predict, they also became easy excuses for lazy or sloppy research. Skinner's idiographic approach (to borrow a term from Gordon Allport) was, in short, aimed at the perfection of control. And, when it came to lever-pressing and other simple responses, he succeeded remarkably. The behavior not only of pigeons and rats but also of psychotics in mental wards and children in the classroom succumbed at times totally to his engineering of circumstances and contingencies. He gained control, but at the cost of abstraction. Skinner (1956) seemed proud to announce that the shapes of cumulative records of responses emitted were so uniform among species ranging from rats to humans that an observer of the records themselves could not distinguish one species from the other. What made the rat a rat, the pigeon a pigeon, or a human a human alluded Skinner completely. The lesson to be taken appears to be that control is indeed possible if the person or animal is reduced by circumstances to the state of a generic animal.

Personality theories often went by other labels, such as "structural dynamic," but remained in the behaviorist mold. The "traits" that they identified merely served as the intervening variables or hypothetical constructs in the S–R model. Gordon Allport, a well-known advocate of such a theory took it for granted that the goals of science "are to understand, predict, and control events" (1965, p. 159), a definition that proves to be redundant since "understanding" is estimated from the ability to predict and control.

Many claimed initially that the cognitive psychology that arose in the 1960s broke the mold. At least it allowed psychologists once again to speak with some legitimacy about presumed mental events. But the claim was easily shown to be mistaken. The information-processing theories that emerged were simply elabo-rate arrangements of intervening variables, and hypotheses about them were still tested by correlating independent and dependent variables. The only change that occurred in the behavioral–functional methods of so-called scientific psychology was their further refinement. The underlying causal S–R model was not challenged. The matter was certainly not improved by the move taken by many cognitive psychologists to a focus on brain processes, which tended only to make persons the helpless victims of their brains and genes.

So, what specifically is wrong with this model that has dominated mainstream psychology since the beginning of the twentieth century? Perhaps the most obvious problem is that it is committed to a conception of causality according to which, given S, R will occur – strike the match and it will light; tap the patellar tendon and the knee will jerk. The repeated failure to demonstrate such an invariant determinism for psychological events more complex than simple reflexes was explained by recourse to multiple causation: it was, in short, understood as a question of the state of the art, not one of erroneous assumptions. But people experience themselves as free agents with a say in how they respond to stimuli. When they are compelled by circumstances to act, they tend to know they are compelled and they resent it. This is what philosophers call intentionality, and there has been no room for intentionality in mainstream psychological theories.

A second obvious problem with the S–R model is that it ignores subjectivity. Again, people live in a world pervaded by subjectivity. But, of course, this theoretical oversight is related to the assumptions about causality: if what we do is caused by external events or their internal equivalents such as brain processes, then whatever is experienced as subjectivity must be epiphenomenal. Where concession has been made to inner experience by mainstream psychology, the events have been considered as simply continuations of the causal chain linking the external events to responses. Subjectivity thus becomes merely a class of events like any other. Is then intentionality an illusion?

A problem that ought to be obvious but appears for many not to have been so is that the causal model isolates the individual in an unnatural way. One sees this most clearly in the structure of the typical psychological experiment in which the subject is placed into cubicle and told to follow instructions. It is taken for granted here that the subject understands the language and knows how to accommodate its meaning. But the theory assumes that only the external events are the determining factors. Where other people are involved, they too are treated as equivalent to other external events, just another set of causes. That relations among people might be qualitatively different from those between people and physical events is not acknowledged. In the statistical model of variables, other people are simply variables that, for the purpose of any particular piece of research, may be held constant and thus excluded from consideration.

What is missing here is the concreteness of the individual life. Persons are abstracted into manipulable things to be predicted and controlled. The generality achieved by psychological theories is achieved through exclusion of other relevant factors. This is nowhere more obvious than in Skinner's proud claim to have achieved results so general that the observer is unable to tell which species produced them. To him, this seemed to reflect a law of nature akin to that of gravitation, thus proving that psychology can be a science just like physics.

But, what if people are really different in principle from physical, or even from merely biological, objects? Surely, to claim that they are qualitatively different is also a claim to generality, but it is a generality that preserves the concreteness of human life, not one that abstracts it out of existence. Moreover, freedom makes no sense in the abstract account of human behavior; it makes sense only in concrete lives in which the question of intentionality and restrictions on it arises. Indeed, making sense itself makes sense only in the concrete existence of human beings living in a context that is historical and societal in nature.[3]

Toward an emancipatorily adequate psychology

The concrete generality that would be required of a potentially emancipatory psychology can only be achieved by a method that is developmental and historical. Categories and concepts would remain indeterminate unless they can be conclusively deduced or derived from more certain categories. As long, for example, as concepts were operationally defined, the psychologist would simply have to pick and choose according to the particular demands of the moment. For instance, behaviorists spoke of motivation as drives and incentives, others spoke of cognitive dissonance, while still others appealed to purposes. Such definitions obviously have something in common, but in the end it will be impossible to reconcile them because they are not based on a shared understanding of just what motivation is, and this can only be deduced from a study of other life processes.

The model for such an analysis was found in Marx's *Capital*, which was based on the logic of Hegel, but it was not simply a matter of replacing political–economic categories and concepts with psychological ones. A fresh analysis on the basis of biological evolution and cultural history would have to be undertaken, but Marx had shown how it might be done and he had provided a valuable account of the societal formations in which the human subject had developed. In fact, the extension of this kind of analysis to human psychology had already been given a substantial start by A. N. Leontyev (Leontjew, 1971, from the original Russian publication in 1959). The focus of such an analysis would be specifically human subjectivity.

The work on categorial reconstruction that started with the writings of Leontyev was carried further by Klaus Holzkamp and Volker Schurig and was eventually published in four books (Holzkamp, 1973, and Schurig, 1975a, 1975b, 1976), with the full theoretical implications appearing in a fifth book, the monumental *Grundlegung der Psychologie* (Holzkamp, 1983). The result is more complex than

can be fairly treated here. Suffice it to say that an evolutionary history of psychological categories was elaborated, beginning with irritability and running through
sensibility, orientation, meaning, emotionality, communication, motivation, and
learning (to name a few), to the characteristics of the fully developed human
psyche.

The human subject arrived on the evolutionary scene in two stages. The first of
these was associated with the systematic manufacture and use of tools. Doubtless
for a very long time, early hominids made and used tools to mediate their relations
to objects in their surrounding world much as many animals, especially primates,
still do. The significant change came, however, when our ancestors began to keep
their tools for future use and to make them in the absence of their intended object.
This had enormous implications for cognition. The toolmaker had to be able to
represent the object to him- or herself and prepare the tool according to that
representation. This was the beginning of the ability to think things through
independently of the circumstances themselves. The tool can then be said to
have become an end in itself, rather than just a means linked directly to an
immediate end. This inversion of means and end in tool making and using also
had significant implications for social relations. It meant that the maker and user
of the tool no longer needed to be the same person. Thus, not only the intended
object of the tool's use had to be mentally represented to the tool maker, his or her
relations to others had also to be represented. This also meant a need to communicate, so the representations of the tool and its object took forms that could be
passed back and forth among participants, that is, they assumed the form of words
and language, verbal now rather then gestural because the hands were occupied by
the tool itself.

In this scenario one can see all the distinctive human traits emerging: conscious
social organization, division of labor, meaning, language, intention, and thought;
all of which have their precursors in animal species but are clearly and qualitatively
more highly developed among human beings.

The second major step took place when this new societal mode of existence
came to dominate the biological. The individual could no longer live outside
society and human biology itself became an object of intentional action. At this
point we no longer speak in terms of evolution but of history. The individual's
relation to the world is now entirely mediated by societal meaning structures,
including not only physical objects but traditions, beliefs, attitudes, etc. Our
relation to the world is no longer "natural." Even something as natural as a tree
is now confronted as an object with a name that carries with it an understanding of
its taxonomy, history, function, value to us, and so forth. This condition of being
mediated by meaning is all the more obvious with objects like hammers, houses,
and computers. There is simply no aspect of our world that is not mediated for us

by societally constructed meanings. Moreover, our actions with respect to these aspects are also mediated. I would not know what to do with a computer unless I commanded the relevant meanings. Moreover, these meanings have been appropriated by me from social practices; indeed, I command them only as a participant in such practice. My individuality, in short, is attained only in society; it is not something that is set off against society. All the things I am able to do are made possible by my relation to the societal structure of which I am a part. But the introduction of meaning also changes the very nature of the individual's relation to the objects of the world; individual action, being now mediated by societal meanings, is now related to its object as a *possibility*. That is, objects no longer evoke responses but offer possibilities for action. This is, of course, what we commonly mean by "free will": every action implies a choice to act, depending on the possibilities offered. This essentially human characteristic is totally obscured by most traditional psychologies, but especially by behaviorism and brain-based cognitivisms.

We now see the subject as an actor with certain powers made possible by his or her position in society. The "problem" of subjectivity can then be seen as hinging on that position. Whether or not I can utilize the possibilities offered by an object or situation will depend on my power to do so. Holzkamp called this power *Handlungsfähigkeit*, which has been translated as "action potence." It can also been translated as "agency," a translation that I now prefer, if only because "action potence" sounds awkward.

Agency is first concerned with the fulfilment of needs: I must feed myself, clothe myself, and house myself. These are some of the possibilities created by the society of which I am a part. What particular possibilities exist for me depends on the stage of historical development of my society. I have possibilities for need fulfilment and personal development now that never existed before. The basic needs of my ancestors were met in very different ways than my needs are for me. But we do not all have equal access to the possibilities created by the current stage of historical development. This brings us back to "position." In the current global economy the issue of position is more obvious than it has ever been. We are able to produce a global surplus food supply, yet there are many who have only the most restricted possibility of satisfying their hunger, and indeed an embarrassingly great many are literally starving to death.

In summary, the position arrived at by Critical Psychology's reconstruction of its understanding of the human subject is decidedly anti-causal, not out of some metaphysical opposition to determinism or an extra-scientific concern to champion free will, but because it is precisely this "looser" connection between the human subject and its world that is revealed in the analysis of evolution, history, and culture. To the human subject, the world presents not determinants but possibilities. The subject is free to relate to the world. Meaning and language create an "epistemic distance" between the subject and the world that makes this possible. This, in turn, is the product of societal existence which is qualitatively distinct from the social existence of any other animal. Societies have histories; social groups do not. The actions of subjects are thus said to be grounded in the premises for action made available by the particular societal–historical context. Grounds for action are therefore, ultimately objective, but more immediately they are always subjective. The choice of action from among possible actions is guided by what Holzkamp regarded as the sole material *a priori* and fundamental axiom of human intersubjectivity, namely that no one acts contrary to his or her own interests as he or she understands them. We are always guided by what we imagine will contribute most to the subjective quality of our lives. In the end, of course, though it may not always be clear to acting subjects, there is no contradiction between the individual and common interests. Our capacity for what is specifically human arises out of the common societal life and its ultimate "good" is necessarily also found there.

Freedom and *Handlungsfähigkeit*

Critical Psychology's conception of freedom is positive. It is the freedom to act in accordance with one's own interests, which are, in the final analysis, consonant with the common interest. In order to understand this, we need, once again, to see how humans are different from rats and pigeons. Rats and pigeons have relations to the world about them that are relatively unmediated. In order to satisfy their needs they deal directly with the objects of their word. They may display social facilitation or rudimentary cooperation at times, but they are generally not dependent on social arrangements. Humans, by contrast, generally satisfy their needs only in relation to others. Only in consciously organized *societal* arrangements do we find the food, shelter, and clothing we need. Unlike rats and pigeons, our relation to the world is mediated by social meanings and practices which we appropriate and become part of in the course of growing up. As such, we are inextricably dependent on other people. We come to see ourselves not as objects but as centers of intentionality, which condition we call subjectivity, and as related to others whom we also recognize as centers of intentionality, which we call intersubjectivity. This societal mediation of our relation to objects creates an asymmetry in which we are not, as supposed by behaviorism, controlled by those objects. Rather, objects have meanings for us, and these meanings offer us possibilities of action. Our relation to objects is thus a possibility relation in which we choose whether, when, and how to act. We control objects; they don't control us. This control Holzkamp calls *Handlungsfähigkeit* or agency, which he defines as "participation in the control of the general process of societal production and reproduction, including the particular requirements relevant to one's own life" (1983, p. 240) or "the exercise of control by the individual over his or her own requirements of life through participation in the control of the societal process" (1983, p. 241). Freedom is the unrestricted power to exercise agency, that is, to satisfy our needs through meaningful participation in societal practice.

While as humans we are subjects in the sense described, we are also *de facto* objects as well. The control that agency gives a person to act on objects can also be directed at other persons. Humans can, in short, be objectified and instrumentalized, which, it will be apparent, is akin to being dehumanized. This necessarily distorts or even annuls individual agency. Such a distortion or annulment is a restriction on freedom and it occurs when power, knowledge, and privilege are unevenly distributed in society. When this happens to an individual or group of individuals within society, there are two options. The first and obvious option is to give up one's own humanity entirely. While this is a possibility, it is rarely exercised or even seen as a viable choice. The more common option is to accept a restricted form of agency (*restriktive Handlungsfähigkeit*) by which one fulfils at least some basic needs through identification with more powerful elements in society, but at the sacrifice ultimately of one's own interests. This is certainly a subjectively functional option – indeed it is firmly rooted in and promoted by capitalist society – but to one extent or another it constitutes a denial of the true societal interest, and to the same extent, owing to the fact that in the final analysis individual interests are identical to the collective societal interest, it puts individuals into a position of hostility toward themselves. This cannot but lead to disturbances of a clinical nature.

It is not possible to describe here the entire rationale and content of this line of theorizing (see, for example, Holzkamp, 1983; Tolman & Maiers, 1991; Tolman, 1994), but it is, I hope, clear from what has been said here that an emancipatory psychology is possible if it begins with the correct conception of human subjectivity as consituted in societal relations. It is also clear that emancipation is not just a psychological affair; in the end there will be no true emancipation without significant changes in the societal structure of power.

Moving on to practice

There can be no question that global capitalism generates an oppressive form of society that, by its very nature, feeds off the unfreedom of the many to support the illusion of freedom for some and ensure the absolute power of the few. Only a revolution can change that, and there is little sign of that in these days of triumphal corporate globalism. There can also be no question that the social sciences, including psychology, as promulgated in our universities and other institutions, have served the ideological function of justifying the status quo. Behaviorist theories and brain-based cognitivisms deny outright the freedom that is the focus of any liberatory thought, while personality theories and the testing industry locate the source of all problems in individuals who are then expected to adjust to the demands of an exploitive and unjust society. Perhaps there is something that can be done about that.

Consider alone how research is carried out in contemporary mainstream psychology. The "subject" of research is brought in to the laboratory and submitted to a procedure carefully designed to provide data untainted by the subject's whims. It is no longer considered ethical to deceive "subjects" but they are seldom fully informed about what use will be made of the data they provide. Outside the laboratory, "subects" are given personalities inventories, attitude questionnaires, or similar instruments on which, once again, they provide data, over the use of which which they have little or no control. Standard research procedures, in short, are calculated to eliminate precisely what is human about the "subjects," their intentionality. They are invariably objectified. The resulting "knowledge" can only be about objects to be judged or manipulated.

Does the critical psychology point to a less objectifying, more human way of doing research? There surely are methodological implications of its revised conception of the psychological subject matter as agency, intentional action, subjectivity, all situated in a societal environment that presents the world to the agent not as stimuli and causes but as possibilities for action. Certainly, any research coming from such a point of view and motivated by a need to understand agency (*Handlungsfähigkeit*) and to make it more effective must reflect a basic equality of those conducting the research and those providing the data. Indeed, the psychologist, or any other social scientist, is also a subject. The interests of both the scientist and the participants must therefore, be ultimately identical. One clear implication of this is that no degree of deception or enforced ignorance can be part of the research strategy. Moreover, the problem must be one the investigation of which truly advances knowledge in the interests of humanity in general, and not just to advance careers.

The scientist does, however, normally start with an advantage, namely possession of the already-existing theoretical knowledge of the problem. At least initially, this represents an effective difference in power between the researcher and the participants. One aim of critical research would then be to reduce or even eliminate this difference. The participant not only provides data and other information but also acquires the power of understanding. Of course, such an approach is not entirely new: it was, for instance, the way psychoanalysis was intended by Freud to proceed. The point now, however, would be to extend this to a research practice in which, on the basis of genuine common interests, subject–participants become co-researchers who help to define the problem and share in the expertise and resulting knowledge.

Members of the Psychology Institute at the Free University of Berlin have initiated a number of projects in the last quarter century aimed at implementing a subject-oriented research program and working through its methodological complications. For instance, in 1977 a research group at the Free University of Berlin undertook a study of early child development that focused on the development of agency and subjectivity. The project was intended to "make possible a realistic pedagogical approach to development in the family in the interest of extending shared developmental possibilities" (Bader et al., 1985, p. 46). In contrast to the usual psychological study of child development in which the psychologists stand outside the parent–child relationship, acquire presumed knowledge about it, and then feed the results back to the parents in the form of counseling and advice, The FUB group, as a pilot project, enlisted the participation of nine expectant parents of six children who would become co-researchers in the project. All participants were initially provided with a set of categories in terms of which the problems encountered could be framed. These categories included activity, agency (*Handlungfähigkeit*), subjectivity, meaning, and subjective and instrumental relations. The focuses of attention included the development of agency and subjectivity in all involved parties, the development of the child's capacity to influence its own conditions, and the pedagogical practices used by the parents. The parents kept diaries of their observations and reflections and the entire group met every 2 weeks to share their experiences. The diaries were reproduced and made available to all participants. Discussions at the meetings were recorded, transcribed, and, again, shared. A total of 70 meetings were held covering the children's first 2 to 3 years, producing over 1000 pages of diaries and another 1000 pages of transcriptions. The results are rather difficult to summarize. Certainly, the participants came out of it with a heightened sense of the consequences of their own actions and of the importance of the immediate contexts of those actions, and with greater sensitivity to the developing action possibilities of the children in influencing the conditions of their own lives. As important for the psychologist–participants were the insights gained about the methodological problems involved in this type of research. These included the participants' development of qualifications and confidence and how to deal with privacy issues and trust. Clearly, more work needs to be done before generalizable scientific knowledge can be confidently claimed as a result.

In a project coordinated by Ute Osterkamp on racism and discrimination, relations between residents, social workers, middle-management, and administrators of refugee centers of the German Red Cross have been analyzed along similar theoretical lines. Certain mechanisms, many of which are at least partially supported by social science, had to be exposed as obstructing the availability of good reasons for mutual solidarity in the interest of improving oppressive living conditions (Osterkamp, 1991). One important finding of this project was the extent to which racist thinking is embedded in our everyday discourse. Racist thinking is grounded in very real anxieties and threats felt by individuals, which are then projected on to members of identifiable other groups. Such projection is often encouraged and seemingly justified by the ways in which, for instance, governmental agencies and the popular press present information and judgments about refugees and other foreigners. But, in the absence of any comprehensive understanding of the actual societal-structural dynamics of racism, blaming others effectively is equivalent to blaming oneself. As Osterkamp observes, racism, closely analyzed, is a form of self-disempowerment (Osterkamp, 1996).

In a project on professional practice (Fahl & Markard, 1993) an attempt was made to identify, among other things, theory-like patterns of reasoning that encourage self-obstruction in psychologists' professional practice, along with ways in which these can be steered toward non-defensive modes of practice.

In all of these projects the task has been to critically analyze the constructs of the science of control, so as to reveal the fixations and reifications that they contain, and to develop and implement theoretical conceptions that can capture adequately reasoned action and the conditions that mediate its functionality. This also implies conceptions of social relations that transcend the instrumentalizing one-sidedness of traditional concepts. The intersubjective context must always be construed in such a way as to make clear that *I* and *the other* not only confront one another, but that *I am the other for the other*, such that what I cause to happen to the other can be seen as also having an effect on me. With theorizing of this sort from the scientific standpoint of the subject, we should be able to understand, at both the conceptual and empirical levels, the manifold ways in which we can create conditions that remove the good reasons for obstructing the realization of possibilities for action and mutually blocking the goals that we and others set ourselves.

NOTES

(1) The words "subjectivity" and "subject" are used here to imply a person's both being and being aware of being the subject of one's own actions, as opposed to being an object of external forces.

(2) The Hawthorne experiments represented but one of many attempts in the early part of the twentieth century to apply social science to the problem of production in industry. They became famous because it seemed that production increased no matter what the experimenters did. This became known subsequently as the "Hawthorne effect" (Mayo, 1933, ch. 3).

(3) Psychoanalysis, which remained outside the mainstream of academic psychology, makes a telling contrast with the dominant behavioral/functional/cognitive psychology. While Freud appears from his *Civilization and Its Discontents* (1930/1975) to have missed the essentially societal nature of human beings in that he took society and individual to be inherently opposed to one another, his theory of the superego captured well the way in which oppressive social relations are internalized, thus making subjects instruments in their own dehumanization. Holzkamp (1991a) saw this as one of the main reasons why Freud remained popular among left-leaning social scientists and others.

REFERENCES

Allport, G. W. (1965). *Letters from Jenny*. New York: Harcourt, Brace & World.

Bader, K., Grüter, B., Holzkamp, K. *et al.* (1985). Subjektentwicklung in der frühen Kindheit: Der Weg eines Forschungprojekts in die Förderungsunwürdigkeit. *Forum Kritische Psychologie*, **17**, 56–81.

Fahl, R. & Markard, M. (1993). Das Projekt "Anlayse psychologischer Praxis" oder: Der Versuch der Verbindung von Praxisforschung und Psychologiekritik. *Forum Kritische Psychology*, **32**, 4–35.

Freud, S. (1975). *Civilization and Its Discontents*. London: The Hogarth Press. (Original work published 1930.)

Holzkamp, K. (1970). Zum Problem der Relevanz psychologischer Forschung für die Praxis. *Psychologische Rundschau*, **21**, 1–22.

Holzkamp, K. (1972). *Kritische Psychologie: Vorbereitende Arbeiten*. Frankfurt/M.: Fischer-Verlag.

Holzkamp, K. (1973). *Sinnliche Erkenntnis: Historischer Ursprung und gesellschaftliche Funktion der Wahrnehmung*. Frankfurt/M.: Campus Verlag.

Holzkamp, K. (1983). *Grundlegung der Psychologie*. Frankfurt/M.: Campus Verlag.

Holzkamp, K. (1991). Psychoanalysis and Marxist psychology. In *Critical Psychology*, ed. C. Tolman & W. Maiers. New York: Cambridge University Press, pp. 81–101.

Leontjew, A. N. (1971). *Probleme der Entwicklung des Psychischen*. Berlin, GDR: Volk und Wissen Verlag.

Mayo, E. (1933). *The Human Problems of an Industrial Civilization*. New York: Macmillan.

Osterkamp, U. (1991). Rassismus und Alltagsdenken. *Forum Kritische Psychologie*. **28**, 40–71.

Osterkamp, U. (1996). *Rassismus als Selbstentmächtigung*. Hamburg: Argument Verlag.

Schurig, V. (1975a). *Naturgeschiche des Psychischen 1: Psychogenese und elementare Formen der Tierkommunikation*. Frankfurt/M.: Campus Verlag.

Schurig, V. (1975b). *Naturgeschiche des Psychischen 2: Lernen und Abstraktionsleistungen bei Tieren*. Frankfurt/M.: Campus Verlag.

Schurig, V. (1976). *Die Entstehung des Bewußtseins*. Frankfurt/M.: Campus Verlag.

Skinner, B. F. (1956). A case history in scientific method. *American Psychologist*, **11**, 221–233.

Staeuble, I. (1968). Faschistoide und kritisch-autonome Haltung: Versuch über die Rolle des Konzepts 'Einstellung zu kritischer Vernunft' in der Vorurteilsforschung. *Zeitschrift für Soziologie und Sozialpsychologie*, **20**, 38–61.

Tolman, C. W. (1994). *Psychology, Society, and Subjectivity: An Introduction to German Critical Psychology*. London: Routledge.

Tolman, C. W. & Maiers, W. (1991). *Critical Psychology: Contributions to an Historical Science of the Subject*. New York: Cambridge University Press.

Watson, J. B. (1924). *Psychology from the Standpoint of a Behaviorist*, 2nd edn. Philadelphia: J. B. Lippincott Co.

Woodworth, R. S. (1929). *Psychology: A Study of Mental Life*. 2nd edn. New York: Henry Holt & Co.

6

Psychopolitical validity in the helping professions: applications to research, interventions, case conceptualization, and therapy

Isaac Prilleltensky, Ora Prilleltensky, and Courte Voorhees[1]

Introduction

What is preventing the advancement of liberation psychiatry? Why is it that after so many volumes of critique, the helping professions are still firmly grounded in traditional medical models (Prilleltensky, 1994; Teo, 2005)? How can we challenge the regnant deficit, reactive, disempowering, and individualistic oriented approaches in psychology, psychiatry, social work, counseling, and allied professions? This chapter is a modest attempt to translate the abundant theoretical critique of the helping professions into practical guidelines for action. In our view, there is a wide gap between the cogent reservations about dominant paradigms and actionable formulations. Unless we manage to convert critique into construction, and deliberation into delivery of new practices, the gap between discourse and action will continue to grow, leaving behind a trail of doubly disaffected practitioners; disaffected with the medical model, and disaffected with critical approaches that fail to suggest convincing alternatives for practice.

We build our case for action around the concept of psychopolitical validity. Following an introduction of the construct and its rationale, we articulate its implications for research, interventions, case conceptualization and therapy. The first two areas of interest apply to all the helping professions, whereas the last two pertain more directly to therapeutic interventions.

What is psychopolitical validity?

Psychopolitical validity is a criterion for the evaluation of understanding and action in professions dealing with oppression, liberation, and well-being. The

Liberatory Psychiatry: Philosophy, Politics, and Mental Health, ed. Carl I. Cohen and Sami Timimi. Published by Cambridge University Press. © Cambridge University Press.

criterion consists of the level of attention given to the role of power in explaining psychological and political phenomena affecting suffering and well-being. The term psychopolitical denotes the inseparable nature of psychological and political dynamics. Affective, behavioral and cognitive experiences cannot be detached from power plays being enacted at the personal, relational, and collective levels of analysis. Similarly, political contexts cannot be understood without an appreciation of the subjective, ideological, and cultural forces shaping power relations. This dialectic accounts for the term psychopolitical. As Oliver recently pointed out:

> We cannot explain the development of individuality or subjectivity apart from its social context. But neither can we formulate a social theory to explain the dynamics of oppression without considering its psychic dimension. We need a theory that operates between the psyche and the social. (Oliver, 2004, p. xiv)

When it comes to the psychological, why focus on power and not, for example, on cognitive distortions or the unconscious? When it comes to the political, why focus on power and not, for example, on values or philosophical ideology? In both cases, the alternatives are valid foci of attention. In fact, they have received wide recognition and literally volumes of attention. What we are still missing in the helping professions is a clear articulation of how power dynamics affect cognitive distortions, the unconscious, values and ideology, and what we can do about it.

Power is a central construct in well-being. In the literature, power is dealt with through a variety of proxies, including sense of control, locus of control, empowerment, self-determination, self-efficacy, feelings of inferiority, authoritarian personality, and others. In most cases, however, power is individualized, subjectivized, and decontextualized. Respectively, this means that power is treated as an attribute of individuals, that it is regarded as a phenomenological perception, and that it can be interpreted regardless of surrounding circumstances. Power contains much explanatory merit that has not been captured yet. By bringing to light the collective dynamics of power, its objective sources, and its contextual variables, we stand a better chance of understanding oppression, liberation, and well-being. In essence, the collective, objective, and contextual variables account for the political side of the psychopolitical equation. The more we situate psychological experiences of power in political dynamics, the richer our understanding of oppression, liberation, and well-being.

In short, psychopolitical validity derives from the simultaneous consideration of power dynamics operating in psychological and political spheres at various levels of analysis, from the personal to the relational to the collective. The more we understand how power influences oppression, liberation, and well-being, the more effective we are likely to be in bringing about a more satisfactory state of affairs for individuals, families, groups, communities, and societies. We can claim that psychopolitical validity is achieved when power has been fully factored into these experiences at the various levels of analyses. When this kind of analysis is applied to research, we refer to *epistemic* psychopolitical validity. When it is applied to interventions, we refer to *transformational* psychopolitical validity.

To be even more precise in our definition of psychopolitical validity, however, we have to offer a precise definition of power. For us, power consists of ten postulates:

(1) *Power refers to the capacity and opportunity to fulfil or obstruct personal, relational, or collective needs.*

(2) *Power has psychological and political sources, manifestations, and consequences.*

(3) *We can distinguish among power to strive for wellness, power to oppress, and power to resist oppression and strive for liberation.*

(4) *Power can be overt or covert, subtle or blatant, hidden or exposed.*

(5) *The exercise of power can apply to self, others, and collectives.*

(6) *Power affords people multiple identities as individuals seeking wellness, engaging in oppression, or resisting domination.*

(7) *Whereas people may be oppressed in one context, at a particular time and place, they may act as oppressors at another time and place.*

(8) *Due to structural factors such as social class, gender, ability, and race, people may enjoy differential levels of power.*

(9) *Degrees of power are also affected by personal and social constructs such as beauty, intelligence, and assertiveness; constructs that enjoy variable status within different cultures.*

(10) *The exercise of power can reflect varying degrees of awareness with respect to the impact of one's actions.*

According to the first tenet, power is an amalgam of ability and opportunity. The aim is to influence a course of events. This definition of power combines aspects of agency, or volitional activity on one hand, and structure or external determinants on the other. Agency refers to ability whereas structure refers to opportunity. The exercise of power relies on the reciprocal determinism of agency and contextual dynamics (Martin & Sugarman, 2000). Agency and contextual dynamics always incorporate psychological as well as political dimensions. Our capacity to act as agents of change for personal or collective benefit depends on subjective, cognitive, behavioral, and affective variables as well as political, economic, and societal factors. In essence, we embrace an ecological view of power (Kelly, 2006).

Power is not tantamount to coercion though, for it can operate in very subtle and concealed ways, as Foucault demonstrated in detailed historical analyses of population control (1979). Eventually, people come to regulate themselves through the internalization of cultural prescriptions. Hence, what may seem on the surface as freedom may be questioned as a form of acquiescence whereby citizens restrict their life choices to coincide with a narrow range of socially approved options. In his book *Powers of Freedom*, Rose (1999) claimed that:

Disciplinary techniques and moralizing injunctions as to health, hygiene and civility are no longer required; the project of responsible citizenship has been fused with individuals' projects for themselves. What began as a social norm here ends as a personal desire. Individuals act upon themselves and their families in terms of the languages, values and techniques made available to them by professions, disseminated through the apparatuses of the mass media or sought out by the troubled through the market. Thus, in a very significant sense, it has become possible to govern without governing *society* – to govern through the "responsibilized" and "educated" anxieties and aspirations of individuals and their families. (p. 88)

Power, then, emanates from the confluence of personal motives and cultural injunctions. It is not just a matter of persons acting on the environment, but it is a matter of individuals coming into contact with external forces that, to some extent, they have already internalized (Kelly, 2006; Oliver, 2004). The implication is that we cannot just take at face value that individual actions evolve from innate desires. Desires grow from norms and regulations. This is not to adopt a socially deterministic position however, for even though a person's experience depends on the prescriptions of the day, agency does play its part. As Martin and Sugarman (2000) claimed that:

While never ceasing to be constructed in sociocultural terms, psychological beings, as reflection-capable, intentional agents, are able to exercise sophisticated capabilities of memory and imagination, which in interaction with theories of self can create possibilities for present and future understanding and action that are not entirely constrained by past and present socio-cultural circumstances. (p. 401)

If our goal is to enhance wellness and fight oppression, awareness of our actions and those of our students, clients, and community partners is crucial. People may be aware of being oppressed, but not of being oppressors. We may wish very strongly, and consciously, to liberate ourselves from social regulations, but we may be buying, less consciously, into oppressive cultural norms. Young women may think that dieting is fashionable and will help them achieve popularity, but with dieting come the risks of eating disorders and perpetuating commercialism and consumerism. Contradictions abound. Humanists, for instance, wished to pro-mote individual well-being without recognizing their contribution to the status quo by individualizing sources of suffering (Prilleltensky, 1994). They wished to advance personal liberation without changing social oppression.

As seen from the foregoing discussion, our conceptualization of power cascades into three subsidiary constructs that also deserve precise definition: oppression, liberation, and well-being. Oppression entails a state of asymmetric power relations characterized by domination, subordination, and resistance, where the dominating persons or groups exercise their power by the process of restricting access to material resources and imparting in the subordinated persons or groups self-deprecating views about themselves (Bartky, 1990; Fanon, 1963; Freire, 1970, 1975, 1994; Memmi, 1968). Oppression, then, is a series of asymmetric power relations between individuals, genders, classes, communities, and nations. Such asymmetric power relations lead to conditions of misery, inequality, exploitation, marginalization, and social injustices.

The dynamics of oppression are internal as well as external. External forces deprive individuals or groups of the benefit of personal (e.g., self-determination), relational (e.g., democratic participation), and collective (e.g., distributive justice) wellness. Often, people internalize these restrictions (Moane, 1999; Mullaly, 2002; Prilleltensky & Gonick, 1996). In short, we define political and psychological oppression as follows:

(1) Political oppression, which is the creation of material, legal, military, economic, and/or other social barriers to the fulfilment of self-determination, distributive justice, and democratic participation, results from the use of multiple forms of power by dominating agents to advance their own interests at the expense of persons or groups in positions of relative powerlessness.

(2) Psychological oppression, in turn, is the internalized view of self as negative, and as not deserving more resources or increased participation in societal affairs, resulting from the use of affective, behavioral, cognitive, material, linguistic, and cultural mechanisms by agents of domination to affirm their own political superiority (Prilleltensky & Gonick, 1996).

Liberation, in turn, refers to the process of resisting oppressive forces. As a state, liberation is a condition in which oppressive forces no longer exert their dominion over a person or a group. Liberation may be from psychological and/or political influences. Following from the previous interpretation of oppression, there is rarely political without psychological oppression, and vice versa (Moane, 1999; Mullaly, 2002).

Building on Fromm's dual conception of "freedom from" and "freedom to" (1965), liberation is the process of overcoming internal and external sources of oppression (freedom from), and pursuing wellness (freedom to). Liberation from social oppression entails, for example, emancipation from class exploitation, gender domination, and ethnic discrimination. Freedom from internal and psychological sources includes overcoming fears, obsessions, or other psychological phenomena that interfere with a person's subjective experience of well-being. Liberation to pursue well-being, in turn, refers to the process of meeting personal, relational, and collective needs. In fact, we define well-being as a positive state of affairs, brought about by the simultaneous satisfaction of personal, relational, and collective needs of individuals, groups, communities, and societies.

Having defined psychopolitical validity (epistemic and transformational), power, oppression, liberation, and well-being, we are now in a position to explore how psychopolitical validity can inform research in the helping professions. Following that, we examine how psychopolitical validity can inform interventions, case conceptualization, and therapy.

How does psychopolitical validity inform research in the helping professions?

At the macro/collective level, oppressive structures and major paradigms are diminishing the well-being of individuals and communities. Structural components of the status quo (i.e., laws, national culture, HMOs) and fundamental paradigms (i.e., the medical model, capitalism, rugged individualism) are often the underlying causes of oppression, barriers to liberation, and bases of the collective gaps in well-being. Macro-level academic incentive structures also reify the status quo with "in the box" research (Stancato, 2000; Tierney, 1997). Without research designs and processes addressing the underlying structural causes of the issues faced by the helping professions on a daily basis, there will be an eternal revolving door of clients needing services and a never-ending stream of research results that either reify or ineffectively face the oppressive status quo.

The accountability for establishing the relevancy of ecological connections and analyzing power differentials in research design currently falls on the *critics* of research practice, not on the researchers carrying out potentially ecologically and psychopolitically invalid work. As no discipline can realistically hope for a top-down mandate for critical reflection on the dominant paradigm of inquiry, the critical researcher is the premier hope for pursuing liberation in research practice (Table 6.1).

By raising the consciousness of research participants through education and increased control over the research process (Freire, 1970), critical researchers will shift needed power to the community (Nelson & Prilleltensky, 2005). It is the responsibility of the researcher to seek out participation, as research participants may have no exposure to their potential part in the research process (Maguire, 1987). Shifting structural norms and incentives toward creating interdisciplinary research teams will yield better triangulation of research data, a

Table 6.1. Applications to research

Stages of wellness/ empowerment ▶ Level of analysis/ intervention▼	Oppression (state):	Liberation (process):	Well-being (outcome):
Macro/collective/ structural/ community	Nomothetic, ameliorative based paradigm of research. Academic research and training structures that reify the status quo.	Shift to culturally conscious, preventative research paradigm. Efforts to build collaborative relationships between disciplines.	Culturally sensitive, preventative, participant driven research. Support for transdisciplinary researchers and teams working in partnership with communities.
Meso/ organizational/ group/relational	Expert-driven research design and implementation. Dehumanization of research participants.	Seek out participation in all aspects of research. Empower research participants through process and as an outcome.	Empowered stakeholders participating in all aspects of the research process. Equalized power between all parties.
Micro/individual/ personal/ psychological (emotional, cognitive, behavioral, spiritual)	Participants seen as "subjects", passive instruments of the researcher. Labeling/diagnostic focus of research.	Increased voice and choice of participants in research. Shift from diagnosis of weaknesses to cultivation of strengths.	Participants seen as expert agents in the research project. Strengths and resiliency of participants identified and supported.

better understanding of oppressive conditions, and create a collaborative atmosphere that welcomes critical reflection on the research questions, process, and outcomes. Only once practical exemplars of participatory research become common will policy and institutional culture shift away from its oppressive roots.

Research that supports the well-being of communities and societies is participatory, culturally appropriate, and pursues well-being over adjustment to existing conditions. This not only requires measuring traditional variables of focus, but also tracking the shifting position of the researcher within the ecological topography of the research setting and the constantly changing power dynamics between all participants (Hesse-Biber *et al.*, 2004). Macro-level structures and paradigms change slowly and with much effort, but enduring transformation at this level will have an effect on many oppressed communities and individuals – often eroding the root causes of countless crises, making collective change a necessary part of liberation.

At the meso/relational level, the interaction between researcher and participants is largely expert-driven (Prilleltensky, 2005) – wherein the researcher is seen as the holder of knowledge and the "subjects" are seen as data. As a result of this relationship, research results accumulate as academic and medical knowledge, not as actionable information available to the communities and individuals that need it most. The dehumanization of participants parallels their disempowerment in other civic and social relationships (Kenig, 1986), making normal research in the helping professions just another cog in the oppressive machine of society.

Liberation and empowerment of research participants must be seen as more than a purely individual endeavor, instead focusing on mutual respect and democratic participation between all stakeholders and researchers (Perkins & Zimmerman, 1995). At the meso-level, liberation research conceptualizes and measures interpersonal and organizational interactions as the units of analysis (Peterson & Zimmerman, 2004), while fostering the development of social power for participants (Speer & Hughey, 1995). By granting voice and choice to participants in all interactions within the research process, participation and empowerment will become a cultural norm in interpersonal research discourse. These elements of liberation also open the door to actionable research outcomes, rather than merely seeking an accumulation of catalogued data.

Research that fosters interpersonal well-being is collaborative, empowering, reflective, and action oriented (Speer & Hughey, 1995). Participants are given a seat at the research table – wherein they have reasonable power over all aspects of the research process and are fully aware of their position, the research purpose, and the actual and potential effects of the research outcomes. The goal of relationships with – and between – participants is to equalize power and organize for the pursuit of well-being.

At the micro/personal level in our traditional research paradigm, participants are seen as mere "subjects" serving only as the passive instruments of the researcher – virtually inanimate points of datum. Traditional research in the helping professions often aims to find individualistic etiology and treatment that fits into a nomothetic, universal framework. This paradigm is the accepted norm in psychiatric research for a number of useful reasons, like determining genetic markers of mental illnesses, compiling effective treatments, and so forth (Blashfield & Livesley, 1999; Raulin & Lilienfeld, 1999). The advantages of this approach alone would be a boon to the helping professions, but the disadvantages often outweigh these achievements. The entire research process has disempowered participants – resulting in habituation to this unacceptable state of affairs, making the oppressive state seem justified and necessary (Montero, 1998).

Although empowerment is an interpersonal process, it is often misinterpreted as a responsibility to foist onto the individual as a means of micro-level transformation (Perkins & Zimmerman, 1995). Increased voice and choice of participants in research is necessary, but this power shift must be facilitated beyond the micro-sphere. In light of the stigmatization, suspicion, fear, and hostility experienced by individuals diagnosed with a psychopathology (Murphy, 1976), we must also challenge the continued taxonomic research paradigm. In order for the oppressive state of affairs to change, the normalcy of traditional research must be deconstructed.

Well-being at the micro-level includes participants as expert agents in the research process, with control over the research questions, processes, and applications. Personal empowerment is strengthened by participants' voice and choice in the research. Their strengths are sought and cultivated, rather than being subjected to systematic labeling and pathologizing. Researchers that support liberation and well-being at the micro-level are actively connected with the lives and experiences of the people that they work with, fostering self-determination and re-humanization of all participants.

How does psychopolitical validity inform interventions in the helping professions?

In this section, we define interventions as organizationally or institutionally based coordinated efforts to affect a single problem or set of issues in a population. This can be a state-run case management of people experiencing homelessness, for-profit community mental health centers, the action component of an action research project to reduce depressive symptoms in a community, or any number of coordinated efforts to aid people in need. What separates interventions from therapy in this context is the coordinated – often meso-level – effort, rather than an individual therapeutic setting.

At the macro/collective level, organizations and practitioners intervening in social and community settings have the collective ability to avoid numerous pitfalls of individual practice, but many interventions still commit the *context minimization error* by ignoring or downplaying enduring contextual factors when more sensitivity to multi-level issues of power and ecological influence are warranted (Shinn & Toohey, 2003). Although many interventions started with a liberatory mission, structural and cultural influences eroded the vision and practice over time. As an example, the community mental health movement fell from its original social mission by the early 1980s due to funding decreases, diminished media attention, and a lack of unified ideals and practice (Kenig, 1986).

The erosion of ideals in interventions paved the way for a top-down process of psychiatric colonization (Table 6.2). Context has taken a back seat to establishing nomothetic responses to mental illnesses in interventions, rather than examining the relevant ecological and psychopolitical factors that weigh heavily on the presentation of mental illness. We know that mental illnesses such as schizophrenia have clearly traceable biological components, but none stand alone as causal (Green, 1998). Many other mental illnesses have tenuous biological or genetic etiology at best, making the wholesale minimization of macro-level influences a dangerous leap of faith (Gorenstein, 1984).

In order to pursue liberation at the collective level, interventions must understand and act upon the cultures and societies that an individual or population is embedded in. To affect the lives of people who are experiencing homelessness and mental illness, a coordinated intervention should not just hand out psychotropic medications, but create or find affordable and sustainable housing, reduce social stigma of the target population, seek to change social policies that create undue economic stress, etc. An intervention that continuously commits the context minimization error not only eschews a mission of liberation, but also aids the status quo by reifying a structure that requires individualized pharmaceutical-induced adjustment to oppression.

Interventions that support well-being at the macro-level utilize professional resources to advocate for structural change and organize populations to achieve their own liberation within society. Such an intervention would prevent and ameliorate the effects of globalization and colonialism, instead of just accepting macrospheric forces as unfortunate givens.

At the meso/interpersonal level, there is an acute tension between Western diagnosis and community culture. Western psychiatry constructs universal causes and cures, while many communities and cultures understand the elements of human interaction missing in Western interventions (Castillo, 1997; Kirmayer, Young, & Hayton, 1998). Fromm (1958) captures the interpersonal issues that are raised by mental illness – often ignored by current interventions: "Mental illness is always a sign that basic human needs are not being satisfied; that there is a lack of love, a lack of reason for being, a lack of justice; that something important is missing and, because of this, pathological trends are developing" (p. 2).

Fabrega (1989) asserts that the biomedical science of the West – touted as pure objective fact – is merely another culturally grounded theory. This "theory" has been used as a biological marker to exclude people from society, à la racism, sexism, and xenophobia. Without needing to refute biological evidence, we must include

Table 6.2. Applications to intervention

Stages of wellness/empowerment ▶ Level of analysis/intervention ▼	Oppression (state):	Liberation (process):	Well-being (outcome):
Macro/collective/structural/community	Top-down process of psychiatric colonization. Decontextualized, culturally insensitive intervention strategies. Deficit based interventions aiming to adjust patients/clients to existing macro-structures.	Increased control and participation of intervention recipients. Inclusion of context and culture in intervention planning. Investigation of client and community strengths, structural change to promote a healthy society.	Partnerships between professionals, communities, and individuals to execute interventions. Culturally and contextually valid strategies. Strengths based focus, social programs and collective cultures that put health over profit.
Meso/organizational/group/relational	Devaluation of local knowledge. Western science and perspective viewed as objective fact. Diagnostic focus creates stigmas for people seeking help.	Wider use of cultural knowledge in the DSM-IV and in intervention planning. Western medical model can be seen as just another culturally bound perspective. Shift to participatory and narrative approaches to rehumanize people seeking help.	Partnerships between professionals and help-seekers to plan and execute interventions. Equal weight given to the advantages of all culturally bound knowledge, whether Western or local. Valued interplay between experience and taxonomic knowledge.
Micro/individual/personal/psychological (emotional, cognitive, behavioral, spiritual)	No ownership by clients of intervention goals, processes, or outcomes. Addiction, low self-esteem and low self-efficacy brought on by oppressive conditions.	Education about and participation in interventions. Consciousness raising and skill building.	Participant knowledge and ownership of the intervention. Individuals with high self-efficacy and esteem participating in interventions, political processes, and organizing.

community-level contextual factors in the formulation and execution of interventions in the helping professions to avoid further marginalization of those seeking help.

Widiger and Clark (2000) note a growing acceptance in mainstream psychiatry of including cultural factors in the diagnosis of psychopathology, as evidenced in the DSM-IV. Although this is a step in the right direction, this shift will likely fall short of advancing well-being without changes in other areas of the medical model. Interventions must move beyond changes in diagnosis to changes in conceptualization of mental and social ills. Local knowledge can be captured in narratives (White & Epston, 1990) or through participatory research (Maguire, 1987) to inform interventions.

At the interpersonal level, well-being includes partnerships between professionals, communities, and individuals to execute interventions (Israel *et al.*, 1998). Pooling the knowledge of all stakeholders alleviates many of the pitfalls of Western diagnosis, while the relationships formed through partnerships reflexively inform the intervention process. Well-being requires awareness and action at the interpersonal level, wherein control is commensurate with stake, and symptoms are recognized as a community issue rather than a purely medical one.

At the micro/personal level, affected stakeholders have little or no ownership of intervention goals, processes, and outcomes. Individuals are labeled, categorized, managed, treated, and pushed through a system that alienates and stigmatizes them (Murphy, 1976). From this vantage, interventions appear to be an organized effort to manage and medicate clients that are seeking help. Individuals may internalize these or other oppressive conditions, potentially leading to disempowerment, addictions, diminished mental health, or myriad other personal issues (Prilleltensky, 2003).

An increase in participation in the intervention process also aids in liberation at the personal level. Power over goals and strategies helps individuals build identity and resist oppression (Prilleltensky, in press). Liberation should also include raising the consciousness of individuals through educational projects (Freire, 1970) and educational components of helping interventions. Individual strengths must be noticed and fostered, as the skills of the individual are an essential part of multi-level liberatory action (Watts *et al.*, 2003).

The well-being of the individual extends beyond mere participant ownership of the intervention. People experiencing wellness are also freely participating in political processes, experiencing enhanced physical health, and have a greater self efficacy (Prilleltensky, 2005). The liberated individual personally experiences the positive state of affairs brought about by their path to well-being, rather than being a passive recipient of collective or interpersonal benefits.

How does psychopolitical validity inform case conceptualization in the helping professions?

In this section we focus on the application of psychopolitical validity and the constructs of oppression, liberation, and well-being to the lives of clients who present for counseling and psychotherapy. We highlight some key problems with traditional approaches to client assessment and case conceptualization and provide an alternative framework that is consistent with empowerment and well-being.

It is probably safe to say that the vast majority of helping professionals have received solid training in assessment and case conceptualization. Most professionals would agree that setting goals and developing an appropriate intervention plan is contingent upon a thorough exploration and understanding of troublesome aspects in the lives of clients. Once a client tells her story and explicates her reason for seeking therapy, a thorough and collaborative exploration of the components of the problem can set the stage for intervention. This typically includes an understanding of overt behaviors, affective components, and cognitions and beliefs associated with presented concerns. Case conceptualization from a cognitive-behavioral framework also includes an exploration of the frequency, intensity, and duration of the problem as well as its antecedents, consequences, and pattern of contributing variables (Table 6.3) (Cormier & Cormier, 1997; Hackney & Cormier, 2005).

Professional literature on case conceptualization emphasizes that a thorough analysis of problem areas should be supplemented with details on client strengths, assets, and resources. However, we venture to say that in most intake interviews, case conceptualization notes, and psychological and psychiatric reports, there is a stark imbalance between the wealth of information denoting problem areas and the dearth of information on client strengths and resources. "Being problem-oriented, the clinician easily concentrates on pathology, dysfunction, and troubles, to the neglect of discovering those important assets in the person and resources in the environment that must be drawn upon in the best problem-solving efforts" (Wright & Lopez, 2002, p. 36). Psychiatry, as a field, has focused on the diagnosis and treatment of mental illness and, as such, has concentrated on the pathological and abnormal components of human functioning. Clinical psychology has followed in the steps of psychiatry in its efforts to develop interventions and best practices that can cure mental illness, or at least minimize its destructive impact on the lives of affected individuals. As a result, there has been a much greater focus on assessing pathology and mental illness than on identifying and amplifying well-being (Maddux, 2002; Seligman, 2002a, b). Seligman (2002a, b) quips that the National Institute of Mental Health (NIMH) formed in 1947 may well have been called the National Institute of Mental Illness, given its almost exclusive focus on mental disorders and neglect of mental health.

Table 6.3. Applications to case conceptualization

Stages of wellness/ empowerment ▶ Level of analysis/ intervention ▼	Oppression (state):	Liberation (process):	Well-being (outcome):
Macro/collective/ structural/ community	Context minimization error: failing to assess for and highlight the role of macro-level systemic factors (i.e., poverty, neighborhood violence) as well as social policies and cultural norms (i.e., xenophobia; blame the victim mentality) that increase problematic functioning and decrease well-being. In a similar vein, failing to assess macro-level factors (i.e., greater gender equality) that enhance well-being.	Highlighting macro-level constraints and their correlation with problematic functioning at the personal, interpersonal and familial level.	Highlighting the interdependence between personal, organizational, and collective well-being. Acknowledging that micro-level interventions are necessary but insufficient and must be supplemented with meso- and macro-level interventions. Must realize that personal well-being cannot be attained in the absence of organization and collective well-being.
Meso/ organizational/ group/relational	Failing to assess for, or giving insufficient weight to, contextual factors and organizational structures (i.e. school climate, work environment) that increase problematic functioning and decrease well-being. Failing to assess for contextual factors and organizational structures that reduce problems and enhance	Identifying meso-level constraints that increase dysfunction and reduce well-being (i.e., bullying at school; an unhealthy work environment). Identifying and amplifying meso-level factors that currently serve as protective factors (i.e., positive school climate; collaborative work environment).	Clear guidelines for meso-level interventions designed to alleviate distress, dysfunction and/or mental illness. Clear guidelines for meso-level interventions designed to enhance well-being, flourishing, and mental health. Clear guidelines for strengthening and building on positive structures.

Micro/individual/ personal/ psychological (emotional, cognitive, behavioral, spiritual)	well-being, as well as factors and structures that have the potential for doing so. Amplifying deficits and dysfunction. Ignoring strengths and resilience. Focusing exclusively on alleviating illness and distress. Overlooking potential for flourishing and well-being.	Assessing ways of building on healthy structures and affecting those that impede well-being. Supplementing problem assessment with situations when said problem was resisted or overcome. Assessing for internalized oppression. Inquiring about health-enhancing relationships and problem-free spheres in the client's life. Assessing for personal strengths, assets, and examples of thriving and well-being.	A balanced assessment process that builds on personal strengths, assets, and resources (i.e., good social skills; perseverance). Clear guidelines for individually based interventions designed to alleviate distress, dysfunction and/or mental illness. Clear guidelines for individually based interventions designed to enhance well-being, flourishing, and mental health.

A case conceptualization that it is largely based on explicating deficiencies of the individual in question misses the mark on several fronts. Not only are personal strengths and assets not given due consideration, but the role of the environment in shaping personal experience and psychological functioning recedes to the background (Wright & Lopez, 2002). Drawing upon research on information processing, perception and social psychology, Wright and Lopez (2002) make a cogent case for how we systematically undermine the potency of the environment in undermining or enhancing mental health and well-being as well as creating pathology or protecting from it, as the case may be. By definition, environment is at the background while individuals are at the foreground, "active, moving in space, commanding attention by their behavior" (p. 32). Furthermore, "where the primary mission of a treatment center is to change the person, assessment procedures will be directed toward describing and labeling person attributes. The danger is that the environment scarcely enters the equation in understanding behavior" (p. 35). To this, we add that environment should not be seen as a single construct. Thus, when it is taken into consideration in the assessment process, it is often at the level of immediate contexts and relationships versus organizational and systemic structures that can impede or enhance well-being. Meso-level organizational structures and macro-level systemic barriers rarely find their way into the process of assessment and diagnosis.

Wright and Lopez (2002) assert that professional tendency to focus on personal dysfunction and undermine the role of the environment can be addressed by adopting a four-front approach to assessment. The four components entail personal weaknesses and deficiencies; personal strengths and resources; environmental lacks and deficiencies; and environmental resources and opportunities. Elsewhere, we suggested a similar assessment process using the acronym ROWS: "Risks" and "opportunities" pertain to the environment whereas "weaknesses" and "strengths" pertain to the person (Prilleltensky & Prilleltensky, 2006).

We further contend that case conceptualization that highlights personal deficiencies, ignores personal strengths, and minimizes environmental barriers, is disempowering, oppressive, and contraindicated with mental health and well-being. This is particularly applicable to marginalized populations that, on a daily basis, have to contend with a host of structural and systemic barriers that are played out in the arena of their personal lives. Bronfenbrenner's ecological theory emphasizes that environment extends far beyond the immediate settings in which a person engages. It includes relationships between arenas, influences of larger settings in which the person may not directly participate, as well as the culture at large (Lemme, 2006). Thus, daily exposure to an unhealthy and oppressive work environment will likely spill over to the home front, just as a board decision to close down an unprofitable plant could lead to dire consequences for particular individuals and families. Factors such as these, however, are rarely taken into consideration when Johnny's parents are summoned to a school conference to discuss his problem behavior or when a previously happily married couple experiences a high level of marital discord. In the words of relationship scientist Ellen Berscheid, sayings such as "love conquers all" are based on romantic beliefs that "close, committed, and loving relationships are impermeable and unsinkable vessels that can sail through any environmental storm with impunity" (Berscheid, 2004, p. 31).

As we stated earlier, psychological and political dynamics are intertwined. As indirect and unrelated as it may seem, the well-being of individuals is highly affected by the distribution of societal resources and by power plays being enacted at the personal, relational, and collective levels of analysis. If our goal is to move from a problem-saturated, person-centered and thus oppressive assessment process toward one that is broad-based, affirming, and liberating, a paradigm shift is in order. We propose an assessment process that will integrate individual-relational, organizational, and systemic factors that can hinder or facilitate well-being. These correspond to the micro-, meso-, and macro-levels of analysis, respectively. Given our focus on case conceptualization, the micro- (personal-relational) level of analysis is most closely related and thus easiest to understand. We suggest, for example, that an empowering assessment process would directly explore client strengths, assets, and examples of thriving and well-being. Some of the recent literature on human flourishing provides operational definitions of symptoms of mental health. Rather than simply assessing for the absence or presence of pathology, health care professionals can assess for indications of mental health as well as assist their clients to move in this direction (Keyes, 2003).

Moving up to the meso-level of analysis, a liberating and empowering assessment process would highlight abuses of power and organizational constraints (i.e., bullying at school; top-down, hierarchical work environment) that interfere with well-being, and explore ways of affecting change. Such an assessment process should result in clear guidelines for interventions, not only at the individual and interpersonal level, but at the organizational level as well. We cannot help a child who is the victim of bullying without dealing with the bullies and the system that allowed the behavior to take place.

As a final example, a liberating assessment process must acknowledge the insidious, almost invisible relationship between cultural norms, power imbalances, and unjust allocation of societal resources on the one hand, and distress and maladaptive functioning at the personal, interpersonal, and familial level, on the other. Thus, an atmosphere of xenophobia and collective anger toward undocumented workers "who are taking our jobs" is likely to permeate the work environment and the school climate and potentially infect marital and family relationships. An undocumented worker who suffers from powerlessness on the job may nonetheless abuse power in his relationship with his wife and children. Internalizing the oppression is also a definite risk, whereby one comes to believe that he is not worthy or deserving of more resources or more control over his life. Next, we explore the implications and applications to counseling and psychotherapy.

How does psychopolitical validity inform counseling and psychotherapy in the helping professions?

An assessment process that is grounded in client deficiencies and problem areas will invariably result in a treatment plan designed to "fix" the individual in question. As long as we consider the problem as residing within the individual client or family unit and limit our goal to the elimination or reduction of problematic functioning, we will design a person-centered treatment plan that is unlikely to consider broad environmental factors or focus on flourishing and well-being. We are not suggesting that maladaptive functioning at the personal level should not be targeted for intervention. Nonetheless, if done in the absence of accentuating client strengths and without proper grounding in interpersonal, organizational, and systemic contexts, it is ineffective at best, and harmful at worse.

The importance of contextualizing personal experience is central to feminism and feminist therapy. "Although we view people as active agents in their own lives and as such, constructors of their social worlds, we do not see that activity as isolated ... rather, we locate individual experience in society and history, embedded within a set of social relations which produce both the possibilities and limitations for that experience" (Acker *et al.*, 1991, p. 135). While written in reference to feminist approaches to research, the above quote has clear implications for therapeutic interventions. The political analysis of psychological distress is at the heart of feminist therapy. This is represented by one of its core principles "the personal is political" and is highly consistent with the construct of psycho-political validity. One of the major goals of feminist therapy is the empowerment of women who are struggling with sexual and other forms of inequalities (Brown, 1994; Watson & Williams, 1992). Nonetheless, its principles and strategies are applicable to multiple sources of inequality and oppression and to therapeutic interventions with women as well as men.

Feminist therapy, along with narrative therapy (Morgan, 2000; White & Epstein, 1990), critical psychology (Prilleltensky, 1997; Prilleltensky & Nelson, 2002), community counseling (Lewis *et al.*, 2003), and multicultural counseling and therapy (Ivey *et al.*, 2002), represent alternative therapeutic paradigms that directly address discrimination, oppression, and other systemic barriers (Table 6.4). As such, they pass the test of psycho-political validity and are consistent with liberation, empowerment, and well-being. In addition to addressing personal and interpersonal sources of distress as well as their extra-personal correlates, these paradigms focus on

Table 6.4. Applications to counseling and psychotherapy

Stages of wellness/ empowerment ▶ Level of analysis/ intervention ▼	Oppression (state):	Liberation (process):	Well-being (outcome):
Macro/collective/ structural/ community	Failing to address macro-level systemic factors (i.e., poverty, neighborhood violence) as well as social policies and cultural norms (i.e., xenophobia; blame the victim mentality) that increase problematic functioning and decrease well-being. In a similar vein, failing to amplify and build upon macro-level factors (i.e., greater gender equality) that enhance well-being.	Provide information and education on the interdependence of personal, organizational, and collective well-being. Develop alliances with groups committed to social justice. Identify problems that are best addressed through social/political action. Work along with stakeholders and allies to lobby legislatures and affect public policy.	Highlighting the interdependence between personal, organizational, and collective well-being. Partner with social movements and other community organizations working to advance the well-being of disadvantaged populations.
Meso/ organizational/ group/relational	Failing to address contextual factors and organizational structures (i.e., school climate, work environment) that increase problematic functioning and decrease well-being. "Helping" clients adapt to flawed structures and organizations without attempting to affect change at the level of the organization.	When appropriate, direct advocacy on behalf of clients in order to help them gain access to needed resources and services. Working to change organizational structures, policies, and practices that increase dysfunction and reduce well-being (i.e., bullying at school; an unhealthy work environment). Amplifying and building on meso-level factors that currently serve as protective factors (i.e., positive school climate; collaborative work environment).	Power-brokers gain a better understanding of environmental constraints and authorize health-enhancing services and resources. Personal and interpersonal change is supplemented with organizational change.

Table 6.4. (cont.)

Stages of wellness/ empowerment ▶ Level of analysis/ intervention▼	Oppression (state):	Liberation (process):	Well-being (outcome):
Micro/individual/ personal/ psychological (emotional, cognitive, behavioral, spiritual)	Targets for intervention narrowly defined as deficits and dysfunction within the person. Client is not encouraged to contextualize problematic functioning within broader systemic factors. Strengths, resilience and potential for flourishing and well-being are not actively pursued.	Problems are contextualized within broader systemic factors (i.e., the personal is political) and internalized oppression is a target for intervention. Focusing on health-enhancing relationships and problem-free spheres in the client's life and looking for situations when the problem does not occur. Targeting factors associated with well-being (self-determination; environmental mastery; optimism; positive relationships; social engagement).	Client comes to understand struggles as emanating from intrapersonal, interpersonal, and extrapersonal sources. Client takes responsibility for own behavior and functioning and works to change whatever is within her control. Client considers possibility for working toward meso- and macro-level changes.

harnessing client strengths and helping clients explore ways of resisting oppressive forces. For example, narrative therapists believe that people make meaning through the stories they tell about their lives. Life stories that are experienced as oppressive and diminishing are often based on "thin conclusions" made about individuals by others in position of power and authority. Once these thin conclusions take hold, there is a tendency to focus solely on gathering evidence that support the problem-saturated stories (Morgan, 2000; White & Epstein, 1990). Narrative therapists help their clients develop alternative stories by which they would like to live their lives. "Just as various 'thin descriptions' and conclusions can support and sustain problems, alternative stories can reduce the influence of problems and create new opportunities for living" (Morgan, 2000, p. 14). This is particularly important as some dominant cultural stories about certain groups are oppressive and diminishing. Rather than making meaning through these stories, clients can create new stories of resistance, empowerment, and liberation.

Micro-level interventions with clients include building on strengths that can serve as protective factors and buffer against dysfunction and adversity. Understanding and nurturing optimism and hope, building social skills and emotional intelligence, and enhancing self-efficacy and environmental mastery are examples of positive interventions designed to enhance well-being rather than simply ameliorate dysfunction (Lewis *et al.*, 2003; Seligman, 2002a). It is also important to remember that marginalized and vulnerable citizens often have to interact with representatives of organizations in positions of power that act as gatekeepers and have a lot of control over the allocation of services and resources. Thus, in accordance with self-efficacy, environmental mastery, and self-determination, therapeutic work with clients can include communication, influencing, and problem-solving skills that can help them become more proficient in negotiating systems and becoming strong self-advocates. This is particularly important given the constant shrinking of the social safety net and fierce competition for dwindling resources.

As effective as they may be, micro-level interventions with individual clients and families are not enough. Clients may well benefit from gaining a host of health-enhancing skills and competencies. Nonetheless, if the source of the dysfunction is in the systems with which they interact, those systems should be the target of intervention. In Ora Prilleltensky's research on disability, a number of participants commented on growing up with a physical disability and attending special schools. Consistently, they commented on the lack of emphasis placed on academic achievement and on the poor quality of education that they received: "There was such an emphasis on students doing things like physiotherapy and so kids would be pulled out of class to go to therapy . . . the level of the school was not the same as it was in the integrated programs . . . it was also like this huge playground . . . there weren't the expectations that you do your homework or that you have any movement toward adult responsibilities or any kind of responsibilities" (Prilleltensky, 2004, p. 110). No one would suggest that the children in question should adapt in order to fit the system. Clearly, the target of intervention here should be the school system and not the individual client. Although assisting from the sideline is generally preferred, it may also be appropriate to help clients gain access to needed resources by directly negotiating for relevant services and resources on their behalf. Mental health professionals can use their effective communication skills and privileged status to intervene with power brokers who can authorize wellness-enhancing services that can make a difference in the lives of vulnerable clients (Kiselica & Robinson, 2001; Lewis *et al.*, 2006).

If we accept the premise of psychopolitical validity that psychological and political dynamics are intertwined, our interventions cannot focus exclusively on the psychological or even the organizational to the total neglect of the political. "Given the impact of the environment on the well-being of clients, counselors need to influence educational, corporate industrial, social, and political systems. They can do this by raising the general awareness of the problems common to their clients, gaining support from policy makers, and encouraging positive community action" (Lewis *et al.*, 2003, p. 34). This might seem like a tall order and a daunting task for many of us in the helping professions who feel that we lack the time and the expertise to affect macro-level forces. After all, social change and systems advocacy are typically not part of the tool-box we painstakingly assembled over the course of our training and internships. In the field of counseling at least, this is becoming increasingly recognized by training programs that are supplementing interventions for personal change with advocacy skills and systems change. Furthermore, there is a growing body of literature that can serve as a roadmap on how this can be accomplished (Kiselica, & Robinson, 2001; Lewis *et al.*, 2003; Prilleltensky & Nelson, 2002). Recently, Lewis, Arnold, House and Toporek (2006) have generated an extensive list of advocacy competencies, much like the multicultural competencies that have become widely accepted by counseling professionals (Sue *et al.*, 1992). Common to all such attempts to operationalize macro-level interventions is the reminder that we don't have to do it all and we don't have to do it alone. But, we have to do it.

Conclusion

L. F. Harrell – one of my (Courte) mentors – shared with me an oft overlooked or ignored reality in the helping professions: There is an inherent contradiction between pursuing well-being and pursuing adjustment to the status quo. Many technologies – i.e. tests, data collection methods, behavioral techniques, etc. – available to researchers, practitioners, and students are neutral until the values of the user are applied (L. F. Harrell, personal communication, 2006). Whether in research, interventions, case conceptualizations, or therapy, we choose the direction that these technologies take. If we follow the path of least resistance, we likely align ourselves with adjustment to the status quo. Only by critically engaging with our institutions, colleagues, disciplinary traditions, communities, clients, etc., will we be able to pursue liberation and well-being. Both goals cannot be pursued simultaneously.

We assert that only through the coordination or combination of research, intervention, case conceptualization, and therapy can we clearly see the oppressive status quo, work toward liberation at all levels, and support well-being for those seeking help and society at large. We must avoid the myopic tendency that led to current paradigms in the helping professions, instead advancing liberation on all fronts.

The optimist assumes that most people entered the helping professions to advance the well-being of individuals, families, communities, and society rather than to advance the continued stratification and power inequality existing across the globe. Following this assumption, the structures that train and support researchers and practitioners have diverted many well-meaning helpers from the path of liberation. Therefore, liberation is not only the work of existing critical helpers or those new to research and practice, but of all who entered their profession for the sake of pursuing well-being that have been forcefully adjusted to the structures of their guild. This structural influence underscores the need for internally focused liberation as well as externally focused efforts. To use a well-known analogy: In the event of a loss of cabin pressure, you must put your oxygen mask on first, then assist those unable to do so themselves.

NOTE

(1) The authors have equally contributed to this chapter and are listed in alphabetical order.

REFERENCES

Acker, J., Barry, K., & Esseveld, J. (1991). Objectivity and truth: problems in doing feminist research. In *Beyond Methodology: Feminist Scholarship as Lived Research*, ed. M. M. Fonow & J. A. Cook. Indianapolis: Indiana University Press, pp. 133–153.

Bartky, S. L. (1990). *Femininity and Domination: Studies in the Phenomenology of Domination*. New York: Routledge.

Berscheid, E. (2004). The greening of relationship science. In *Close Relationships*, ed. H. Reis & C. Rusbult. New York: Psychology Press, pp. 25–34.

Blashfield, R. & Livesley, W. J. (1999). Classification. In *Oxford Textbook of Psychopathology*, ed. T. Millon, P. Blaney, & R. Davis. New York: Oxford University Press, pp. 3–28.

Brown, L. S. (1994). *Subversive Dialogues: Theory in Feminist Therapy*. New York: Basic Books.

Castillo, R. (1997). Toward a client-centered paradigm: a holistic synthesis. In *Culture and Mental Illness*, ed. R. Castillo. Pacific Grove, CA: Brooks/Cole, pp. 261–281.

Cormier, C. & Cormier, W. (1997). *Interviewing Strategies For Helpers: Fundamental Skills and Cognitive Behavioral Interventions*. New York: Brooks/Cole.

Fabrega, H., Jr. (1989). Cultural relativism and psychiatric illness. *Journal of Nervous and Mental Disease*, **177**(7), 415–425.

Fanon, F. (1963). *The Wretched of the Earth*. New York: Grove Press Inc.

Foucault, M. (1979). *Discipline and Punish*. Harmondsworth, UK: Penguin.

Freire, P. (1970). *Pedagogy of the Oppressed*. New York: Continuum.

Freire, P. (1975). Cultural action for freedom. *Harvard Educational Review Monograph*, **1**.

Freire, P. (1994). *Pedagogy of Hope*. New York: Continuum.

Fromm, E. (1958). The influence of social factors on child development. *La PrensaMedica Mexican*, **23**, 227–228.

Fromm, E. (1965). *Escape From Freedom*. New York: Avon Books.

Gorenstein, E. (1984). Debating mental illness: implication for science, medicine, and social policy. *American Psychologist*, **39**, 50–56.

Green, M. (1998). Neurodevelopmental model of schizophrenia. In M. Green, *Schizophrenia From the Neurocognitive Perspective: Probing the Impenetrable Darkness*. Boston: Allyn and Bacon, pp. 1–21.

Hackney, H. L. & Cormier, C. (2005). *The Professional Counselor : A Process Guide to Helping*, 5th edn. New York: Pearson Education Inc.

Hesse-Biber, S. N., Leavy, P., & Yaiser, M. L. (2004). Feminist approaches to research as a process: reconceptualizing epistemology, methodology, and method. In *Feminist Perspectives on Social Research*, ed. S. N. Hesse-Biber & M. L. Yaiser. New York: Oxford University Press, pp. 3–26.

Israel, B. A., Schulz, A. J., Parker, E. A., & Becker, A. B. (1998). Review of community based research: assessing partnership approaches to improve public health. *Annual Review of Public Health*, **19**, 173–202.

Ivey, A., D'Andrea, M., Ivey, M., & Simek-Morgan, L. (2002). *Counseling and Psychotherapy: A Multicultural Perspective*, 5th edn. Boston: Allyn and Bacon.

Kelly, J. (2006). *Becoming Ecological: An Expedition into Community Psychology*. New York: Oxford University Press.

Kenig, S. (1986). The political economy of community health. *Medical Anthropology Quarterly*, **17**(5), 132–134.

Keyes, C. L. M. (2003). Complete mental health: an agenda for the 21st century. In *Flourishing: Positive Psychology and the Life Well-Lived*, ed. C. L. M. Keyes and J. Haidt. Washington: American Psychological Association.

Kirmayer, L., Young, A., & Hayton, B. (1998). The cultural context of anxiety disorders. In *Meanings of Madness*, ed. R. Castillo. Pacific Grove, CA: Brooks/Cole, pp. 167–178.

Kiselica, M. S. & Robinson, M. (2001). Bringing advocacy counseling to life: the history, issues, and human dramas of social justice work in counseling. *Journal of Counseling and Development*, **79**(4), 387–397.

Lemme, B. (2006). *Development in Adulthood*, 4th edn. New York: Pearson.

Lewis, J., Arnold, M., House, R., & Toporek, R. (2006). *Advocacy Competencies*. http://www.counseling.org/Publications/.

Lewis, J. A., Lewis, M. D., Daniels, J. A., & D'Andrea, M. J. (2003). *Community Counseling: Empowering Strategies For a Diverse Society*, 3rd edn. Pacific Grove, CA: Brooks/Cole-Thomson Learning.

Maddux, J. E. (2002). Stopping the madness: positive psychology and the deconstruction of the illness ideology and the DSM. In *Handbook of Positive Psychology*, ed. C. R. Snyder & S. J. Lopez. New York: Oxford University Press, pp. 13–25.

Maguire, P. (1987). *Doing Participatory Research: A Feminist Approach*. Amherst, MA: University of Massachusetts.

Martin, J. & Sugarman, J. (2000). Between the modern and the postmodern: the possibility of self and progressive understanding in psychology. *American Psychologist*, **55**, 397–406.

Memmi, A. (1968). *Dominated Man: Notes Towards a Portrait*. New York: Orion Press.

Moane, G. (1999). *Gender and Colonialism: A Psychological Analysis of Oppression and Liberation*. London: Macmillan.

Montero, M. (1998). Dialectic between active minorities and majorities: a study of social influence in the community. *Journal of Community Psychology*, **26**(3), 281–289.

Morgan, A. (2000). *What is Narrative Therapy? An Easy-To-Read Introduction*. Adelaide, South Australia: Dulwich Centre Publications.

Mullaly, B. (2002) *Challenging Oppression: A Critical Social Work Approach*. Toronto: Oxford.

Murphy, J. (1976). Psychiatric labeling in cross-cultural perspective. *Science*, **191**, 1019–1028.

Nelson, G. & Prilleltensky, I. (2005). *Community Psychology: In Pursuit of Liberation and Well-Being*. New York: Palgrave Macmillan.

Oliver, K. (2004). *The Colonization of Psychic Space: A Psychoanalytic Theory of Social Oppression*. Minneapolis: University of Minnesota Press.

Perkins, D. D. & Zimmerman, M. A. (1995). Empowerment theory, research, and application. *American Journal of Community Psychology*, **23**(5), 569–579.

Peterson, N. A. & Zimmerman, M. A. (2004). Beyond the individual: toward a nomological network of organizational empowerment. *American Journal of Community Psychology*, **34**(1/2), 129–145.

Prilleltensky, I. (1994). *The Morals and Politics of Psychology: Psychological Discourse and the Status Quo*. Albany, New York: State University of New York Press.

Prilleltensky, I. (1997). Values, assumptions, and practices: assessing the moral implications of psychological discourse and action. *American Psychologist*, **52**(5), 517–535.

Prilleltensky, I. (2003). Understanding and overcoming oppression: towards psychopolitical validity. *American Journal of Community Psychology*, **31**, 195–202.

Prilleltensky, I. (2005). Promoting well-being: time for a paradigm shift in health and human services. *Scandinavian Journal of Public Health*, **33**, 53–60.

Prilleltensky, I. (in press). The role of power in wellness, oppression, and liberation: the promise of psychopolitical validity. *Journal of Community Psychology*.

Prilleltensky, I. & Gonick, L. (1996). Polities change, oppression remains: on the psychology and politics of oppression. *Political Psychology*, **17**, 127–147.

Prilleltensky, I. & Nelson, G. (2002). *Doing Psychology Critically: Making a Difference in Diverse Settings*. New York: Palgrave.

Prilleltensky, I. & Prilleltensky, O. (2006). *Promoting Well-Being: Linking Personal, Organizational, and Community Change.* New York: John Wiley & Sons.

Prilleltensky, O. (2004). *Motherhood and Disability: Children and Choices.* New York: Palgrave Macmillan.

Raulin, M. & Lilienfeld, S. (1999). Research strategies for studying psychopathology. In *Oxford Textbook of Psychopathology*, ed. T. Millon, P. Blaney, & R. Davis. New York: Oxford University Press, pp. 49–78.

Rose, N. (1999). *Powers of Freedom: Reframing Political Thought.* New York: Cambridge University Press.

Seligman, M. E. (2002a). Positive psychology, positive prevention, and positive therapy. In *Handbook of Positive Psychology*, ed. C. R. Snyder and S. J. Lopez. New York: Oxford University Press, pp. 3–9.

Seligman. M. E. (2002b). *Authentic Happiness: Using the New Positive Psychology to Realize Your Potential for Lasting Fulfillment.* New York: The Free Press.

Shinn, M. & Toohey, S. M. (2003). Community contexts of human welfare. *Annual Review of Psychology*, **54**, 427–459.

Speer, P. W. & Hughey, J. (1995). Community organizing: an ecological route to empowerment and power. *American Journal of Community Psychology*, **23**(5), 729–748.

Stancato, F. A. (2000). Tenure, academic freedom and the teaching of critical thinking. *College Student Journal*, **34**(3), 377–82.

Sue, D. W., Arredondo, P., & McDavis, R. J. (1992). Multicultural counseling competencies and standards: a call to the profession. *Journal of Counseling and Development*, **70**, 477–486.

Teo, T. (2005). *The Critique of Psychology: From Kant to Postcolonial Theory.* New York: Springer.

Tierney, W. G. (1997). Tenure and community in academe. *Educational Researcher*, **26**(8), 17–23.

Watson, G. & Williams, J. (1992). Feminist practice in therapy. In *Gender Issues in Clinical Psychology*, ed. J. M. Ussher & P. Nicholson. London: Routledge, pp. 212–236.

Watts, R., Williams, N. C., & Jagers, R. J. (2003). Sociopolitical development. *American Journal of Community Psychology*, **31**(1/2) 185–194.

White, M. & Epston, D. (1990). *Narrative Means to Therapeutic Ends.* New York: Norton Press.

Widiger, T. & Clark, L. A. (2000). Toward DSM-V and the classification of psychopathology. *Psychological Bulletin*, **126**(6), 946–963.

Wright, B. A. & Lopez, S. J. (2002). Widening the diagnostic focus: a case for including human strengths and environmental resources. In *Handbook of Positive Psychology*, ed. C. R. Snyder & S. J. Lopez. New York: Oxford University Press, pp. 26–44.

7

Class exploitation and psychiatric disorders: from status syndrome to capitalist syndrome

Carles Muntaner, Carme Borrell, and Haejoo Chung

Psychiatric epidemiologists were among the first scientists to document that the poor suffer from a higher rate of psychiatric disorders than the affluent. Psychiatric disorders and, more precisely, psychiatric research have propelled many studies on social class and psychiatric disorders which reflect the humanistic concerns of psychiatrists. These studies were motivated by a desire to improve the living conditions of workers, immigrants, and racial or ethnic minorities (e.g., Blazer et al., 1994; Eaton et al., 2004; Jacobi et al., 2004; Lahelma et al., 2005; Regier et al., 1988; Roberts & Lee, 1993). The absence or poor quality of psychiatric care for poor working class, immigrant, or racial and ethnic minority populations (Muntaner et al., 1995a; Alegria et al., 2000; Cohen et al., 2006) raised a related set of concerns about the implications of economic inequality for the treatment of psychiatric disorders.

The psychiatric and public health perspective on social class has been characteristically "pragmatic" (e.g., Asthana et al., 2004). Following the ethos of public health and medical care, the goal has been to "act upon the world" to reduce suffering and increase well-being (Navarro & Muntaner, 2004). Psychiatric disorders, which have a major worldwide impact on disability, are the leading cause of disability among women and, by 2020, are expected to become the main cause of years lost to disability (Murray & Lopez, 1996). Overall, the relevance of social class to psychiatry stems from the strength of the association between social class and psychiatric disorders and the severe consequences that working class life has for the quality of life of psychiatric patients (Fryers et al., 2005; Melzer et al., 2003; Poulton et al., 2002; Stansfeld et al., 2003).

Most psychiatric research is thus grounded in the medical world with its associated materialism and realism. It is within this context of professional pragmatism and technology that several findings on the relation between social class

Liberatory Psychiatry: Philosophy, Politics, and Mental Health, ed. Carl I. Cohen and Sami Timimi.
Published by Cambridge University Press. © Cambridge University Press.

and psychiatric disorders have emerged within the last century. This literature can inform social scientists interested in psychiatry because of the clinical relevance of categories which correspond to the most severe forms of disorders seen by psychiatrists. In spite of its narrow conceptualization of stratification (e.g., as in the popular "status syndrome"; Marmot, 2004), this relatively simple literature on the relations between social class stratification and psychiatric disorders provides important findings that have proved quite robust across time and place. However, we need to inform research on the social inequality and psychiatric disorders by looking beyond education or prestige ranks, such as the urgent need of patients that cannot afford medical care or new drugs in neoliberal states like the USA (Chung & Muntaner 2006) and, crucially, to consider the explanations for social inequalities (e.g., Geyer *et al.*, 2001).

In this chapter we review the recent evidence on the relation between social stratification, social class, and psychiatric disorders, arguing for the need to distinguish between the concepts of social stratification and social class proper in social psychiatry. Next, we venture into uncharted territories in social class and psychiatric disorders by introducing the concept of exploitation. We note a paradox in this area of knowledge: at least in the USA, social scientists often adopt the role of social psychologists while epidemiologists and psychiatrists take on the role of social scientists. We end by emphasizing the need for greater cross-fertilization between Neo-Marxian and Neo-Weberian class analyses and psychiatry in the study of social inequalities in psychiatric disorders.

The status syndrome: the empirical association between social strata and psychiatric disorders

There is a strong inverse association between economic inequality – based on conventional rank indicators – and psychiatric disorders (Eaton & Muntaner, 1999; Muntaner *et al.*, 2004a). The evidence is particularly strong to support the association between economic inequality, measured in terms of income, educational credentials, or occupational social class (often referred to as indicators of "socioeconomic status"), and the most frequent forms of psychiatric illnesses, such as depression, anxiety disorders, and substance use disorders (Eaton & Muntaner, 1999). For example, a comprehensive meta-analysis of prevalence and incidence studies on socioeconomic position and depression indicated that persons with low educational attainment or low income are at higher risk of depression (Lorant *et al.*, 2003). In the United States, individuals with annual household incomes of less than $20 000 per year were found to have a prevalence of major depression in the past month that was twice as high as that for individuals with annual household incomes of $70 000 or more (Blazer *et al.*, 1994). Studies of US metropolitan areas have found even larger differences (with odds ratios of 11 to 16) between high- and low-income respondents' risks of depression (Eaton, 2001). In a 13-year follow-up study that used psychiatric interviews as a method of assessment, poverty was found to increase the risk of depression by 2.5 times (Eaton *et al.*, 2001). In the same study in east Baltimore, respondents who did not receive income from property were ten times more likely to have an anxiety disorder than were those who obtained some income from property (Muntaner *et al.*, 1998).

With regard to occupational social class, the prevalence of depression in the past 6 months among those employed in household services was 7%, almost three times that of executive professionals (2.4%) (Roberts & Lee, 1993). More recent studies show that blue-collar workers are between 1.5 and 2 times as likely to be depressed as white-collar workers (Eaton *et al.*, 2004). Similar risk increases have been reported with a 1-year follow-up period (Eaton *et al.*, 2004). Being born to parents employed in manual labor occupations confers almost twice the risk of depression for women and almost four times the risk of depression for men compared with those born to at least one parent not in the working class (Eaton *et al.*, 2004). In addition to depression, similar two- to three-fold differences in prevalence between high and low occupational strata have been reported in the United States for substance use disorders, alcohol abuse or dependence, antisocial personality disorder, anxiety disorders, and all psychiatric disorders combined (Eaton, 2001; Eaton *et al.*, 2004; Regier *et al.*, 1988). Internationally, even larger differences have been found – up to a four-fold higher current prevalence of common psychiatric disorders among "working-class" respondents compared with their middle-class counterparts (Regier *et al.*, 1988).

Poverty is also a consistent risk factor for multiple psychiatric disorders, including depression, anxiety disorders, antisocial personality, and substance-use disorders (Eaton *et al.*, 2004; Eaton & Muntaner, 1999). Cross-sectional and longitudinal studies have found consistent associations between area poverty and psychiatric disorders. In addition, most income inequality studies have shown an association between income inequality and high rates of psychiatric disorders (Muntaner *et al.*, 2004a; Wilkinson & Pickett, 2006).

The proximal determinants of psychiatric disorders: the contribution of psychiatric epidemiology to social psychiatry

The challenge for psychiatrists and social scientists alike is to use concepts from stratification research to explain these patterns. There is currently a heated controversy on the relative importance of "neo-material" determinants (contemporary physical or biological risk or protective factors) and "psychosocial" determinants, such as perceptions of relative standing in the income distribution, for explaining socioeconomic gradients in health in wealthy countries (Lynch *et al.*, 2000; Muntaner, 2004; Pearce & Davey Smith, 2003). In brief, "neo-material" scholars claim that most social inequalities in health are determined by "material" (socially determined physical and chemical) risk and protective factors linked to poverty and inequality, such as poor housing, poor diet, drugs, environmental and workplace hazards, injuries, poor transportation, lack of access to quality health care, or physical violence (Lynch *et al.*, 2000). Psychosocial scholars, on the other hand, stress the role of perceptions of inequality, social capital, perceptions of job stress, or social isolation (Wilkinson, 2005). Research supports both types of explanations.

Neo-material indicators of economic inequality, such as owning a car or a house, and indices of deprivation have recently been incorporated into research on the social epidemiology of psychiatric disorders (Lewis *et al.*, 1998, 2003; Weich & Lewis, 1998). For example, in a national survey of United Kingdom households, an independent association was found between housing tenure and access to a car, on the one hand, and neurotic disorder (including some anxiety disorders) and depression, on the other (Lewis *et al.*, 2003; Weich & Lewis, 1998). Also, an analysis of the British Household Panel Survey found that low material standard of living was associated with risk for depression and anxiety disorders (Lewis *et al.*, 1998). A geographic area deprivation index, including housing tenure and car ownership, has been associated with the prevalence and persistence of risk for depression. Although deprivation indicators suggest that absence of material goods increases the risk of psychiatric disorders, research has yet to uncover the specific mechanisms linking material factors to depression or anxiety (e.g., food insecurity, bad diet; poor housing, fear of being evicted, homelessness; noise, pollution, dirt, physical violence, extreme temperatures at work or in the community; unsafe working conditions, physical overwork, exhaustion, lack of sleep; poor transportation; poor health, chronic diseases; unmet health care needs).

Studies have also provided cross-sectional and prospective evidence of an association between psychosocial factors, such as perceived job demands and perceived financial hardship, on the one hand, and depression, symptoms of depression, or anxiety disorders, on the other (Eaton *et al.*, 2001; Weich & Lewis, 1998). Since the mid-1970s' Whitehall studies, there have been a large number of studies showing that the effects of social stratification on psychiatric disorders are partially mediated by psychosocial factors such as "job autonomy" or "lack of control" (Marmot, 2004). A substantial amount of this evidence in social epidemiology comes from the Whitehall studies themselves and constitutes the foundation of the "status syndrome" (Marmot 2004). In addition, in social science, a large number of studies have shown compatible results although "material" risk factors and biomedical indicators are less likely to be included in those studies (e.g., Turner *et al.*, 1995;

see the *Journal of Health and Social Behavior* in the last 20 years). Therefore, social scientists might be over-stating the importance of psychosocial factors because they do not usually include measures of material resources.

A common limitation of most "psychosocial" studies is an over-reliance on self-report measures of both psychosocial risk factors and psychiatric disorders outcomes (including questionnaires and lay administered diagnostic interviews), coupled with an infrequent use of clinical diagnostic interviews (e.g., due to lack of psychiatric training), to assess psychiatric disorders. Such methods produce vulnerability to self-report bias (persons might have a tendency to report both "stress" and "psychiatric disorder" without having either). Even in prospective studies that take into account reverse causation it is difficult to rule out the possibility that features of the material environment (physical and biological exposures) are confounded with a respondent's perceptions (Macleod *et al.*, 2002). Nevertheless, the reported associations of job insecurity or remaining in a downsized organization with symptoms of anxiety and depression suggest that psychosocial exposures can have independent effects on psychiatric disorders (Ferrie *et al.*, 2003). Thus, epidemiology's emphasis on the material and objective as well as on the psychosocial and subjective can help refine both methods and explanations in social psychiatry. The implications of this ongoing debate are important for social psychiatry models and methods: (1) the potential neglect of material resources in the determination of psychiatric disorders would force a reappraisal of sociological "stress" models; and (2) evidence of self report bias or confounding as noted above would imply more emphasis on objective assessment of exposures, and less emphasis on self reports.

Class structure and psychiatric disorders

Although there have been relatively few empirical studies on social class, the need to study social class proper has been noted by epidemiologists and social scientists alike (Krieger *et al.*, 1997; Muntaner & O'Campo, 1993). Thus, while social stratification refers to the ranking of individuals in some economic (e.g., income), political (e.g., power within organizations) or cultural (education) continuum, social class deals with the social relations (owner, worker, self-employed; manager, supervisor, worker; professional, technician, unskilled worker) that generate economic, political and cultural inequalities in a social system (Muntaner *et al.*, 1998). Most research on social inequalities in psychiatric disorders relies on indicators of social stratification (e.g., the "status syndrome") and does not include any analysis of social class relations (Muntaner & Lynch, 1999). Nevertheless, social class positions based on employment relations (e.g., workers, managers, employers) can be powerful determinants of population health via processes such as the exposure to risk or protective factors such as social and health services or income (Bartley & Marmot, 2000). In a series of studies (e.g., Borrell *et al.*, 2004; Muntaner *et al.*, 1995; Muntaner *et al.*, 2003; Muntaner *et al.*, 1998; Muntaner & Parsons, 1996), we have examined the relationship between social class and psychiatric disorders within a Neo-Marxian framework which emphasizes class employment relations (Wright, 2005).[1] To illustrate the conceptual and empirical importance of this approach to class analysis, we underscore the conceptual differences between social stratification and class approaches and provide empirical support for the unique relation between class and psychiatric disorders.

Social stratification usually refers to the ranking of individuals along a continuum of economic attributes such as income or years of education. These rankings are known as "gradient" indicators in epidemiology (Muntaner *et al.*, 2004a). Most researchers use several measures of social stratification simultaneously because single measures have been insufficient to explain social inequalities in the health of populations. There is little doubt that measures of social stratification are important predictors of patterns of morbidity from psychiatric disorders (Eaton *et al.*, 2004; Lynch & Kaplan, 2000). However, despite their usefulness in predicting psychiatric disorders outcomes, these measures do not reveal the social mechanisms that explain how individuals come to accumulate different levels of economic (and political or cultural) resources (Muntaner & Lynch, 1999).

Class inequality, which includes relations of property and control over the labor process, is also associated with psychiatric illness. Social class, understood as social relations linked to the production of goods and services (Krieger *et al.*, 1997) is conceptually and empirically distinct from social stratification/socioeconomic status (SES). Moreover, social class is associated with psychiatric disorders over and above SES indicators. (Borrell *et al.*, 2004; Muntaner *et al.*, 2003; Muntaner *et al.*, 1998; Wohlfarth, 1997; Wohlfarth & van den Brink, 1998). One study found a small overlap between SES and social class measures, although the association between social class and depression could not be accounted for by SES (Wohlfarth, 1997). Other studies have found initial evidence of a non-linear relationship between social class and psychiatric disorders, as would be predicted by social class models but not by SES models (Muntaner *et al.*, 2003; Muntaner *et al.*, 1998). Low-level supervisors (who do not have policy-making power but can hire and fire workers) have higher rates of depression and anxiety than both upper-level managers (who have organizational control over policy and personnel) and front-line employees (who have neither). Control over organizational assets is determined by the possibility of influencing company policy (making decisions over number of people employed, products or services delivered, amount of work performed, and size and distribution of budgets) and by sanctioning authority over others in the organization (granting or preventing pay raises or promotions, hiring, and firing or temporarily suspending subordinates). The repeated experience of organizational control at work would protect most upper-level managers against mood and anxiety disorders. Low-level supervisors, on the other hand, are subjected to "double exposure": the demands of upper management to discipline the workforce and the antagonism of subordinate workers, while exerting little influence over company policy. This "contradictory class location" (Wright, 1996) may place supervisors at greater risk of depression and anxiety disorders than either upper management or non-supervisory workers. The bottom line is that this finding was predicted by the "contradictory class location" hypothesis but was not predicted or explained by indicators of years of education or income gradients. The gradient ("SES") hypothesis would have led to the expectation that supervisors, because of their higher incomes, would present *lower* rates of anxiety and depression than workers.

According to the example above, the theoretical and explanatory power of social class stems from social relations of ownership or control over productive resources (i.e., physical, financial, and organizational). Social class relations have important consequences for the lives of individuals. The extent of an individual's legal right and power to control productive assets determines an individual's abilities to acquire income. And income determines in large part the individual's standard of living. Thus the class position of "business owner" compels its members to hire "workers" and extract labor from them, while the "worker" class position compels its members to find employment and perform labor. Social class provides an explicit relational mechanism (property, management) that explains how economic inequalities are generated and how they may affect psychiatric disorders.

In a recent study we further examined the relationships between measures of social class (Wright's social class indicators, i.e., relationship to productive assets) and indicators of psychiatric disorders (Borrell *et al.*, 2004). We tested this scheme using the Barcelona Health Interview Survey, a cross-sectional survey of 10 000 residents of the city's non-institutionalized population in 2000. Health-related variables included self-perceived health (taping mostly psychiatric disorders), nicotine addiction, eating behaviors and injuries. Findings revealed that, contrary to conventional wisdom, health indicators are often worse for employers than for managers, and that supervisors often fare more poorly than workers. Our findings highlight the potential health consequences of social class positions defined by relations of control over productive assets. They also confirm that social class taps into parts of the social variation in health that are not captured by conventional measures of social stratification. Property relations, which figure prominently in both Marxian and Weberian traditions, do not, however, exhaust the theoretical spectrum of class concepts. Another, untapped, notion is that of class exploitation.

Marxian class analysis: class exploitation and psychiatric disorders

Although property relations might be important predictors of psychiatric disorders (Eaton & Muntaner, 1999; Wohlfarth, 1997), they do not capture the underlying mechanism in the Marxian class tradition, namely exploitation (Wright, 1996). According to that tradition, a measure of social class should not only capture property relations but the domination of the "exploited" by the "exploiter" and the extraction and appropriation of labor effort (Resnick & Wolff, 1982; Wright, 1996). In fact, most Neo-Marxian measures of social class are exchangeable with Neo-Weberian measures of employment relations because they capture only property relations. That is, both sets of indicators tap into employment relations or labor market exchanges such as "employer" or "employee," but do not capture the amount of labor effort extracted from the "employee" by the "employer," which forms the basis of "exploitation" as a social mechanism in the classic Marxian tradition (Muntaner et al., 1998; Wright, 2005). To follow that tradition, indicators of class exploitation should take into account that: (1) the material welfare of a class causally depends on the material deprivation of another; (2) this causal relation in (1) involves the asymmetrical exclusion of the exploited class from access to certain productive resources (e.g., property rights); and (3) the causal mechanism that translates the exclusion in (2) into differential welfare involves the appropriation of the fruits of labor of the exploited class by those who control the access to productive resources (i.e., the exploiter class) (Wright, 1996). Thus we can observe that most Neo-Marxian measures of social class measure (1) and (2) in the form of property relations, but do not capture the appropriation of labor effort. In a recent study (Muntaner et al., 2004) we found an association between class exploitation and depression using organizational level indicators that capture both property relations and the extraction of labor effort (for profit ownership, managerial domination, lack of wage increases). These indicators were strong predictors of depressive symptoms in these studies. They are different from employment relations indicators in that they capture social class exploitation at the organizational level (i.e., the combination of for profit ownership, managerial pressure and lack of wage increases taps into high levels of extraction of labor effort and low compensation, or higher exploitation, as compared to the residual category).

In sum, our argument is that there are a number of class constructs that can illuminate the relation between economic inequality and psychiatric disorders. There a numerous, literally hundreds of measures of mental health and psychiatric disorders in the literature (see Buro's *Psychiatric Measurement* volumes). On the other hand, the social part of the equation remains vastly underdeveloped, with researchers using only a handful of measures (income, education, occupation).

The paradox of epidemiology, social psychiatry and the sociology of mental disorders

In spite of their pragmatic, often non-theoretical approach to social factors, psychiatric epidemiology and social psychiatry (both part of public mental health) have now and then tackled structural inequalities. A strong concern for social justice and reducing inequalities (race, gender, poverty) could explain the strong interest in social inequalities in health among epidemiologists. The contemporary definition of public health – as organized efforts by society to improve the health of populations – implicitly acknowledges both social determinants and collective responsibility for the public's health (Last, 1995).

Public mental health is thus faced with the obligation to improve the health of groups affected by social inequality – that is, public health officials have the responsibility to improve the psychiatric disorders of populations that due to economic, political, or cultural inequalities have a high rate of psychiatric disorders. In these disciplines it is understood that a society's unequal distribution of economic, political, or cultural resources will generate worse psychiatric disorders among the relatively poor, powerless, and with less credentials (Navarro & Muntaner, 2004). Furthermore, it is widely recognized that inequalities in property generate an intergenerational transmission of poverty that has disproportionately affected African-Americans in the USA (Conley & Bennett, 2001). Other acknowledged sources of economic inequality involve political inequalities that preclude immigrants from obtaining equal rights, while confining them to economic, political, and cultural subordination. And cultural factors such as racism, ideology, or ignorance that can lead to labor market discrimination and residential segregation with negative economic, political, and cultural consequences for people of various races and ethnicities, nationalities, religions, age groups, sexual orientations, gender, diseases or disabilities, and social classes.

It is within this public health ethos of reversing inequalities associated with the social movements of the 1960s and 1970s that recent research focuses on the interactions between class, gender and race/ethnicity and psychiatric disorders (Artazcoz et al., 2004; O'Campo et al., 2004; Outram et al., 2004). Although generalizations are often inaccurate in social epidemiology, overall, this body of research on the triad of class, gender, and race tends to find worse psychiatric disorders among members of the groups exposed to the three forms of inequality (Krieger et al., 2006). Epidemiologists have also been leaders in topics that overlap with the more structural concerns traditionally associated with sociology and mainstream economics such as the study of the psychiatric disorder effects of new forms of labor market arrangements (Artazcoz et al., 2005; Kim et al., 2006), the effects of social class across the lifespan (Breeze et al., 2001), or the contextual effects of neighborhood economic inequality on psychiatric disorders (Eibner et al., 2004; Muntaner et al., 2004a; Muntaner et al., 2004b; Schneiders et al., 2003; Stafford & Marmot, 2003; Wainwright & Surtees, 2004). Because these studies are often published outside psychiatry, their contributions to theories of social inequality in psychiatric disorders remain under-recognized.

There is thus a curious paradox that looms large in the literature on the sociology of psychiatric disorders. It is not uncommon to observe that (1) epidemiologists and public health researchers without a Ph.D. in social science are those who bring a sociostructural perspective to health inequalities (e.g., Krieger et al., 1997; Muntaner et al., 1998); (2) in spite of some notable exceptions (Kohn & Schooler, 1983), social scientists have been devoted to sociopsychological rather than sociostructural explanations (Pearlin, 1989; Thoits, 2005). Yet social scientists are leaders in psychiatric epidemiology and public mental health without bringing a particular sociological content to their work (Kessler et al., 1994). A detailed historical, professional, and institutional analysis (e.g., are health researchers trained to be critical in general so they dare to approach thorny issues such as "class" when they shift to social inquiry? Do medicine, public health, and psychiatry attract conservative social scientists? Why did social psychology have more influence on the sociology of psychiatric disorders than the sociostructural perspective?), will be needed to sort out the merit of these propositions. They suggest, however, the need for more sustained attention to structural explanations in psychiatric epidemiological research.

Given the soundness of the methods and the robustness of the findings in psychiatric epidemiology and social psychiatry, one might be tempted to conclude that deeper sociological insights are superfluous to such applied disciplines. Why not just raise the minimum wage or increase welfare assistance to the poor as primary prevention? The answer is not so simple, as implicit social models permeate both psychiatric epidemiology and social psychiatry with sharp differences in their policy implications (Muntaner et al., 2000).

More specifically, underlying most research on economic inequality and psychiatric disorders we find competing implicit social models of what constitutes desirable social and health policies. Two opposing views of the social inequalities in psychiatric disorders are prominent (Muntaner et al., 2000). The first is that behavior is a matter of individual agency or volitional control, accounting for the disproportionate burden of psychiatric illness among workers, women, and minorities. This view holds that most social outcomes, including psychiatric disorders, reflect personal autonomous choices and that therefore there is little that society, as a whole, is obliged to do for people who are afflicted by psychiatric disorders (Muntaner & Lynch, 1999). In one study (Link et al., 1995), for example, educated "liberals" respected the autonomy and individual rights of homeless persons but felt little obligation to do anything to improve their situation.

In contrast, the "structural" view focuses on social relations of class, race, ethnicity, and gender inequality as determinants of individual behavior and psychiatric disorders (Muntaner *et al.*, 2000). The policy implications of this view include collective responsibility for those whose psychiatric disorders are negatively affected by class, gender, and racial and ethnic inequalities in access to economic, political, and cultural resources. For example, a recent ethnographic study of African-American and white working-class men concluded that African-American men have a greater sense of collective responsibility and are less prone to use individual responsibility as an explanation for personal outcomes than are their white counterparts (Lamont, 2000). Western European and US whites are more likely to use individualistic attributions for the outcomes of persons in social situations – personal attributes are seen as the cause of personal outcomes, as opposed to the features of the situation (Nisbett, 2003). The implication is that, unless we make social-structural inequalities explicit, we cannot use social science to choose between competing policy perspectives.

Although most studies in social inequalities in psychiatric disorders (Eaton *et al.*, 2004) use stratification indicators that eschew social structure (i.e., the set of economic, political and cultural relations in a given social system) (Muntaner & Lynch, 1999), there is nowadays sufficient evidence to suggest that class, gender, and racial/ethnic inequalities in psychiatric disorders stem from social structures, rather than solely from personal choices or individual attributes. Thus in studies using employment relations indicators social class have been found to predict psychiatric disorders over and above mere stratification indicators (for review see Muntaner *et al.*, 2004a). The implication is that structural social class measures are useful in social psychiatry not only because they provide a social mechanism (e.g., the relation between supervisor and supervisee), but because they can be strong predictors of psychiatric disorders (Muntaner *et al.*, 2004a).

From status syndrome to capitalist syndrome: the role of class exploitation in social psychiatry

The evidence on the inverse association between measures of social stratification such as income and education and common psychiatric disorders is well established. Yet little is known about the relation between the social processes that generate economic inequalities and psychiatric disorders. Recent research points to the need for social psychiatry to delve into the social relations that produce social inequalities in psychiatric disorders, not only into the micro social processes linking social interactions to psychiatric disease (e.g., service utilization, stigma). Social mechanisms generating economic inequalities such as relations of production, property relations, or exploitation are too central to social systems to be addressed exclusively by clinicians. Class analysis input will be ultimately essential to the advancement of our understanding of the relation between economic inequality and psychiatric disorders. Greater class analytic (e.g., Neo-Marxian class exploitation) insight into research on social inequalities in psychiatric disorders would give social psychiatry more depth; would allow testing of alternative models for the social production of psychiatric illness, which now are not accessible due to focus on the outcomes of social structure (e.g., income inequalities); and would ultimately yield deeper causal models that might lead to effective policy interventions.

NOTE

(1) Most of the measures we have used in our studies do not distinguish the Neo-Marxian conceptualization of social class from the Neo-Weberian conceptualization, a framework that focuses on class as employment relations but does not contemplate exploitation as a central mechanism. We discuss the importance of adding indicators of exploitation below.

REFERENCES

Alegria, M., Bijl, R. V., Lin, E., Walters, E. E., & Kessler, R. C. (2000). Income differences in persons seeking outpatient treatment for mental disorders: a comparison of the United States with Ontario and The Netherlands. *Archives of General Psychiatry*, **57**, 383–391.

Artazcoz, L., Benach, J., Borrell, C., & Cortes, I. (2004). Unemployment and mental health: Understanding the interactions among gender, family roles, and social class. *American Journal of Public Health*, **94**(1), 82–88.

Artazcoz, L., Benach, J., Borrell, C., & Cortes, I. (2005). Social inequalities in the impact of flexible employment on different domains of psychosocial health. *Journal of Epidemiology and Community Health*, **59**(9), 761–767.

Asthana, S., Gibson, A., Moon, G., Brigham, P., & Dicker, J. (2004). The demographic and social class basis of inequality in self reported morbidity: An exploration using the health survey for England. *Journal of Epidemiology and Community Health*, **58**(4), 303–307.

Bartley, M. & Marmot, M. (2000). Social class and power relations at the workplace. *Occupational Medicine: State of the Art Reviews*, **15**, 73–78.

Blazer, D. G., Kessler, R. C., McGonagle, K. A., & Swartz, M. S. (1994). The prevalence and distribution of major depression in a national community sample: The national comorbidity survey. *American Journal of Psychiatry*, **151**, 979–986.

Borrell, C., Muntaner, C., Benach, J., & Artazcoz, L. (2004). Social class and self-reported health status among men and women: What is the role of work organisation, household material standards and household labour? *Social Science and Medicine*, **58**(10), 1869–1887.

Breeze, E., Fletcher, A. E., Leon, D. A., Marmot, M. G., Clarke, R. J., & Shipley, M. J. (2001). Do socioeconomic disadvantages persist into old age? Self-reported morbidity in a 29-year follow-up of the Whitehall study. *American Journal of Public Health*, **91**(2), 277–283.

Cohen, A., Houck, P. R., Szanto, K., Dew, M. A., Gilman, S. E., & Reynolds, C. F. (2006). Social inequalities in response to antidepressant treatment in older adults. *Archives of General Psychiatry*, **63**(1), 50–56.

Conley, D. & Bennett, N. G. (2001). Birth weight and income: Interactions across generations. *Journal of Health and Social Behavior*, **42**(4), 450–465.

Chung, H. & Muntaner, C. (2006). Political and Welfare State determinants of population health: an analysis of wealthy countries *Social Science Medicine*, **63**(3), 829–842.

Eaton, W. W. (2001). *The Sociology of Mental Disorders, 3rd edn.* London, UK: Praeger.

Eaton, W. W. & Muntaner, C. (1999). Socioeconomic stratification and mental disorder. In *A Handbook for the Study of Mental Health: Social Contexts, Theories and Systems*, ed. A. V. Horwitz & T. L. Scheid. New York, NY: Cambridge University Press.

Eaton, W. W., Muntaner, C., Bovasso, G., & Smith, C. (2001). Socioeconomic status and depression. *Journal of Health and Social Behavior*, **42**, 277–293.

Eaton, W. W., Buka, S., Addington, A. M. *et al.* (2004). Risk factors for major mental disorders. A review of the epidemiologic literature. Retrieved January 24th, 2005, from http://apps1.jhsph.edu/weaton/MDRF/main.html.

Eibner, C., Sturn, R., & Gresenz, C. R. (2004). Does relative deprivation predict the need for mental health services? *Journal of Mental Health and Policy Economics*, **7**(4), 167–175.

Ferrie, J. E., Shipley, M. J., Stansfeld, S. A., Davey Smith, G., & Marmot, M. (2003). Future uncertainty and socioeconomic inequalities in health: the Whitehall ii study. *Social Science Medicine*, **57**, 637–646.

Fryers, T., Melzer, D., Jenkins, R., & Brugha, T. (2005). The distribution of the common mental disorders: social inequalities in Europe. *Clinical Practical Epidemology and Mental Health*, **1**, 14.

Geyer, S., Haltenhof, H., & Peter, R. (2001). Social inequality in the utilization of in- and outpatient treatment of non-psychotic/non-organic disorders: a study with health insurance data. *Social Psychiatry and Psychiatric Epidemiology*, **36**(8), 373–380.

Jacobi, F., Wittchen, H. U., Holting, C. *et al.* (2004). Prevalence, co-morbidity and correlates of mental disorders in the general population: results from the German Health Interview and Examination Survey (GHS). *Psychological Medicine*, **34**(4), 597–611.

Kessler, R. C., McGonagle, K. A., Zhao, S. *et al.* (1994). Lifetime and 12-month prevalence of DSM-III-R mental disorders in the United States. *Archives of General Psychiatry*, **51**, 8–19.

Kim, I. H., Muntaner, C., Khang, Y. H., Paek, D., & Cho, S. I. (2006). The relationship between nonstandard working and mental health in a representative sample of the South Korean population. *Social Science Medicine*,

Kohn, M. L. & Schooler, C. (1983). *Work and Personality: An Inquiry into the Impact of Social Stratification*. Norwood, NJ: Ablex Pub. Corp.

Krieger, N., Williams, D. R., & Moss, N. E. (1997). Measuring social class in us public health research: concepts, methodologies, and guidelines. *Annual Review of Public Health*, **18**, 341–378.

Krieger, N., Waterman, P. D., Hartman, C. *et al.* (2006) Social hazards on the job: workplace abuse, sexual harassment, and racial discrimination – a study of Black, Latino, and White low-income women and men workers in the United States. *International Journal of Health Services*, **36**(1), 51–85.

Lahelma, E., Martikainen, P., Rahkonen, O., Roos, E., & Saastamoinen, P. (2005). Occupational class inequalities across key domains of health: results from the Helsinki health study. *European Journal of Public Health*, **15**(5), 504–510.

Lamont, M. (2000). *The Dignity of Working Men*. New York, NY: Russell Sage.

Last, J. A. (1995). *Dictionary of Epidemiology*. New York: Oxford University Press.

Lewis, G., Bebbington, P., Brugha, T. *et al.* (1998). Socioeconomic status, standard of living, and neurotic disorder. *Lancet*, **352**, 605–609.

Lewis, G., Bebbington, P., Brugha, T. *et al.* (2003). Socio-economic status, standard of living, and neurotic disorder. *International Review of Psychiatry*, **15**, 91–96.

Link, B. G., Schwartz, S., Moore, R. *et al.* (1995). Public knowledge, attitudes, and beliefs about homeless people: Evidence for compassion fatigue. *American Journal of Community Psychology*, **23**(4), 533–555.

Lorant, V., Deliege, D., Eaton, W., Robert, A., Philippot, P., & Ansseau, M. (2003). Socioeconomic inequalities in depression: a meta-analysis. *American Journal of Epidemiology*, **157**(2), 98–112.

Lynch, J. W. & Kaplan, G. A. (2000). Socioeconomic position. In *Social Epidemiology*, ed. L. F. Berkman & I. Kawachi. New York: NY: Oxford University Press, pp. 76–94.

Lynch, J. W., Smith, G. D., Kaplan, G. A., & House, J. S. (2000). Income inequality and mortality: Importance to health of individual income, psychosocial environment, or material conditions. *British Medical Journal*, **320**, 1200–1204.

Macleod, J., Davey Smith, G., Heslop, P., Metcalfe, C., Carroll, D., & Hart, C. (2002). Psychological stress and cardiovascular disease: Empirical demonstration of bias in a prospective observational study of Scottish men. *British Medical Journal*, **324**, 1247–1251.

Marmot, M. (2004). *The Status Syndrome*: How Social Status Affects our Health and Longevity. New York: Times Books.

Melzer, D., Fryers, T., Jenkins, R., Brugha, T., & McWilliams, B. (2003). Social position and the common mental disorders with disability: Estimates from the national mental survey of Great Britain. *Social Psychiatry and Psychiatric Epidemiology*, **38**(5), 238–243.

Muntaner, C. (2004). Commentary: social capital, social class, and the slow progress of psychosocial epidemiology. *International Journal of Epidemiology*, **33**(4), 674–680.

Muntaner, C., & Lynch, J. (1999). Income inequality, social cohesion, and class relations: a critique of Wilkinson's neo-Durkheimian research program. *International Journal of Health Services*, **29**(1), 59–81.

Muntaner, C. & O'Campo, P. J. (1993). A critical appraisal of the demand/control model of the psychosocial work environment: epistemological, social, behavioral and class considerations. *Social Science Medicine*, **36**(11), 1509–1517.

Muntaner, C. & Parsons, P. E. (1996). Income, social stratification, class, and private health insurance: a study of the Baltimore metropolitan area. *International Journal of Health Services*, **26**(4), 655–671.

Muntaner, C., Anthony, J. C., Crum, R. M., & Eaton, W. W. (1995a). Psychosocial dimensions of work and the risk of drug dependence among adults. *American Journal of Epidemiology*, **142**(2), 183–190.

Muntaner, C., Wolyniec, P., McGrath, J., Pulver, A. E. (1995b). Differences in social class among psychotic patients at inpatient admission. *Psychiatric Services*, **46**(2), 176–178.

Muntaner, C., Eaton, W. W., Diala, C., Kessler, R. C., & Sorlie, P. D. (1998). Social class, assets, organizational control and the prevalence of common groups of mental disorders. *Social Science Medicine*, **47**(12), 2043–2053.

Muntaner, C., Eaton, W., & Diala, C. (2000). Socioeconomic inequalities in mental health: A review of concepts and underlying assumptions. *Health*, **4**, 89–15.

Muntaner, C., Borrell, C., Benach, J., Pasarin, M. I., & Fernandez, E. (2003). The associations of social class and social stratification with patterns of general and mental health in a Spanish population. *International Journal of Epidemiology*, **32**(6), 950–958.

Muntaner, C., Eaton, W. W., Miech, R., & O'Campo, P. (2004a). Socioeconomic position and major mental disorders. *Epidemiology Reviews*, **26**, 53–62.

Muntaner, C., Li, Y., Xue, X., O'Campo, P., Chung, H. J., & Eaton, W. W. (2004b). Work organization, area labor-market characteristics, and depression among U.S. nursing home workers: a cross-classified multilevel analysis. *International Journal of Occupational Environmental Health*, **10**(4), 392–400.

Murray, C. J. & Lopez, A. D. (1996). Evidence-based health policy – lessons from the global burden of disease study. *Science*, **274**(5288), 740–743.

Navarro, V. & Muntaner, C. (2004). *Political and Economic Determinants of Population Health and Well-being: Controversies and Developments*. Amityville: The Baywood Publishing Company.

Nisbett, R. E. (2003). *The Geography of Thought*. New York, NY: The Free Press.

O'Campo, P., Eaton, W. W., & Muntaner, C. (2004). Labor market experience, work organization, gender inequalities and health status: results from a prospective analysis of US employed women. *Social Science Medicine*, **58**(3), 585–594.

Outram, S., Mishra, G. D., & Schofield, M. J. (2004). Sociodemographic and health related factors associated with poor mental health in midlife Australian women. *Women Health*, **39**(4), 97–115.

Pearce, N. & Davey Smith, G. (2003). Is social capital the key to inequalities in health? *American Journal of Public Health*, **93**(1), 122–129.

Pearlin, L. I. (1989). The sociological study of stress. *Journal Health and Social Behavior*, **30**(3), 241–256.

Poulton, R., Caspi, A., Milne, B. J. *et al.* (2002). Association between children's experience of socioeconomic disadvantage and adult health: a life-course study. *Lancet*, **360**, 1640–1645.

Regier, D. A., Boyd, J. H., Burke, J. D. Jr. *et al.* (1988). One-month prevalence of mental disorders in the United States. Based on five epidemiologic catchment area sites. *Archives of General Psychiatry*, **45**(11), 977–986.

Resnick, S. & Wolff, R. D. (1982). Classes in marxian theory. *Review of Radical Political Economics*, **13**(4), 1–18.

Roberts, R. E. & Lee, E. S. (1993). Occupation and the prevalence of major depression, alcohol, and drug abuse in the United States. *Environmental Research*, **61**(2), 266–278.

Schneiders, J., Drukker, M., van der Ende, J., Verhulst, F. C., van Os, J., & Nicolson, N. A. (2003). Neighbourhood socioeconomic disadvantage and behavioural problems from late childhood into early adolescence. *Journal of Epidemiology and Community Health*, **57**(9), 699–703.

Stafford, M. & Marmot, M. (2003). Neighbourhood deprivation and health: Does it affect us all equally? *International Journal of Epidemiology*, **32**(3), 357–366.

Stansfeld, S. A., Head, J., Fuhrer, R., Wardle, J., & Cattell, V. (2003). Social inequalities in depressive symptoms and physical functioning in the Whitehall II study: exploring a common cause explanation. *Journal of Epidemiology and Community Health*, **57**(5), 361–367.

Thoits, P. J. A. (2005). Differential labeling of mental illness by social status: A new look at an old problem. *Journal of Health and Social Behavior*, **46**(1), 102–119.

Turner, R. J. Wheaton, B., & Lloyd, B. (1995). The epidemiology of social stress. *American Sociological Review*, **60**, 104–225.

Wainwright, N. W. & Surtees, P. J. G. (2004). Area and individual circumstances and mood disorder prevalence. *British Journal of Psychiatry*, **185**, 227–232.

Weich, S. & Lewis, G. (1998). Material standard of living, social class, and the prevalence of the common mental disorders in Great Britain. *Journal of Epidemiology and Community Health*, **52**(1), 8–14.

Wilkinson, R. (2005). *The Impact of Inequality*. New York: The New Press.

Wilkinson, R. G. & Pickett, K. E. (2006). Income inequality and population health: a review and explanation of the evidence. *Social Science and Medicine*, **62**(7), 1768–1784.

Wohlfarth, T. (1997). Socioeconomic inequality and psychopathology: are socioeconomic status and social class interchangeable? *Social Science Medicine*, **45**(3), 399–410.

Wohlfarth, T. & Van Den Brink, W. (1998). Social class and substance use disorders: the value of social class as distinct from socioeconomic status. *Social Science Medicine*, **47**(1), 51–58.

Wright, E. O. (1996). *Class Counts*. Cambridge: Cambridge University Press.

Wright, E. O. (2005). *Approaches to Class Analysis*. Cambridge: Cambridge University Press.

8

Ecological, individual, ecological? Moving public health psychiatry into a new era

Kwame McKenzie

This chapter uses the history of public health theories of disease causation as a back drop to investigating a new concept, social capital, which attempts to help us understand and compare societies. In its short life so far the original concept of social capital which was floated decades ago has been caught up in a tide of optimistic social renewal, and vaunted as the great new idea. It has punched well above its weight given the relative dearth of research on the topic because it is a "good idea" and so ripe for media spin. As a societal level construct it offers significant challenges to routine psychiatric thinking. To understand these challenges, I will offer an introduction to the concept of social capital and the literature on its associations with mental health and illness. I will include comment on the machinations that the research community have used to make sense and to make use of the concept. I will finish with some thoughts on what this story tells us about the state of the art of social psychiatry and how social capital could help us understand the social course of illness.

Public health causation and risk

The first true public health physicians were the Sanitary Movement in nineteenth-century England.

Infectious diseases were the scourge of the population. They were a significant contributor to the differential life expectancy between rich and poor: there was a significant difference in mortality rates between rich and poor persons. Doctors did not know what caused infections, but they viewed the deteriorated state of the slums in London and concluded that poverty was an important factor. Because of this focus, the conditions of poverty, not the people or what they did, were the targets for public health interventions. Politicians in concert with the rich were concerned that the diseases produced by poverty could spread to them. Improving the built environment, and especially improving the sewerage systems of the slums, became a priority not just for the poor but also for the rich.

Liberatory Psychiatry: Philosophy, Politics, and Mental Health, ed. Carl I. Cohen and Sami Timimi.
Published by Cambridge University Press. © Cambridge University Press.

Society was connected. The fate of one group was bound to the fate of others. Public health was politics and politics was about improving the environment so that people could thrive. Medical and political power generally agreed that action was needed by doctors and government to improve the environment for the poor.

Dr. John Snow's investigation of cholera in London in the mid nineteenth century is considered the founding study of modern epidemiology (see http://www.johnsnowsociety.org for background information). The demonstration that epidemiological mapping could identify specific environmental sources of disease and that this could lead to an intervention that worked (the removal of the water pump handle from Broad Street stopped the outbreak) undermined the idea that a non-specific environmental influence such as poverty was the vector for cholera. This eventually led to the hypothesis that infectious diseases were caused by micro-organisms, and to the discovery of specific bacteria and viruses. It also moved the focus of causation away from the wider social environment and heralded the advent of germ theory. The environment was seen as important in promoting the risk of infection rather than being causal itself. It was a vector that increased the likelihood of being infected. Killing germs or stopping people catching them became the focus of public health action.

With antibiotics and better sanitation, the death toll from infections decreased. However, the mortality gap between the rich and the poor remained. Thus the fundamental social cause of the disparity was no longer infections; rather it was thought to be due to access to power, knowledge of the causes of illness, and the ability to avoid or prevent illness (Link & Phelan, 1996). With the decline in infectious disease, new illnesses drove the mortality disparity. In high income countries, the focus of public health moved to chronic diseases such as cardio-vascular disease, respiratory problems, and tumors, most of which displayed a significant class gradient.

The analysis of chronic diseases was subtler, with cause and effect more difficult to demonstrate. Rather than catching a disease, you developed it – sometimes over a life-course due to multiple exposures. Lifestyle seemed to increase your risk of becoming ill and the risk of not getting better. Causation was more obscure, with many factors being contributory causes rather than being sufficient by themselves to make one ill. The view now was that there is a web of causation, even though it was very difficult to find the spider (Krieger, 1994).

Risk factor analysis became the order of the day and manipulating risk factors became the role of public health. This ended a journey from the environment being the primary etiological concern to the individual and their lifestyle being most important. Causation had become increasingly individualized. This mir-rored changes in the political discourse from collectivism and central planning to small government and choice.

But risk factor analysis at the individual level has a number of problems. Even the most straightforward of risk factors like cigarette smoking has a social context which has to be taken into account. Anti-smoking campaigns have to understand how communities work if they are to be effective. Moreover, the growth of cities, the rise in pollution, and more recently the advent of global warming, has put the spotlight on place as an important factor in disease.

In addition, new statistical methods have come on stream. Multi-level analysis, which was borrowed from educationalists trying to allow for effects of the collective school environment when investigating a child's academic performance, allowed epidemiologists to partition the impact of individual factors associated with the development of an illness from collective/ecological risk factors.

With this new-found interest came the development of "new" concepts of how societies worked. One such concept is social capital.

The rise of social capital

The first known mention of social capital was in the early twentieth century. Lyda Hanifan was interested in the impact of rural community centers on the development of goodwill in the USA and coined a new term "social capital" (Hanifan, 1920). As with many new ideas, this went pretty much unnoticed.

Modern interest in the concept of social capital has stemmed from Jane Jacobs' book – *The Death and Life of Great American Cities* (Jacobs, 1961). She believed that, in any population, there would be a group of people who had forged neighborhood networks. These networks she considered to be a city's social capital.

Others built on this theory. Pierre Bourdieu studied different forms of capital and considered that social capital was an individual's social networks and how they allowed differential access to resources. Conversely, Coleman, who was interested in child relationships, emphasized social capital as being in the relationships between people. He believed that social capital was useful for the cognitive and social development of children and young people (see McKenzie & Harpham, 2006).

Social capital was popularized by the Harvard Professor Robert Putnam (1993). Putnam had noted that democracy worked better in Italy in areas where there was better social cohesion. He began to wonder what the effects of social cohesion were and what other benefits there might be. He also wondered how social cohesion could best be measured.

His "bowling alone" (Putnam, 2000) concept was essentially that being involved in clubs outside work was an important way of developing the dense networks that are a facet of cohesive societies. America was no longer developing these networks and, if anything, rather than bowling alleys being full of teams playing in leagues, they were full of people and families bowling alone. He demonstrated that, in the USA, the mean number of club meetings that an individual went to in 1 year had decreased from 12 in 1975 to 6 by 1995. This mirrored a fall from 55% in 1965 to 35% in 1995 in the number of people in a national survey who endorsed the box: "Most people can be trusted." Worryingly, the drop in trust among high school students was more precipitous, moving from 44% in 1975 to 22% in 1995.

These levels of trust and club membership were very different across US states and Putnam hypothesized that differences in these proxy measures of social capital would be reflected in various health and social indices. Other researchers tested these hypotheses. Professor Ichiro Kawachi in the Department of Public Health at Harvard investigated links between measures of social capital such as trust and individual and societal health in US states (Berkman & Kawachi, 2000 and Kawachi *et al.*, 1997). An impressive list of associations between social capital and health and societal functioning was assembled. The level of social capital was negatively associated with the level of crime in an area and the level of perceived physical ill-health. It was positively associated with educational attainment, life expectancy, economic activity, and the functioning of government (McKenzie & Harpham, 2006). The results seemingly demonstrated that life was better in those US states with higher levels of social capital.

Social capital took off and became one of the big ideas of the 1990s. There were different responses to this increased interest in the connectedness of society. In the USA, President Bill Clinton met Putnam and paid lip service to the need to develop social capital, while in the UK Margaret Thatcher stuck to her belief that "There was is no such thing as society; just individuals and families." Social capital was ignored in the UK at government level until Tony Blair came to power in 1997. His Government adopted the language of social capital, although like the Clinton government many of their over-arching policies destroyed it. A non-exhaustive list of government offices with "social capital programs" included: the Cabinet Office, Department for Education and Skills, the Department for International Development, the Department of Health, the Foreign and Commonwealth Office, the Home Office, and the Office of the Deputy Prime Minister.

The new optimism and belief in the importance of community was transmitted to the populace. The British Social Attitudes survey is an annual survey of a representative sample of the British population, and includes a question on whether people in general "Help each other or go their own way." In 1984 the percentage of people who thought people helped each other was just over 40% and it dropped to its low point of just under 30% before the 1997 election. It rose from then to 2000 when current available records end (see http://www.statistics. gov.uk/STATBASE).

What is social capital?

The most commonly used definition of social capital in the health sciences originates from Robert Putnam (Putnam, 1993) and consists of five principal characteristics:

(1) Community networks, voluntary, state, personal networks, and density.
(2) Civic engagement, participation, and use of civic networks.
(3) Local civic identity-sense of belonging, solidarity, and equality with local community members.
(4) Reciprocity and norms of co-operation, a sense of obligation to help others, and confidence in return for assistance.
(5) Trust in the community.

This definition goes beyond conventional social network theory. Local civic identity and trust could be considered descriptions of groups rather than just of individuals and thus reflect ecological social capital. The impact of civic identity and trust on health could be considered to have individual psychological correlates but also ecological effects. For instance, individuals with both high and low levels of trust could benefit if the community in general had high levels of trust and civic identity and therefore invested in community facilities that everyone had access to. Though an individual's access to community facilities would be important, the actual level of facilities that are available is governed by the overall level of trust in the community, not by the level of trust or civic identity of the individual in question. The overall level of trust and civic identity in a community is the important factor in the provision of infrastructure rather than that of any individual under consideration. It is this general level of trust, identity, fraternity, and networks that Putnam identifies.

Types of social capital

As interest in the concept has increased, so have attempts further to refine levels and types of social capital. As with the gross definition of social capital, there is ongoing debate about the accuracy of these subtypes. However, they are important as they propose that social capital is multidimensional. They also rely, as do most of the hitherto discussed definitions, on a triad of factors that are the essential building blocks of social capital: *relationships, norms, and trust*. These exist between, as well as within, groups and institutions.

We can consider social capital to have at least three dimensions: structural/cognitive, bonding/bridging, horizontal/vertical.

Structural and cognitive social capital

Structural social capital describes the relationships, networks, associations, and institutions that link people and groups together. Cognitive social capital consists of values, norms, reciprocity, altruism, and civic responsibility, sometimes called "collective moral resources."

Bonding and bridging social capital

Social capital can be considered as bridging (inclusive) or bonding (exclusive). Bonding social capital is inward focused and characterized by homogeneity, strong norms, loyalty, and exclusivity. It is intra-group and relies on strong ties. It can be thought of as the type of social capital that a family unit has or that which is found in small close knit migrant groups who need mutual support. Bridging social capital is outward focused and links different groups in society. The ties between people are weaker and some would consider bridging social capital to be more fragile. An individual's social networks reflect their bridging social capital. Bridging social capital is generally considered to be a positive thing. It acts as a sociological superglue binding groups in the community together and so can facilitate common action.

Horizontal and vertical social capital

A final dimension on which social capital can be split is horizontal and vertical. Horizontal social capital describes social capital between people in similar strata of society and vertical social capital describes social capital that provides integration between people in different strata of society. Essentially, horizontal social capital can be considered to include the bonding social capital, bridging social capital, cognitive, and structural social capital that is confined to particular social class. Vertical social capital can be seen as the degree of integration of groups within a hierarchical society that allows them to influence policy and access justice and resources from those in power. It can be seen as a type of bridging social capital with structural components referring to the organizational integrity, penetration and effectiveness of the State and cognitive elements reflecting group identity (Woolcock, 1998).

Measuring social capital

As would be expected in a growing area with competing theories, there are many different tools available to measure social capital. Though tools are available, many have not been validated and few capture all the dimensions. However, there are more fundamental questions; for instance, if we are measuring context, what context should we measure? What is a community? Is it geographical or psychological or functional (e.g. a work or religious community)? If it is geographical, what size area should we measure and who should define it, the community or policy makers? Social capital has been measured at a number of different sizes of population and area including; US state level, UK electoral ward, and on particular housing estates. Which of these is correct or should we be using different size areas depending on the social context?

The belief that social capital primarily resides in the neighborhood has been perpetuated in the empirical work. However, the assumption that communities are generally place based may be erroneous and this issue needs further attention. For example, a refugee living in a stable neighborhood of a large city may find support in the city-wide refugee community from the same country far more important than the neighborhood community. Many faith groups find their faith community more important than their residential community, especially if they are in the minority in their geographic area. Moreover, socially excluded groups such as those suffering from mental illness may link with each other through support groups, which are increasingly based on telephone lines and the internet.

It is an open question as to whether the concepts of social capital developed for spatial communities are applicable in non-spatial communities and what kind of impact it has on community members. There is a need for further research into the nexus between the individual, the neighborhood community, and the non-spatial communities to which they belong. There is also a need to define and refine concepts of community and what is the appropriate unit of ecological analysis.

But before we get too carried away with the hype about new non-spatial societies, we may want to reflect on the fact that geographically based associative behavior has been present and important in all the major studies conducted thus far. Moreover, people are likely to continue to belong to a number of different communities both geographical and non-spatial. The rise of the latter may diminish but not extinguish the importance of the former. We should remember that area-based government and health services are likely to find area-based policy easier to promote.

What is good for one group in society may not be good for another. The possibility of a differential impact of social capital on subgroups is well recognized. All the different dimensions of social capital discussed earlier could vary according to the group in question. For example, relatively immobile groups such as children and the elderly may be more affected by neighborhood social capital than groups who have high mobility. Similarly, minority groups or new arrivals to a town may find some strong forms of social capital impenetrable and exclusionary in nature.

Social capital, ecological variables and the causes of mental illness

Social capital has provided a new problem for social psychiatry. Much of the original enthusiasm in the concept was because it was ecological and helped explain the effects of societal structure. Psychiatry has a long history of interest in societal structure. Durkheim (1951) was among the first to postulate that the structure of a society rather than the individuals *per se* was an important factor in the rate of mental illness. Similarly, Faris and Dunham's (1939) landmark work in Chicago postulated that the organization of a city had important influences on mental health.

However, as the world and illness has been seen in increasingly individual terms, such work has been sidelined by mainstream psychiatry. This has mirrored moves away from the study of society to the study of "families and individuals." Social capital exemplifies how this thinking influences research. Rather than developing ecological work, the most notable early discussions about social capital have been disagreements about whether it is the property of individuals or whether it is the property of groups of society (McKenzie & Harpham, 2006).

Individual or ecological?

The sociologist Bourdieu's view of social capital may be considered to reflect an assumption that it is a property of an individual. A person's individual social relationships allow differential access to resources (e.g. health care and education) and these relationships define social capital (Bourdieu, 1986).

Social capital has also been considered as ecological (for a review, see McKenzie *et al.*, 2002). It would thus relate to groups or areas rather than to individuals. Those who follow this definition see social capital as being embodied in relationships between individuals, between groups, and between groups and abstract bodies such as the state. The problem that many people have with the individual definition is that it is unclear where the existing and well-researched concepts of social support and social networks stop and social capital begins. If social capital is simply a measure of an individual's access to social networks or social support, then it is not really a new concept.

There has been a significant body of research into the links between access to social support and illness. Mortality rates for those with few social relationships have been shown to be many times higher than for those with larger social networks. Social support protects against a variety of other illnesses and low levels of social networks are correlated with an increased risk of accidents, suicides, and cardiovascular disease. The lack of a supportive confiding relationship is a risk factor for depression, and Durkheim (1951) found that married men had a lower prevalence of neurosis than single men. Social support is believed to buffer an individual against both chronic and acute stress through the provision of emotional, informational, and instrumental support. The socially isolated individual lacks this support and suffers the consequent disadvantages.

If social capital is the property of an individual, it could be considered as acting in a similar manner. Its effects on health could be due to preventing isolation, alienation, and lack of access to social support. If this is true, then individual social capital may be a proxy variable for access to the active ingredient – social support and social networks. It would be unclear whether anything is to be gained by employing a new term such as social capital as a proxy variable rather than using more accurate descriptions of the factors under observation – accessed social support or social networks. Some researchers who analyze social capital at the individual level have extended the concept to include measures of trust, sense of belonging, and civic engagement. This goes further than social support and networks, so in these cases social support is not merely being used as a proxy for the older concepts.

With such problems, the easiest way forward is to say that you have a multi-faceted variable that can be measured at a number of different levels. Social capital may work at an individual level and at various ecological levels depending on the grouping (family, extended family, community, town, etc.). The actions and mechanisms at different levels would be different and there would need to be an investigation of how these worked. This would also reflect newer models of causation and prevent individuals making illogical arguments when trying to work out how society impacts on the individual.

It is important to differentiate between individual and ecological because the mechanisms through which these factors work are different. Too often researchers make inferences about the individual from ecological analyses (ecological fallacy), or about the community from analyses at an individual level (atomistic fallacy) (Diez-Roux, 1998). It is not that these two levels are unrelated, but there does need to be clarity in the investigation, the use of research, and in the subsequent generation of hypotheses for the mechanisms considered to be responsible for any association.

It is perhaps easier to understand these problems by considering the case of smoking and premature death. Those who smoke have an increased risk of developing a variety of cancers and cardiovascular disease. The rates of illness in groups who smoke have increased. In order to build an evidence-based strategy to decrease the impacts of smoking on health, we may want initially to investigate the mechanisms through which smoking has its effects. The mechanisms can be interrogated in a number of ways and at a number of levels. For instance:

Molecular level – how do nicotine and tar affect the contents of a cell?

Metabolic level – how do cell death and disruption affect other bodily systems?

Individual level – why does the individual smoke, why can the individual not stop, what can the individual do to decrease the risk that smoking causes?

Group level – why do certain social groups smoke more than others?

Societal level – why do some societies smoke more than others and what can be
    done legislatively to decrease the rate of harm from smoking?

All these investigations have the same aim: to investigate the mechanisms linking
smoking to illness, but the analytical tools needed, theory, and scientific rules at
each level are different as are the inferences that can be made from the research.
Using the tools and methodology of molecular biology to investigate societal
level factors is unlikely to work very well. Similarly, we are unlikely to understand
an individual's metabolic pathophysiology by using systems theory of group
dynamics. Investigating smoking legislation and tariffs may give you an indication of why the rate of smoking is higher in one country than another; it may give
information on why there are consequent increases in, for instance, cardiovascular illness in one area or another; but it does not give information on an
individual's risk of harm if he is a smoker or why one person smokes and another
does not.

This is clear if we consider smoking, but it is surprising how often authors of
excellent ecological epidemiological work investigating social capital attempt to
explain their findings in terms of individual risk and the actions of individuals
instead of considering group risk or the interaction between groups of individuals.

There is an underlying question for those who conduct research on individual social capital: why would anyone want to reduce social capital to the individual level alone? One answer would be that it is difficult for mental health
researchers to consider forces that are outside their clinical expertise. They work
with individuals and, at most, families and so this is what they investigate. There is
little in the way of public health psychiatry or prevention in high income countries
that dominate research in this field, and so grand societal concepts are not
considered to be what "they do."

The problem is that, for many psychiatric diseases, risk factor analysis and
multifactorial models of illness at an individual level have proved unsatisfactory.
Certainly, biological risk factor analysis has not proved useful in understanding
the rates of illness or their prognosis. For psychotic illnesses such as schizophrenia,
the most important risk factor on a population level is not identifiable familial
predisposition, it is not obstetric complications, and it is not cannabis misuse, it is
being born and brought up in a city. The risk increases with the size of the city. The
"city" is likely to be a proxy variable, but a proxy variable for what? It could be a
proxy for some form of environmental biological toxin, but it is more likely that it
is the way we live in cities and the way we set up society.

Other ecological factors such as income inequality give testimony to the importance of the perception of society in the development of illnesses that were thought
to be biological in aetiology (Boydell *et al.*, 2004). Moreover, a number of recent
findings demonstrate the importance of the perceived structure of a society in the

incidence of psychosis. For instance, one study investigated cases of schizophrenia between 1986 and 1997, using the Maastricht Mental Health Case Register in the Netherlands. A multilevel analysis was conducted to examine the independent effects of individual-level and neighborhood-level variables. They found that the incidence rate of schizophrenia was higher in single mothers who were living in areas where more people were married than in areas where there were more single mothers. This effect persisted after the authors tried to adjust for other possible explanations and individual factors that may have increased psychosis risk. Thus, there was clear impact for a feature of societal structure on the rate of schizophrenia. One possible conclusion is that any increased vulnerability to developing schizophrenia through socioeconomic factors or decreased social buffering in the single mother group was exacerbated by living in areas that were perceived as hostile.

Other studies have demonstrated the "ethnic density effect," where the rates of mental illness in ethnic minorities are higher in areas where there are fewer ethnic minorities. In South London the rate of psychosis is doubled in areas low in ethnic minorities compared with areas high in ethnic minorities. It is unclear why this should be and there have been hypotheses as to whether this reflects decreased social support or increased exposure to racial abuse. But, for the purposes of this discussion, it raises the same issue, the possibility that the shape of the environment and the perceived fit of different communities within it are important for rates of mental illness (Boydell *et al.*, 2001).

This thesis has posed problems for social psychiatry. Social psychiatry is considered by some not to be hard science. Partly because of this, psychiatrists have generally used it to develop interventions and understand family dynamics that are out of the reach of molecular biologists, geneticists, and scanners. Epidemiological studies have identified risk factors such as season of birth effects on incidence rates of psychosis and differences in rates of mental illness and recovery in different countries, but these concepts have quickly been given individual and, "better still," biological explanation before they have been accepted. It is hard not to produce errors in logic when trying to shoehorn causal explanations of rate differences (ecological) into the dominant individual paradigm (Diez-Roux, 1998).

Given that it is the most important risk factor for psychosis and an important risk factor for depression, should we devote our efforts to finding out what the active ingredient in a city is which affects mental health, or do we need to spend more time understanding what a city is and how it works?

So does social capital have an effect on mental health and if so how?

There are essentially three perspectives in the public health literature on how social capital has an effect on health.

The first is a "social support" perspective, which argues that informal networks are central. They improve an individual's welfare and this is transmitted as increased rates of well-being in a community. Another theory is the "inequality" paradigm. This posits that widening economic disparities are a societal cancer. They erode a sense of social justice, decrease social inclusion and produce a society that is full of fear. This heightened anxiety has an impact on life expectancy as well as health more generally. The third is a "political economy" approach, which sees the primary determinant of poor health outcomes as the socially and politically mediated exclusion from material resources (Cullen & Whiteford, 2001; McKenzie & Harpham, 2006).

Although some see social capital as an important lens through which to investigate community structure, others see it as a way of blaming the poor for their ill-health. They see it ending up in the: "we will help the poor help themselves" camp, rather than the "we will decrease the gap between rich and poor" camp.

However, much of this is premature for mental health. The most recent comprehensive review of the association between social capital and mental illness gave a necessarily complex assessment of the state of the art (De Silva et al., 2005). When studies that considered social capital to be an individual level variable were reviewed overall, there was strong evidence for an inverse association between the level of cognitive social capital and common mental disorders. There was less evidence for an inverse association between cognitive social capital and child mental illness, and combined measures of social capital and common mental disorders. The ecological studies were diverse in methodology, populations investigated, and mental illness outcomes, making them difficult to compare. The review concluded that "The strength of the current evidence, in particular that from studies measuring ecological social capital, is inadequate to inform the need for development of specific social capital interventions to combat mental illness. A program of further research is urgently required" (De Silva et al., 2005).

Individual level studies were more numerous because of easy access to secondary data to analyses. The positive results would be expected, given the closeness of their underlying hypothesis to the social support literature.

More socially inclusive bridging social capital, which links different groups together, rather than bonding social capital, which is exclusive, seem to be important for mental health. However, it is unclear whether, in general, ecological social capital benefits mental health.

What can we learn from the short history of social capital and mental health?

It is much too early to come to any real conclusions about the impact of social capital. What the story indicates is that social psychiatry moves with the times.

There has been a general move from the investigation of societies to the investigation of individuals. Making sense of society is difficult and doctors feel more at home with individual mechanisms and interventions as this fits neatly with the doctor–patient paradigm. Public health psychiatry and prevention are therefore relegated to the second division in importance. Moreover, social psychiatry is seen as not being hard science, and it is not surprising that more new age theories such as the connectedness of society are considered unhelpful. In addition, as the world ditches as much of the old collectivism as possible and we move towards a brave new material world, medicine is bound to follow. Or is it?

In the rest of medicine, society and context are being considered increasingly important (Krieger, 1994; Diez-Roux, 1998). In psychiatry our inability to offer effective treatment, rather than just symptom amelioration argues for giving precedence for prevention over attempts at cure. With individual risk factors so weak at a population level and with the impact of society so strong – at least 30% of the variance in incidence of schizophrenia is due to being born and brought up in a city and rates of common mental disorders are far higher in cities than in the countryside – understanding and advocating the improvements needed in the way we construct our society would seem one of the most important issues for psychiatry.

Psychiatry with its history of Durkheim and Faris and Dunham used to be at the vanguard of new thinking in the understanding and importance of society. Public health, with the sanitary movement, and societal psychiatry, with Durkheim started by thinking ecologically. Over a hundred years later their concepts have endured while other theories of causation have come and gone. Perhaps we can learn from this.

Social capital and emancipation

One of the most important findings in social capital research is that social efficacy is good for your health. Indeed, one way of measuring social capital is to ask people whether their area is the sort of area that can organize to fight off the closure of a fire station, or hospital, or is the sort of place where people look out for each other. It is easy to imagine that these sorts of neighborhoods are the sorts of places where a cohesive community can stand up for their rights. These are the sorts of communities that can make their voice heard. They are the sorts of communities that Governments consult with rather than do things to. They are the sorts of communities that offer social support to their members, pay for social safety nets and invest in human capital. They police health norms and their intergenerational bonds offer conduits for health messages. Not surprisingly, they are the sorts of places where the incidence of a number of illnesses and mortality rates is relatively low when compared with communities of equal socioeconomic standing.

Communities with high social efficacy could offer a model for the democratization of mental health. If these communities are better able to articulate their illness models, this could improve the relevance of diagnostic categorization. If these communities were able to counterbalance some of the drive towards the individualization of illness and suffering, we could end up with a more balanced armamentarium of treatment, moving towards true social model treatment. Moreover, the social networks that are available for investigation could offer deeper insights into the causes of mental illness.

Theoretically, areas with high social efficacy could be healthier communities and could allow the development of alternative conceptualizations and treatments of mental illness. However, we do not live in such a theoretical world. Unfortunately, in general, areas with high social efficacy tend to be socially rigid. They are great places to be if you are considered worthy but they are difficult places to be if you are considered unworthy. The price of social support in part is social participation and those who do not contribute can have problems. Those who are considered challenging or different also have problems.

Areas high in social capital may decrease your risk of developing some mental illnesses. This could be through social support, policing of deviance such as teenage sex and pregnancy and drug taking, wider family support decreasing parental separation, investment in education and a better built environment. However, it is not clear that high social efficacy areas are always good places to be once you have developed a mental illness. A simple way to demonstrate social efficacy is to make sure that those considered deviant are dealt with, be they law breakers or mentally ill. In high social capital areas people with mental illness are more likely to be re-admitted to hospital, homeless mentally ill are more likely to attempt suicide but of interest is the fact that those who are considered deserving – war veterans – get better treatment (McKenzie & Harpham 2006).

Initially, societal psychiatrists thought that social capital would simply be a force for good (McKenzie et al., 2002). Now things are less clear. The challenge is to find a model that would develop high social efficacy communities that are tolerant of mental ill-health. But in the meantime understanding the possible impacts of an area's social capital on the social course of an illness may be useful in making more simple decisions such as where to place a community-based rehabilitation unit. By situating them in an area with low social capital, patients may be at risk; however, in situating them in an area with high social efficacy, clients may be victimized.

Conclusions

The history of public health was ecological, but society seems to have become more individualistic and so have our paradigms for understanding illness causation. In psychiatry this has not proved efficacious. The idea of social capital has grown faster than its evidence. In some ways it was an idea in the right place and the right time, but in other ways it could be regarded as an idea that tried to explain a void in the biomedical model. Social capital is a powerful concept which seems to be relevant in illness rates and outcome but it may be that its utility lies in understanding what is going on rather than in developing interventions.

REFERENCES

Berkman, L., Kawachi, I. (2000). Social cohesion, social capital, and health. In *Social Epidemiology*. New York, Oxford: Oxford University Press.

Bourdieu, P. (1986). *Forms of Capital*. New York: Free Press.

Boydell, J., Van Os, J., McKenzie, K. *et al.* (2001). Incidence of schizophrenia in ethnic minorities in London: ecological study into interactions with environment. *British Medical Journal*, **323**, 1336–1338.

Boydell, J., Van Os, J., McKenzie, K., & Murray, R. M. (2004). The association of inequality with the incidence of schizophrenia an ecological study. *Social Psychiatry and Psychiatric Epidemiology*, **39**(8), 597–599.

Cullen, M. & Whiteford, H. (2001). Interrelation of social capital with mental health. *Mental Health Strategy*. Commonwealth of Australia.

De Silva, M., McKenzie, K., Harpham, T., & Huttly, S. (2005). Social capital and mental illness: a systematic review. *Journal of Epidemiology and Community Health*, **59**(8), 619–627.

Diez-Roux, A. V. (1998). Bringing context back into epidemiology: variables and fallacies in multilevel analysis. *American Journal of Public Health*, **88**(2), 216–222.

Durkheim, E. (1951). *Suicide*. New York: Free Press.

Faris, R. E. L. & Dunham, H. W. (1939). *Mental Disorders in Urban Areas*. Chicago: University of Chicago Press.

Hanifan, L. J. (1920). *The Community Center Boston*. Silver Burdett.

Jacobs, J. (1961). *The Death and Life of Great American Cities*. London: Penguin.

Kawachi, I., Kennedy, B. P., Lochner, K. *et al.* (1997). Social capital, income inequality, and mortality. *American Journal of Public Health*, **87**, 1491–1498.

Krieger, N. (1994). Epidemiology and the web of causation: has anyone seen the spider? *Social Science Medicine*, **39**(7), 887–903.

Link, B. G. & Phelan, J. C. (1996). Understanding sociodemographic differences in health – the role of fundamental social causes. *American Journal of Public Health*, **86**(4), 471 473.

McKenzie, K. & Harpham, T. (2006). *Social Capital and Mental Health*. London: Jessica Kingsley Publishers.

McKenzie, K., Whitley, R., & Weich, S. (2002). Social capital and mental illness. *The British Journal of Psychiatry*, **181**, 280–283.

Putnam, R. (1993). *Making Democracy Work: Civic Traditions in Modern Italy*. New Jersey: Princeton University Press.

Putnam, R. (2000). *Bowling Alone: The Collapse and Revival of American Community*. New York: Simon & Schuster.

Whitley, R. & McKenzie, K. (2005) Social capital and psychiatry: review of the literature. *Harvard Reviews in Psychiatry*, **13**(2), 71–84.

Woolcock, M. (1998). Social capital and economic development: towards a theoretical synthesis and policy framework. *Theory and Society*, **27**(2), 151–208.

9

Children's mental health and the global market: an ecological analysis

Sami Timimi

Introduction

Prescriptions of psychotropic medication to children and adolescents have shown a phenomenal increase in most Western countries. For example, the amount of psychotropic medication prescribed to children in the United States increased nearly fourfold between 1985 and 1994 (Pincus *et al.*, 1998). Researchers analyzing prescribing trends in nine countries between 2000 and 2002 found significant rises in the number of prescriptions for psychotropic drugs in children, were evident in all countries – the lowest being in Germany where the increase was 13%, and the highest being in the UK where an increase of 68% was recorded (Wong *et al.*, 2004). Of particular concern is the increase in rates of stimulant prescription to children. By 1996 over 6% of school-aged boys in America were taking stimulant medication (Olfson *et al.*, 2002) with children as young as two being prescribed stimulants in increasing numbers (Zito *et al.*, 2000). Recent surveys show that, in some schools in the United States, over 17% of boys are taking stimulant medication (LeFever *et al.*, 1999) and it is now estimated that about 10% of school boys in the United States take a stimulant (Wallis, 2006). In the UK prescriptions for stimulants have increased from about 6000 in 1994 to over 350 000 children by 2004 (Woolf, 2005), suggesting that we in the UK are rapidly catching up with the USA.

How did such a dramatic change occur? Is this increase in the numbers of children getting diagnoses like attention deficit hyperactivity disorder (ADHD), autism, and childhood depression due to a change in the way we think about the behaviors and emotional experiences of children (often simplified and de-politicized by talking about "better identification")? Does the increase reflect a "real" increase in adverse behavior and emotional experiences in young people? Either way, central to understanding a change in the way we think about (and hence deal with), and what is causing increases in adverse behavior and emotional experience,

Liberatory Psychiatry: Philosophy, Politics, and Mental Health, ed. Carl I. Cohen and Sami Timimi.
Published by Cambridge University Press. © Cambridge University Press.

is an engagement with issues of context (socioeconomic, cultural and political). The current simplistic biological/genetic explanations put forward for conditions such as ADHD cannot explain these changes, unless we are to accept that there was a biological disorder all along but it is only recently that we have "discovered" it. If this were true, why are we still unable to locate what this biological abnormality is and how to find it in any individual we suspect of having this "biological" condition? Nor can this explain why it is only recently (in the last few decades) and in the industrialized north that certain behaviors and emotional experiences of young people have come to be viewed as problematic, particularly when we take into account that certain treatments (such as stimulants for ADHD) were "discovered" and first used on children over 70 years ago (Timimi, 2005a).

In approaching the task of trying to understand why this increase is happening, I will first contextualize current theory and practice through reference to the particular conditions within which child psychiatry was born and started to grow up (its history), followed by a brief critique of the notion of "development" on which so much child and adolescent mental health theory and practice relies. Following this, I will briefly explore how a context rich ecological analysis helps provide new theoretical directions and finally I will present the implications of this analysis for both theory and practice in child and adolescent psychiatry.

A brief history of Western child psychiatry

An understanding of childhood deviance requires an understanding of "normal" childhood and child-rearing practices. Every culture defines what it means to be a normal child, how children should look and act, what is expected of them, and what is considered beyond their capabilities. Any given society may not explicitly discuss or even acknowledge their particular definition, but they will act on their assumptions in their dealings with children (Calvert, 1992). Thus child psychiatry's history is intimately bound with the history of childhood in the West over the past century (both in the influence "folk" understanding of childhood had on child psychiatric theory and, more latterly, the influence of child psychiatric theory and practice on "folk" understanding of childhood).

In late-nineteenth-century Europe and North America something of a perceived crisis was occurring in the social structures of the time, and children were often at the heart of the resulting political debates. Prior to the nineteenth century there were few voices raised against child labor. For most children, laboring was held to be a condition that would teach them numeracy, economics, social, and moral principles (Hendrick, 1997). During the course of the nineteenth century, a new construction of childhood was being put together where the wage-earning child would no longer be considered to be the norm. There are several explanations for this fundamental change including the scale and intensity of exploitation of children and the scale and intensity of the industrialization process itself. The campaigners for reform had their roots in eighteenth-century psychological, educational, and philosophical developments and wished to promote a childhood that they considered more suitable for "civilized" and Christian nations. With the growth of the first mass working class political movements that were also complaining about the brutalization and dehumanization of their children, the ruling classes became concerned about unstable social conditions and issues relating to public order became matters of national security (Pearson, 1983). In addition, the growing economic success of industrial capitalism resulted in a growing demand for a semi-skilled, skilled and educated work force, lessening the economic need for child labor and increasing the demand for education (Zelizer, 1994).

In their approach to reform many made the implicit assumption that, in the long run, only education would prevent the dangerous classes from continually reproducing their perceived malevolent characteristics. The birth of the idea of "willing obedience" through education was another step towards the coming of age of industrial democracy where the idea of "rule by consent" was to become the norm (Pearson, 1983). For the reformers the idea of effective schooling now became paramount. The reconstruction of the factory child through the prism of dependency and ignorance was a necessary precursor to mass education in that it helped prepare opinion for shifts in the child's identity from wage earner to school pupil and for a reduction in the income of working class families that would result from the loss of the child's earning. It further paved the way for an important new development; that of introducing the state into the parent/child relationship. Not only had the reformers put aside the financial hardships many working class families would suffer as a result of the ending of the child laborer, but in addition they depicted the parents of such families as collaborators in the exploitation of their own children and so introduced a new way regulating family feeling too; if children were useful and produced money, they were not being properly loved (Zelizer, 1998).

By the late nineteenth century, partly under the impact of schooling and partly as a result of growing concern about poverty and its possible political consequences, a prolonged and unprecedented public discussion about the physical and mental condition of children began. One development above all others turned children into attractive research subjects, namely the opportunities afforded to investigators by the now compulsory mass schooling. School made children available to professionals such as sociologists, psychologists, and doctors, all of whom sought to do scientific surveys of pupils (Sutherland, 1984). Now children found themselves being examined under the influence of science. Mass schooling revealed the extent of mental and physical handicap amongst pupils which, together with a growing anxiety about racial degeneration and the effects of poverty, led a variety of professionals, parents, and politicians, to become concerned about the quality of the child population leading to a great interest in the subject of human development (Wooldridge, 1995).

In the nineteenth century, the standards for classifying children as disordered were much less nuanced, the standards of normality much broader, and the mechanisms for social and individual surveillance that we take for granted today simply did not exist, and therefore the mental well-being of children was not part of the remit of most psychiatrists. A few psychiatrists, however, did deal with children during the era of the large asylums of the nineteenth century, where children were occasionally admitted alongside adults. Physicians favored removal of some children from their homes to establish control unhindered by parental and family interference (Parry-Jones, 1990). However, at this point in history, child and adolescent psychiatry as a discipline had not been established and it was rare for problematic behavior in children to be viewed through a medical/psychological lens.

By the early twentieth century child welfare was achieving a new social and political identity, with a shift in emphasis toward maximizing children's potential (Baistow, 1995). This was thought politically to be in the national interest. At that time in Western society, policy was being developed that stressed the importance of national efficiency with an emphasis on education, racial hygiene, responsible parenthood, social purity, and preventative medicine (Hendrick, 1994). In each of these areas the state was becoming more interventionist through legislation. Both the state and charitable welfare organizations were now making a number of assumptions mainly derived from the rise of "psycho-medicine," about what constituted a proper childhood (Cunningham, 1995).

The inter-war period saw further significant refinements of the conceptualization of childhood through the influence of early developmental psychology and the birth of child psychiatry in the child guidance movement (Wooldridge, 1995; Hendrick, 1997). A properly functioning family was deemed essential for mental health, and the role of the mother in rearing emotionally balanced children was emphasized. Children were now being viewed through a more psychological lens with their inner life of emotions, fantasies, dreams, instincts, and unconscious conflicts being explored. A more understanding, liberal, and tolerant attitude towards children was encouraged by these European professionals (Rose, 1985). By the 1930s, child guidance clinics had become important propagandist institutions through radio talks, popular publications, and lectures that promoted certain views of happy families and happy children, which were dependent upon a new tolerance of and sympathy for the child (Rose, 1985) – a view that would finally catch the cultural imagination in the post-Second World War West.

In the years after the Second World War, the West's attitude to child-rearing changed, from viewing relations between adults and children primarily in terms of discipline and authority, to that of permissiveness and individual rights (Jenkins, 1998). In addition, whilst the pre-war model prepared children for the workplace within a society of scarcity, the post-war model prepared them to become pleasure-seeking consumers (along with their parents) within a prosperous new economy (Wolfenstein, 1955).

Shifting economic structures was also leading to profound changes in the organization of family life. Suburbanization and the economic demands of successful market economies were resulting in greater mobility, less time for family life, and a breakdown of the extended family. Many families (particularly those headed by young women) were now isolated from traditional sources of child-rearing information. In this context childrearing guides took on an unprecedented importance, allowing for a more dramatic change in parenting styles than would have been conceivable in a more rooted community, and greater ownership by professionals of the knowledge base for the task of parenting (Zuckerman, 1975).

The new child-centered permissive culture was a godsend to consumer capitalism. Childhood could now be successfully commercialized and an industry of consumer goods for children developed (Weinman-Lear, 1963). As permissive "fun morality" was exploited and childhood was commercialized, children gained access to the world of adult information and entertainment, resulting in a blurring of boundaries between what is considered adulthood and what is considered childhood, and leading to children coming to be viewed as, in effect, miniature adults (Jenhs, 1996).

Also following the traumas of the Second World War and the evacuation process for children in Britain, prominence began to be given to the effects of early separation of young children from their mothers. This construction was reinforced by the development of attachment theory by the British psychoanalyst John Bowlby (1969, 1973). The evacuation was to reveal the extent of urban poverty and slum housing, the tenacity of ordinary working class families in sticking together, and the existence of what was coming to be known as the "problem family."

Child psychiatry after the Second World War began to examine the mother–child relationship and the family context. The anthropologist Gregory Bateson and his team (Bateson *et al.*, 1956) first applied systems ideas to patients with "schizophrenia," hypothesizing that the distorted thought processes of the "schizophrenic" were the result of the family's complex and contradictory transaction and communication patterns. The family was now viewed as a system with its own properties that often resisted change. Thus it was "observed" that, if the "identified patient" improved, the rest of the family could become destabilized (Laing & Esterson, 1964). Within this new frame it seemed logical that, if individual pathology developed within the family, then its very breeding ground needed to be treated resulting in the birth of the field of family therapy (Asen, 2006). Family therapy's focus soon shifted, away from an interest in families containing adult schizophrenic members, to working with families containing problematic children and adolescents – and problematic parents (Haley, 1979). Whilst the early pioneers (e.g. Ackerman, 1967) were preoccupied with unconscious processes, therapists largely replaced psychoanalytical ideas with rather concrete but also pragmatic models (Minuchin & Fishman, 1981).

Toward the end of the last century, child and adolescent psychiatry in the West began to move away from reliance on these more systemic models, toward more internalized biopsychological models of classification and intervention due to a number of reasons which I discuss later in this chapter.

Views of development

Each culture has its own vision of child development, and many ancient cultures (such as can be found in Islamic and Hindu writings) have described complex developmental stages for children (Timimi, 2005a). In the West professionals concerned with children such as child psychologists, psychiatrists, and pediatricians have put much energy in trying to discover the apparently natural and universal ways in which children are supposed to develop from birth through to adulthood.

In traditional Western writing on development and "developmental psychopathology" (the discipline of analyzing what's happening when development goes wrong), a particular approach to knowledge is taken, which, for historical and cultural reasons, is based on Western beliefs regarding the "knowability" of the physical world; a form of science that is modeled on the physical sciences. An underlying assumption is that the general laws of developmental change are present in the world and can be discovered by appropriate research (Karmiloff-Smith, 1992). Systematic experimentation, observation, and appropriate measurement are taken to represent the means to this end. This positivism tends to be accompanied by the belief that developmental change is a natural, biological process (Morss, 1990). The line of argument is also a functionalist one; that is, it treats the activity of children as an adaptation to a relatively stable environment.

Developmental psychology was one of the first branches of psychology to be established, precisely because childhood was seen as the prime location to investigate how nurture impinged on nature. Unlike the natural scientists, psychologists and psychiatrists have never had any clear idea of how the processes they study actually operate and how the molding together of nature and nurture actually happens. What we are left with is a metaphor for a process and not the process itself. Psychologists and psychiatrists therefore, can only speculate in vague terms about the way their theories actually operate (Stainton-Rogers & Stainton-Rogers, 1992). Borrowing ideas from the natural sciences meant that genetic material was now held to have the power to specify not only how things are made (for example, having blue eyes or tall stature) but also behavior (behavioral genetics) and a whole host of experiences and beliefs.

One of the strongest stories of modernism is that, if we want to know about something, all we need to do is measure it. Guided by this recipe, developmental psychologists and psychopathologists have employed those direct means of investigation, for example, by using psychometric tests (such as those used to measure a child's intelligence) and diagnostic questionnaires (for example, to diagnose anxiety or depression). The answers to these questionnaires cannot tell us anything directly about any quality of the child, only about a hypothetical property of the child (for example, the child's intelligence) as constructed by the designer of the test. Yet psychological tests purport to be direct indicators of fixed and stable properties (traits) of a child or to diagnose "real" medical conditions in a child (such as autism). The use of measurement has beguiled many into assuming that they are finding out some truth about what the child being tested is like. Yet all such tests achieve is to replace one unknown (the child) with another set of unknowns (the traits out of which the child is assumed to be constituted). As soon as we probe further to find out about what these tests and traits mean, we find that they too are subjects about which more tests and debates are written (Stainton-Rogers & Stainton-Rogers, 1992)!

Much state intervention into its citizens' lives is rationalized in terms of the "developmental needs" of particular age groups. At the same time, much of the entrepreneurial effort of the private sector is directed at the re-definition of those needs in terms of the products and services it wishes to sell. That children have certain characteristics, that adults have others, and that it is natural to grow from one to the other are messages that we receive from all forms of modern communication (Burman, 1994). Morss (1996) points out not only the limits and constraints of child developmental knowledge, but also its cultural specificity, its bio-determinism, the impact it has had upon how our culture deals with children (for example, the impact of developmental theories in education and social work practice), and the constraints it puts upon our ability to develop a broader understanding of children and their problems.

Kessen (1979) notes the historical dimension involved in how we situate the knowledge that we use. He notes that, if adult treatment and perception of children in the Middle Ages or in the nineteenth century was in any way historically dependent and a product of those times, then it must also be historically dependent today. It is inconsistent, for example, to treat child labor in the nineteenth century as somehow a historically dependent, unnatural state for children while at the same time neglecting the role of present day circumstances in defining childhood. If child labor happened as a consequence of economic conditions, then it follows that present-day treatment of children must also be relevant to present-day economic and social circumstances.

Within the developmental discourse, there is a constant subtext that is saying there is a superior and inferior position. Development says to the child, the parent, and the teacher this is your future and, if you do not reach it, you are, in some senses, inferior (Morss, 1996). It is not just children who are said to develop but also peoples and economies (Sachs, 1992; Rahman, 1993). Development is about modern hierarchies of superiority and inferiority. Developmental explanations instil the notion of individual competitiveness; from the moment you are born, you will have developmental milestones thrust upon you. As parents, we are desperate to see our children achieve these age-bound expectations. Development of our children is under constant professional surveillance starting with health visitors and community pediatricians and moving on to general practitioners, nursery nurses, teachers, and a whole range of specialists (including child psychiatrists). We are concerned when our children seem to be falling behind and we are constantly encouraging them to achieve these expectations. If we are not concerned and not encouraging, presumably we are neglecting.

And what of the children themselves? If there is a belief that these are natural, unfolding processes for which professionals must be involved in helping children achieve, does this not encourage competitiveness from a very early age? How much do the children get caught in these parental and professional anxieties? How relaxed can children be, from the moment they are born, to just be, as opposed to having to do something to ease these cultural anxieties? When these anxieties cannot be comforted and there is a perception that a child has strayed from their pre destined development path, what is to blame? Developmental psychopathology literature has generally pointed toward the mother for blame and more recently toward the child's genes. In a culture where families have shrunk and fathers seem to disappear and relinquish duty and responsibility in ever-increasing numbers, mothers have to shoulder not only the responsibility for caring for their family (a role given much lower status in Western culture than many non-Western cultures), but also the responsibility for things going wrong. In a final stab from the developmental discourse, mothers are then denied credit for their work when things do go well, as children are then simply seen as achieving their biological destiny.

Current developments in child psychiatry and its relationship to neoliberalism

In any culture, people come to acquire their subjective selves through incorporation of values, beliefs, and practices that sustain the desired social relationships of that culture (Althusser, 1969). In a capitalist, market-driven economy, mass consumption is vital to maintenance of the system and therefore, becomes an important part of our self and consciousness. This has led necessarily to the domination of market values, which penetrates all aspects of social life and subjects them to their logic (Amin, 1988). This philosophy pushes to the limit of absurdity an opposition between humankind and nature. The goal of finding an ecological harmony with nature disappears as nature, the human body, and mind (among other things), all come to be viewed as potential commodities to be manipulated for monetary (profit) ends. Thus even personal relations and the self become objects of consumption (Broughton, 1986) like the stereotype consumer wife comparing the whiteness of her sheets with those of her neighbors, the subjects of consumer societies constantly compare their own inadequacies with those of others. This practice of self-examination causes a cult of self-awareness. In doing so, it can create inner qualities, including whatever passes for personal growth with every day one seeking to make oneself a better product – new, improved, best, and brightest yet (Timimi, 2005a). Reliance on consumerism has also led to a kind of "growth fetish," whereby Western culture and politics are obsessed with an ideology that demands never-ending growth and expansion. Yet, despite several decades of sustained economic growth, population surveys show we are no happier and rates of dissatisfaction are increasing. Growth not only fails to make people contented; it destroys many of the things that do through weakening social cohesion (Hamilton, 2003). This also has a class-specific character with the plight of the poorest being viewed as self-inflicted, with the poor constantly confronted with their shortcomings by advertising that tells them they are "deficient" without this or that latest accessory (Rabin, 1994).

The social/political function of the psychiatrist, as this profession developed in the industrialized north, was that of providing a form of social control for society's non-criminal misfits. Whether this task was carried out humanely or not, has and continues to be debated. Lack of therapeutic success, limited resources, and enlightenment hope that scientific progress was to free mankind from all manner of suffering (a dynamic that helped doctors gain the upper hand in the interdisciplinary battle over "ownership" of the "insane"), resulted in psychiatrists having to bear responsibility for a section of society, whose needs challenged the entrepreneurial, antiwelfare zeitgeist with the seemingly impossible task of bringing these "patients" back into the realms of "normal" behavior.

The social/political role of the psychiatrist has naturally changed as the political and socioeconomic climate of their natural host culture (the industrialized north) has changed. The beginning of the "psychopharmacology" era following discovery that chlorpromazine could calm some psychotic patients, eventually dovetailed nicely into the broader neoliberal political aims of late twentieth-century economies, with the worship of the market as the guiding philosophy on which social, economic, and political development rests. Now psychiatry could begin to fulfil a new role. Not only was it (arguably falsely) portrayed as more potent in delivering back to society, those who had fallen off its rails (using cocktails of medication whose effects are likened to that of insulin in diabetes), but also medicalization could now serve a whole new purpose. Not only does narrow medicalization obscure social/political and other environmental causes of mental distress (thereby effectively letting governments and their institutions "off the hook"), but also "mentalizing" the ups and downs of life, previously viewed as normal responses to difficult circumstances, provides the opportunity to create new roles for doctors and allied professions, the opportunity to create new, potentially enormous markets (most notably for the drug industry), and another means by which to convince the population that they are inadequate in some way (thereby spurring them on to consume more products). This growth in the role and political/economic function of the psychiatrist has also led to increasing blurring of boundaries between criminality and mental health, and increasingly visible roles for psychiatrists in coercive social control, whether this is through the increasing demands for psychiatric reports in court proceedings, psychiatric "treatments" in prisons, the emergence of new eugenics suggesting biological causes of criminality, or the move toward greater powers for involuntary psychiatric "treatment" in the community.

It is this expanded remit of psychiatry and its relationship to socioeconomic developments that is of particular relevance to child psychiatry. Whilst the origins of child psychiatry is in a movement that was delving into the inner world of the child, mother–child relationships, and the dynamics of the family, it is the advent of this new broader role for psychiatrists that created the ideal conditions for psychiatry to expand as rapidly as it has into the pathologizing of young people and the social control of the young through psychiatric technologies (such as drugs and behavior therapy).

The widespread establishment of right-wing monetarist policies in Western economies at the same time as further individualizing through ideals of growth, market expansion, and wealth creation, has had a profound effect on the managed healthcare system in the USA. With the managed healthcare system being the bread and butter of the majority of psychiatrists and pediatrician's work, when the more labor-intensive psychotherapies lost favor with healthcare insurers, doctors soon realized they could make more money by going down the psychopharmacology route than the psychotherapy one. Managed healthcare has meant an economic system has come to be built around DSM IV diagnoses, with diagnoses offering an easy way to organize the economic system of psychiatric healthcare. In order to obtain a legitimate ticket to a service, you need a DSM IV diagnosis. Thus DSM IV has become more than a mental health diagnostic manual; it is a legal, financial, and ideological document, driving thinking about all sorts of emotions and behaviors, including those of our children, toward ever more medicalized notions.

The greater medicalization of American child and adolescent psychiatry together with its cultural power has resulted in child psychiatry in the UK itself changing enormously in the last 10 years. Thus, the UK's professional discourse has similarly become convinced that there are more personal and professional rewards to be gained by it adopting a more medicalized American style approach (e.g., Goodman, 1997). This has helped construct the field of "neuro-developmental" psychiatry, which the public, trusting such high status opinions, has come to view as real.

An ecological analysis

Thus far I have tried to contextualize current theory and practice in child psychiatry by briefly reviewing its history, critiquing the central notion of "development" and examining the relationship between theory and practice and the values of modern neoliberal market economies. This led to me to suggesting that the greater medicalization of childhood reveals an important shift in the practice of psychiatry toward greater "commodification" of emotions and behavior, and which follows the global shift to neoliberalism and greater penetration of market values.

Classification systems in psychiatry rely on a positivist reductionist focus on internal sickness and disease states as the location of the "pathology" to be diagnosed and from which treatment programs can then be planned. Although the classification systems we use (ICD 10, DSM IV) set out to be descriptive and atheoretical, the choice of focus implies a choice of construction that will automatically favor internal bio-psychological models of causation and treatment at the same time as rending more context-rich systemic frameworks as largely irrelevant. The result of structuring our theory base and consequently practice around an "internalizing" classification system, is that analysis of "sickness" and "disorder" by social groupings (such as class, gender, race, nationality, political system, economy, age, sexual orientation etc.) rarely happens and, when it does, it occupies a hierarchically inferior position (in other words the primary interest is in an internal "disease state" and differential rates of diagnosis by social grouping is often put down to under-/over-diagnosis, or the outcome of having the disorder). This has the effect of de-politicizing mental health. Our role as psychiatrists is to take mad, unhappy, or badly behaved people, diagnose what's going wrong "inside" them, treat it, and send them back into society, hopefully with them feeling happier and behaving in a more socially acceptable manner; it is not our role to question how the way that society functions could be causing or exacerbating madness, unhappiness, or bad behavior.

An ecological perspective attempts to reverse the hierarchy and propose that an examination of the broader social, political, and economic context may shed new light on how we understand and consequently deal with madness, unhappiness, or bad behavior. This requires an examination of the way context shapes both how meaning is constructed and as a causal agent. In relation to children, given their dependence on adults for many aspects of their well-being, it would seem obvious that a thorough examination of context is always necessary. However, as I have described above, such is the logic of current psychiatric nosology, a stripping away of context is exactly what has happened in child psychiatry as it got incorporated into adult psychiatric theory and practice, with little of the opposite occurring (i.e., adult psychiatry incorporating the more systemic thinking that used to be found in child psychiatry).

Let's take gender for example. The gender distribution for psychiatric disorders in pre-adolescent children is in the region of three to four boys to every girl (mainly made up of behavioral disorders such as Attention Deficit Hyperactivity Disorder (ADHD), Oppositional Defiant Disorder (ODD), and Autistic Spectrum Disorders (ASD)). Such a gender distribution that seems to sweep across the entirety of psychiatric disorders found in the primary school years implies either that boys are biologically weaker or "disabled" in some way, or that (from a sociocultural perspective) we have come to be more troubled by boys' than girls' behavior (or, of course, a combination of both). From the sociocultural perspective, what is likely to be involved is a complex interplay between: shifting ideas of masculinity and femininity, the role and position of men and women in society, and the relentless progress of the project of "individualism."

As new educational and psychological authorities were developed to meet the new imperatives of social adjustment, the boundaries between normality and pathology were problematized. Psychologists, psychiatrists, and pediatricians began "discovering" apparent manifestations of a vast range of disorders among the children they surveyed. These developments in the way we think about childhood and its problems interact with the rapid political, economic and social changes seen in the last few decades in the West, some of the hallmarks of which are: the movement into smaller family and social networks, decreasing amounts of time that parents spend with their children, aggressive consumerism preying on children's desire for stimulation, greater involvement of professionals in childrearing activities (and advice on childrearing), and a sense of panic about boys' development (Timimi, 2005a).

Free market capitalism can be seen as the most complete and organized example of a political, social, and economic system based on the values of masculinity that the world has ever seen. Its social and psychological values are based on aggressive competitiveness, putting the needs of the individual above those of social responsibility, an emphasis on control (rather than harmony), the use of rational (scientific) analysis, and the constant pushing of boundaries. Such a system produces gross inequalities (both within and between nations), has reduced the status and importance of nurture, and therefore the esteem attached to the role of mother. As a consequence, more and more women are brought into the workplace – both to increase the workforce needed to service the market economy's demand for continuous growth, and to give women the self esteem taken away from them as the role of motherhood lost its status. This movement out of the family sphere and into the public sphere has not been matched by a corresponding reverse movement of men out of the public sphere into more family and nurturing roles (quite the contrary in fact).

At the same time as there has been a movement of adults out of the family; there has been a movement towards childcare becoming a professional (mainly female) activity. Thus, what appears to be happening in the psychological space of childhood is an increasing feminization in many aspects, particularly educational ones. There is now a large body of literature that supports the notion that educational methods currently used in most Western schools (such as continuous assessment and socially oriented work sheets) are favored more by girls than boys (Burman, 2005). This is then mirrored in national exam results where girls are now consistently achieving higher grades than boys even in some traditionally "male" subjects like Maths and Science. Boys also dominate the special needs provision where they are marked out as having disproportionately high (again in the region of 4 to 1) problems with poor reading and poor behavior. With schools under market economy, political pressure to compete in national league tables, and boys coming to represent a liability, it is hardly surprising that boys have come to be seen as the "failed" gender, provoking anxiety in their (primarily female) carers and teachers (Timimi, 2005a).

The feminization of certain aspects of the masculine capitalist culture we live in has also had an impact on the working environments our education is preparing us for. Ideas such as cultivating "emotional intelligence" in management and working relations started to become more popular in the 1990s (Gordo-Lopez & Burman, 2004). Far from an enlightened move toward a nurturing and caring society, this is part of developing "better" ways to motivate the workforce and manipulate the consumer. Thus modern Western culture demands more convoluted and complicated forms of socializing (in an image-obsessed age) than in the past (or in many other cultures) in the context of the diminishing size of families (resulting in more intense emotional contact between members of these smaller units, and less opportunity for learning to negotiate differing types of relationships that contact with the wider range of people that extended families provided).[1]

Such an ecological analysis throws up some interesting questions in relation to common child psychiatric disorders. For example, Professor Baron-Cohen (2004) has recently put forward convincing evidence that the biological component of ASD is that of the "extreme male brain," suggesting that the male brain is more geared to "systematizing" while the female brain is more geared to "empathizing," with ASD sufferers being at the extreme end of the "systematizing" spectrum, hence the reason why we get ASD diagnosed more in boys than girls. Although there are many problems with the narrowness of such a construct, if we were to take this theory at face value, it still leads to important questions that Professor Baron-Cohen doesn't ask; particularly that of why "systematizing" boys are seen as more problematic nowadays than "empathizing" girls. In relation to ASD this leads to an interesting paradox. One of the core features in the diagnosis is a lack of empathy. However, improving the "emotional intelligence" of the workforce is for the purpose of using "empathy" to successfully exploit and manipulate your customers and workforce into doing what you wish. It seems strange that people who find it difficult to understand emotional nuances but who can be compassionate are pathologized, yet those who can use an understanding of others' emotional state to manipulate them for selfish ends are what the market value system needs and rewards.[2]

Looking at ASD through a more ecological framework also reveals how many aspects of the construct are culture specific. For example, poor eye contact is meant to be another diagnostic feature, yet the Japanese are very wary about establishing eye contact with relative strangers or seniors. Similarly, in Levine *et al.*'s study (1994) of the Gusii tribe in Kenya, it was observed that, according to their traditions, mothers must make a conscious effort not to make eye contact with their children as they believe it can cause "over-stimulation" particularly in the early years of the child's life. In many ancient cultures, reading and writing, even where they existed, were not as favored as much by the wise as rote memorization (a typical way of learning for a "systematizing" brain), which for sacred religious reasons could not deviate from the original even by as much as one word. In societies that value such things it is not hard to imagine that a person lacking socializing abilities might still be considered special and even holy for possessing such a unique ability. Indeed, many ASD characteristics are not at all dissimilar to devoted religious lifestyles, for example, seeking solitude, vows of silence, non-materialistic values, lack of personal relationships, and daily following of rituals (Timimi, in press).

Similar analysis can be made through an ecological exploration of gender relations in ADHD. The scale of the increase in diagnosis of ADHD and medication use for this is extraordinary. The gender gap in the child population diagnosed with ADHD is matched by a significant and opposite differential among adults initiating the labeling process. While young males form the majority of those labeled with ADHD, it is overwhelmingly adult females, their mothers and teachers, who make the first determination that a child's behavior falls outside the normal range of what little boys are expected to do. Though this differential reflects the adult female's more immediate involvement in the day-to-day care of children, mothers and fathers frequently disagree on the "pathological" nature of their son's behavior. Surveys of stimulant use in the United States has shown that its use is highest in prosperous white communities where education is a high priority, where the educational achievement of both sexes is above the national average and, most importantly, where the gender gap in educational achievement favoring females is at its highest. This distinctive pattern lends no support to the idea that ADHD represents a congenital abnormality requiring small children to be treated with powerful psychotropic drugs. The ecological pattern is more consistent with the view that ADHD can be seen as a barometer of social anxiety about boys' development, with stimulants being used as a tool for rearing and educating them (Hart *et al.*, 2006).

Whatever part of conditions such as ADHD is biological, how we construct meaning out of this is a cultural process. For example, Brewis and Schmidt (2003) carried out a study in a middle-class, Mexican school of over 200 pupils. Using standard diagnostic criteria, they found that about 8% of the children could be diagnosed as having ADHD, yet there was only one child in that school with the diagnosis. Through interviews with parents and teachers they discovered that these carers regarded ADHD-type behaviors as within the boundaries of behaviors viewed as normal for these children's ages.

Conclusion and new directions for child and adolescent mental health

In this chapter I have tried to contextualize current theory and practice in child and adolescent psychiatry by briefly reviewing its history, critiquing the central notion of "development," examining the relationship between theory and practice and the values of neoliberalism, and demonstrated how new directions for theoretical investigation can be found by taking a more context rich "ecological" approach.

Deconstructing ideological assumptions helps us critically examine the theoretical assumptions that underlay current practice. An ecological analysis then helps us understand how context may contribute both to the meaning we give children's behavior and emotional experience and to highlight potential social causes of emotional and behavioral difficulties. This is all very well, but what can we do about all of this, particularly in the context of steadily rising numbers of young people presenting with psychosocial problems (Rutter & Smith, 1995), and with the accusation that much of our current theory and practice is not suitable for the developing world (Timimi, 2005b)?

The following are my brief suggestions for a new "manifesto" for child and adolescent psychiatry:

New theoretical directions

New forms of research should be encouraged, particularly those that combine the qualitative and the quantitative, use more naturalistic (such as clinic-based) settings, and encourage cross-disciplinary theoretical and methodological approaches. Current reliance on a narrow conception of "evidence-based medicine" cannot progress theory, as it is essentially "parasitic" relying on the flawed assumptions of the current diagnostic system. Adoption of a more open and diverse model of child development that recognizes that different cultures have different versions of child development has the potential to reduce the amount of pathologizing of childhood that currently occurs in Western medical practice. This would mean the medical and psychological professions actively engaging in the questioning the universal validity of the concepts and rating questionnaires they use.

New models of practice

We need more context-rich approaches to practice that take full account of each child's unique ecological context. Taking full account of context opens up new opportunities for interventions that capitalize on potential resources, rather than just trying to rid the child of their internal disease state. All communities have resources, whether that is within the immediate family, extended family, religious community, schools, and other institutions, that may well have positive suggestions and interventions to offer. Ideas from other systems of medicine can be utilized. For example, Ayurvedic medicine sees illness as a disruption in the delicate somatic, climactic, and social system of balance. Causes are not located as such but are seen as part of a system out of balance with symptoms viewed as being a part of a process rather than a disease entity (Obeyesekere, 1977). Such an attitude based on balance with nature (as opposed to controlling it) has resonance with new approaches that include lifestyle interventions focusing on aspects such as diet, exercise, and family routines (Timimi, 2005a).

Promoting public health

The rise in the rates of prescription of psychotropic medication for children and adolescents may also be the result of an increase in what might be loosely termed psychosocial suffering amongst children in Western society. Medicalizing this can render the psychosocial causes invisible (Timimi, 2004). As socially respected practitioners, we have a responsibility to understand that we bring a cultural value system into our work. We cannot be dispassionate bystanders. Our actions will ripple out into the wider local community. We need to consider the ethics of our actions and be able to take a long-term socially responsible perspective. In this respect, I believe there should be a moratorium in place on the prescribing of psychotropic medication for all but the most seriously affected (for example, it could be decided that medication would only be initiated within adolescent inpatient units). The current evidence suggests that our increasing reliance on psychotropic medication may well have caused more harm than good in terms of lack of efficacy, dangerous side effects, increased circulation of potential drugs of abuse, and its long-term sociocultural effects (Timimi, 2004, 2005a; Jackson, 2005). Alternatives for promoting better child and adolescent mental health include better nutrition, more support for parents (particularly those isolated from support), and creation of community orientated support around schools (such as parent advice/support groups).

Legislative

In an ideal world, global politics would be moving away from aggressive consumerist, market economies towards a more socialist, ecologically friendly economic system centered more on pro-social values, such that the drive for psychiatry to assist in commodifying emotions and behavior would not be so powerful. In the meantime, I suggest we need a moratorium on the mass prescription of psychotropic drugs to the under-18s whilst the evidence on safety and effectiveness is re-evaluated, all links between child and adolescent psychiatry and the drug companies severed, support for efforts aimed at fighting global child poverty, family-friendly business practices to allow more time for parents with their children to be encouraged, wilfully absent parents criminalized, and policies that promote more social equality supported.

NOTES

(1) A relevant counter argument to this is that certain technologies such as the internet have created new, previously unavailable opportunities for potentially global social networks. These new networks are helping create new "hybrid" cross-cultural identities and subcultures – most notably amongst today's youth. Fuller exploration of this is beyond the scope of this chapter; however, these "virtual" social networks are not aspects of the younger children's lives that I am mainly referring to, and whether and in what way they are adequate substitutes for face-to-face contact remains to be explored.

(2) It should be noted here that I am not referring to the classical definition of autism, most notably that of Kanner, which describes a rare disorder found in severely disabled and impaired individuals (Frith, 1989). The group I am here referring to are those who are attracting the more recent expanded notion of "Autistic Spectrum Disorders," which seems to be following similar epidemiological dynamics as other childhood behavioral disorders

such as ADHD – increasing numbers receiving the diagnosis, predominantly male, often related to school based problems, and with rather "fuzzy" boundaries in its definition.

REFERENCES

Ackerman, N. W. (1967). *Treating the Troubled Family*. New York: Basic Books.

Althusser, L. (1969). *For Marx*. Harmondsworth: Penguin.

Amin, S. (1988). *Eurocentrism*. New York: Monthly Review Press.

Asen, E. (2006). Systemic approaches – critique and scope. In *Critical Voices in Child and Adolescent Mental Health*, ed. S. Timimi & B. Maitra. London: Free Association Books.

Baistow, K. (1995). From sickly survival to realisation of potential: child health as a social project. *Children in Society*, **9**, 20–35.

Bateson, G., Jackson, D., Haley, J., & Weakland, J. (1956). Toward a theory of schizophrenia. *Behavioural Science*, **1**, 251–264.

Baron-Cohen, S. (2004). *The Essential Difference*. London: Penguin

Bowlby, J. (1969). *Attachment and Loss, Volume 1, Attachment*. London: Hogarth Press.

Bowlby, J. (1973). *Attachment and Loss, Volume 2, Separation*. London: Hogarth Press.

Brewis, A. & Schmidt, K. (2003). Gender variation in the identification of Mexican children's psychiatric symptoms. *Medical Anthropology Quarterly*, **17**, 376–393.

Broughton, J. (1986). The psychology, history and ideology of the self. In *Dialectics and Ideology in Psychology*, ed. K. Larsen. Norwood, NJ: Ablex.

Burman, E. (1994). *Deconstructing Developmental Psychology*. London: Routledge.

Burman E. (2005). Childhood, neo-liberalism and the feminization of education. *Gender and Education*, **17**, 351–367.

Calvert, K. (1992). *Children in the House: The Material Culture of Early Childhood, 1600–1900*. Boston: Northeastern University Press.

Cunningham, H. (1995). *Children and Childhood in Western Society Since 1500*. London: Longman.

Frith, U. (1989) *Autism: Explaining the Enigma*. Oxford: Blackwell.

Goodman, R. (1997). An over extended remit. *British Medical Journal*, **314**, 813–814.

Gordo-Lopez, A. & Burman, E. (2004). Emotional capital and information technologies in the changing rhetoric around children and childhoods. *New Directions in Child Development*, **105**, 63–80.

Haley, J. (1979). *Leaving Home: Therapy for Disturbed Young People*. San Francisco: Jossey Bass.

Hamilton, C. (2003). *Growth Fetish*. Crows Nest: Allen and Unwin.

Hart, N., Grand, N., & Riley, K. (2006). Making the grade: The gender gap, ADHD, and the medicalization of boyhood. In *Medicalized Masculinities*, ed. D. Rosenfeld & C. Faircloth. Philadelphia: Temple University Press.

Hendrick, H. (1994). *Child Welfare England 1870–1989*. London: Routledge.

Hendrick, H. (1997). Constructions and reconstructions of British childhood: An interpretive survey, 1800 to the present. In *Constructing and Reconstructing Childhood: Contemporary Issues in the Sociological Study of Childhood*, ed. A. James & A. Prout. London: Falmer Press.

Jackson, G. (2005). *Rethinking Psychiatric Drugs*. Bloomington: Author House.

Jenhs, C. (1996). *Childhood*. London: Routledge.

Jenkins, H. (1998). Introduction: childhood innocence and other modern myths. In *Children's Culture Reader*, ed. H. Jenkins. New York: New York University Press.

Karmiloff-Smith, A. (1992). *Beyond Modularity: A Developmental Perspective on Cognitive Science*. Cambridge, MA: MIT Press.

Kessen, W. (1979). The American child and other cultural inventions. *American Psychologist*, **34**, 815–820.

Laing, R. D. & Esterson, A. (1964). *Sanity, Madness and the Family*. London: Tavistock.

LeFever, G. B., Dawson, K. V., & Morrow, A. D. (1999). The extent of drug therapy for attention deficit hyperactivity disorder among children in public schools. *American Journal of Public Health*, **89**, 1359–1364.

LeVine, R. A., Dixon, S., LeVine, S., *et al.* (1994). *Child Care and Culture: Lessons from Africa*. Cambridge: Cambridge University Press.

Minuchin, S. & Fishman, H. C. (1981). *Family Therapy Techniques*. Cambridge, MA: Harvard University Press.

Morss, J. R. (1990). *The Biologising Of Childhood: Developmental Psychology And The Darwinian Myth*. Hove: Lawrence Erlbaum Associates.

Morss, J. R. (1996). *Growing Critical: Alternatives To Developmental Psychology*. London: Routledge.

Obeyesekere, G. (1977). The theory and practice of psychological medicine in Ayurvedic tradition. *Culture, Medicine and Psychiatry*, **1**, 155–181.

Olfson, M., Marcus, S. C., Weissman, M. M., & Jensen, P. S. (2002). National trends in the use of psychotropic medications by children. *Journal of the American Academy of Child and Adolescent Psychiatry*, **41**, 514–521.

Parry-Jones, W. L. (1990). Juveniles in 19th century Oxfordshire asylums. *British Journal of Clinical and Social Psychiatry*, **7**, 51–58.

Pearson, G. (1983). *Hooligan: A History of Respectable Fears*. London: Macmillan.

Pincus, H. A., Tanielian, T. L., & Marcus, S. C. (1998). Prescribing trends in psychotropic medications. *Journal of the American Medical Association*, **279**, 526–531.

Rabin, L. (1994). *Families on the Frontline: American Working Class Speaks About the Economy, Race and Ethnicity*. New York: HarperCollins.

Rahman, A. (1993). *People's Self-Development*. London: Zed Press.

Rose, N. (1985). *The Psychological Complex: Psychology, Politics and Society in England 1869–1939*. London: RKP.

Rutter, M. & Smith, D. (1995). *Psychosocial Disorders in the Young: Time Trends and their causes*. Chichester: John Wiley and Sons.

Sachs, W. (1992). *The Developmental Dictionary*. London: Zed Press.

Stainton-Rogers, R. & Stainton-Rogers, W. (1992). *Stories of Childhood: Shifting Agendas Of Child Concern*. Hassocks: Harvester.

Sutherland, G. (1984). *Ability, Merit and Measurement Mental Testing and English Education*. Oxford: Clarendon Press.

Timimi, S. (2004). Rethinking childhood depression. *British Medical Journal*, **329**, 1394–1396.

Timimi, S. (2005a). *Naughty Boys: Anti-social Behaviour, ADHD and the Role of Culture*. Basingstoke: Palgrave Macmillan.

Timimi, S. (2005b). Effect of globalisation on children's mental health. *British Medical Journal*, **331**, 37–39.

Timimi, S. (2007). Autism in context. In *Typical or Atypical Development? Child Psychiatry and Applied Psychology Perspectives*, ed. A. Hosen. Edwin Mellen Press: In press.

Wallis, C. (2006). Getting hyper about Ritalin. *Time Magazine*. February 10th.

Weinman-Lear, M. (1963). *The Child Worshipers*. New York: Pocket.

Wolfenstein, M. (1955). Fun morality: an analysis of recent child-training literature. In *Childhood in Contemporary Cultures*, ed. M. Mead & M. Wolfenstein. Chicago: The University of Chicago Press.

Wong, I. C., Murray, M. L., Camilleri-Novak, D., & Stephens, P. (2004). Increased prescribing trends of paediatric psychotropic medications. *Archives of Disease in Childhood*, **89**, 1131–1132.

Wooldridge, A. (1995). *Measuring the Mind*. Cambridge: Cambridge University Press.

Woolf, M. (2005). One in 20 suffers attention disorder. *The Independent*. January 15th.

Zelizer, V. A. (1994). *Pricing The Priceless Child: The Changing Social Value Of Children*. New York: Basic Books Inc.

Zito, J. M., Safer, D. J., Dosreis, S., Gardner, J. F., Boles, J., & Lynch, F. (2000). Trends in prescribing of psychotropic medication in pre-schoolers. *Journal of the American Medical Association*, **283**, 1025–1030.

Zuckerman, M. (1975). Dr. Spock: the confidence man. In *The Family in History*, ed. C. Rosenberg. Philadelphia: University of Pennsylvania Press.

10

Postcolonial psychiatry: the Empire strikes back? Or, the untapped promise of multiculturalism

Begum Maitra

Introduction

"But the history of all cultures is the history of cultural borrowings."

(Said, 1993, p. 261)

On arriving in Britain in the early 1980s I discovered that I had unexpectedly entered a sort of cultural "limbo" of immigrant doctors and nurses from British ex-colonies, many of which (such as Bangladesh, Mauritius, Sri Lanka, the islands of the Caribbean) had, until then, registered only dimly on our awareness. I began to see how profoundly the view of the world that I had grown up with in India was dominated by the preoccupations of the "white" West (Britain, Europe, and the United States of America), or by the Indian response to these. The nature and legacy of these historical relationships seemed to make "objectivity," highly prized by our professional trainings, impossible when considering culture. This chapter tracks some of the responses of immigrant professionals such as myself, from the earliest stages of bewilderment, through anger at what we learned to identify as "racism," and into the relief of contemporary debates about ethnicity and multi-culturalism that a social constructionist viewpoint has introduced. It hopes to draw attention to those subjects that seem impossible to discuss in professional settings, obstructed as much by external realities of discrimination based on "ethnic" categories and the uncertainties of professional survival, as by fears about ourselves and our undiscovered prejudices. It also hopes to raise specific questions about the legacies of a particular part of British history, namely, its colonial relationship with parts of the world that currently provide significant numbers of the mental health workforce in Britain, in the belief that these are relevant to understanding how the practice of psychiatry is inevitably re-shaped in an increasingly multicultural Britain.

Liberatory Psychiatry: Philosophy, Politics, and Mental Health, ed. Carl I. Cohen and Sami Timimi.
Published by Cambridge University Press. © Cambridge University Press.

"Doctors," "nurses," "patients"

Despite critiques of how mental health practice addressed cultural difference, such as *Aliens and Alienists* in 1982 by Lipsedge and Littlewood (1997, 3rd edn.), the responsibility for difficulties in understanding and addressing unfamiliar patterns of distress continue to be attributed to immigrants, their linguistic difficulties, their failure to "acculturate" to British norms, or the alleged ill-effects of their cultures of origin.[1] Personal experience suggested that immigrant doctors tried hard to suppress their disquiet about such matters, but, as an incident early in my (re[2])training at a psychiatric hospital outside London foretold, there seemed little prospect of avoiding conflicts around cultural difference.

As we sat writing clinical notes in an acute psychiatric ward one morning, an older South Asian colleague (also re-training in psychiatry as I was), jiggling a crossed leg furiously as he considered the matter and apparently oblivious to the presence of a number of white female nurses, observed that "these English ladies" (our patients) were "terribly shameless." The immodesty of their dress and evident immorality of their social habits, he felt certain, were responsible for the pattern of psychiatric presentations we were seeing. The collective hiss of outrage from the nurses, followed by a sudden emptying of the office, genuinely puzzled him for a few moments before he shrugged it off, unable to see any connection between his comments and their actions. He may, had he referred to newly acquired information about "British" cultural practices, have attributed their departure to a collective need, for example, for a cigarette break.

Regrettably, what such moments of acute discomfort promote in both immigrant and indigenous professional groups is a strong impulse to distance oneself both from the offender, and the offending point of view, especially when it is believed to be "cultural" in origin. Discussion is discouraged by a welter of unspoken, and often unconscious, "boundaries" separating the domains, public from private, professional from personal, individual from shared, in cultural and social systems with very different goals. Before the specter of "political correctness" attached itself to exploration of all forms of difference, and the recent willingness to explore indigenous (British) social codes (Fox, 2004), the responsibility for gaffes, or worse, appeared to the immigrant anxious for social acceptance by their British colleagues, to lie squarely with her/him. Acceptance, often framed in oblique comments,[3] provided brief reassurance before other, presumably less acceptable, cultural differences marred this benign dream of a shared, culture-free universe of proper beliefs and behavior. It soon became apparent that both the initial shame, as well as the relief (not to say, gratitude) at "acceptance," were restrictive and misleading if "difference" was to be kept in focus.

While women everywhere might be well acquainted with male chauvinism and with the particular brand of offensive paternalism that sees itself as protecting women from themselves, the framework of sexism identifies only one of the several dimensions in play in this vignette. What adds a surreal quality to such multi-cultural encounters is that the ambiguity inherent in everyday interpersonal communications is unpredictably multiplied by simultaneous and contradictory perceptions, confounded by differences of history as much as by language, culture, gender, and social class. Among the effects of globalization on British culture, and its unavoidable imprint on mental health practice, is this recursive relationship of individual narratives of history and hierarchy. Other contemporary assaults on established hierarchies and relationships – between center and periphery, elite and commoner, ruling (policy makers and the writers of history) and "subaltern" class – that may at first glance appear irrelevant to the field of mental health, are nevertheless central to a consideration of mental health policy, practice and workforce in the twenty-first century. A consumer model of "service delivery" that tailors "products" (e.g., service provision) to user demand and satisfaction is fast replacing the medical positivist criterion of patient/illness outcomes. While it may appear to restore some of the balance of power between professional and lay public, it is unlikely to dispel the urge to mythologize professional power and expertise (Maitra, 2006a). Indeed, the hierarchical relationships between academia, policy makers and service providers in mental health provide an excellent example of the inherent contradictions within a group's relationship with those it considers mentally ill or deviant and the systems and professionals it delegates to take responsibility for them.[4]

The motivations underlying this chapter are both undisguisedly personal, and born of a longstanding discomfort with the rigidity of Western boundaries between personal and professional. The personal motive is the wish to step away from the confusions promoted by these interlocking hierarchies of race, gender and prestige in order to consider how the personal "subaltern"[5] experience of minority ethnic professionals might provide fresh insights into mental health politics. The chapter will focus on specific questions that, while deeply familiar to other immigrant professionals like the author, have been haunted by fears of betrayal – whether of one's personal cultural group or self, one's professional independence, or the freedom to make and break affiliations based on intellectual tastes, irrespective of cultural and professional hierarchies. Having briefly addressed the limitations of "race" thinking, along with racism and antiracism, in describing the mental health arena in Britain, this chapter will address the less comfortable questions raised by the changing "ethnic" profile of the mental health workforce, speeded up by global transfers of personnel and ideas. Recent publications about overseas recruitment of consultant psychiatrists, and a study of white patients and their minority ethnic psychiatrists indicate covert tensions and unexpected benefits. On the other hand, Western cultural norms continue to be "imported" into non-Western social and cultural contexts, whether by returning graduates of Western psychiatric trainings keen to "modernize" their country's mental health services, or by a renewed yearning for Western "scientific expertise" among the ex-colonies prompted by the explosion in global travel and employment opportunities. A selection of papers and a vignette about clinical dilemmas reveal the unforeseen dangers of these yearnings.

Why a focus on racism is not enough

It might appear that "prejudice" (or racism) is sufficient explanation for the negative constructions that, as in the vignette we started with, one group might impose on another. A range of measures has been proposed in the hope that these would provide sufficient guarantees against recurrence. These include antiracism or racism-awareness trainings, provision of information about "cultural diversity" in the hope that such information will instill "respect" for the lifestyle choices of other cultural groups, and organizational policies to address discrimination. Framed by category-ridden understandings of "ethnicity," "rights," and "equity," and embedded in the contemporary culture of indemnity and compensation, there is little evidence that these measures do more than send cultural misunderstanding and resentment underground.

Racism, like ethnicity, is oddly elusive, not because discrimination on the basis of racial difference is difficult to identify, but because the meanings and operational significance of power, and perceptions of "oppression" shift with context and, even more unpredictably, with biographical history. Was the South Asian doctor in the vignette we started with "oppressing" women,[6] or white women? Could his apparent denigration of white women justify a charge of "racism" against him? How much of the apparent contempt in his words might be attributable to distortion – from cultural styles of emotional and verbal expression, simple errors of language (including those motivated by "unconscious" attitudes)? Or, if we knew more about him, would we interpret his comments as compensating for feelings of immigrant vulnerability, as attempts to re-instate himself nearer the top of some familiar hierarchy of professional men? Or, even as "unconscious" attacks (or defense, perhaps against desire) on white women and nurses, both groups he may have resented feeling inferior to in an "ethnic" hierarchy? What significance would we accord to his personal history, his relationships with authority, and the insidious psychological imprint of colonization on the repertoires of masculinity among South Asian men, and between them and "white" men (Sinha, 1995)? Could it be argued that the residual psychological impact of colonial relationships – between the "feminized" South Asian subject (man) and his white master, and its visible repercussions as increasing injustices against South Asian women – have some part in present-day

South Asian attitudes towards women and sexuality? In describing the important place of women's movements in the nationalist resistance to colonial powers, Said (1993) suggests the close links between the dominations of race and gender, and that overturning colonial domination, through the achievement of independence, often allowed the displacement of the orthodoxies and injustices based on gender.

Does a focus on the history of black/white relationships provide useful answers to contemporary relationships between the groups? Bains (2005) noted that, in the 1970s, Black American mental health professionals rejected the idea that long-standing oppression had caused damage and distortion to the Black American psyche, seeing this as an attempt to justify their "oppressed" status. In Britain today public discourse about "racial discrimination" puts forward both poles of the argument – namely, that racism, individual and institutional, is fundamental to black–white relationships and continues to pose a significant risk to the former, and that "black people" (almost exclusively) possess the skills to combat the effects of racism.[7]

Whether or not all "black" groups experience racism and respond to it in similar ways, what these beliefs about racism imply is that there is not much more to be "understood" about the power relationships between the two groups. The inviolate status of "black identity," and "black pride," that buttress this separatist stance make any attempt to continue the debate appear problematic, and at least weakening if not actively damaging to this particular stand against racism. The limitations of this particular form of resistance is obvious in Said's (1993, p. 276) warning about the risks of "essentialization,"

> ... to accept nativism is to accept the consequences of imperialism, the racial, religious, and political divisions imposed by imperialism itself. To leave the historical world for the metaphysics of essences like *négritude*, Irishness, islam or catholicism is to abandon history for essentializations that have the power to turn human beings against each other; ....

What impact does this stance have on black/white professional relationships, and on white professionals and their capacity to work with non-white clients? Personal experience suggests a rather depressing picture of white professional responses ranging from anxiety, apology, and a tendency to placate black colleagues who are perceived as "angry," to hostile silences that erupt in unpredictable conflict, often displaced onto unrelated areas. Both sides retire convinced of the impossibility of open discussions on "race." Whether disguised as humor or expressed more directly, white professionals may charge black colleagues with using the "racism card" to gain unfair advantage. Should this be brushed off as yet more evidence of white racism? The conscious utilization of a weakness to gain an advantage is neither unusual nor ineffective in such longstanding "wars," but it leaves neither side unmarked. For both white and black it risks an increasing imprisonment in attitudes of rage and self-defence, with little differentiation necessary between real, imagined, remembered, or re-interpreted historical insults. These categories are even less meaningful for the growing number of those who cannot neatly define themselves as one or the other, black or white, whether due to parentage, or ties of affection or experience.

Mental health practice in Britain

In response to continuing complaints about discrimination against minority ethnic groups (and some more than others), the emphasis remains on getting the numbers right, i.e., employing more minority ethnic staff. In a recent proposal NHS Employers (2005) suggest "positive action." While "positive discrimination" remains illegal positive action, as this document attempts to define it, seeks to "support groups in society which have been disadvantaged in the past" by helping to "address some of the imbalances which still exist between staff in the NHS and the communities we serve." The question of how one might address past disadvantage without a closer look at its exact nature, and presumably its particular effects on mental health, never really gets asked. Another recent drive to "eradicate discrimination in the Mental Health Services" (DoH, 2005) proposes the appointment of "community development workers" who will "engage communities in planning services."

In the now familiar style (act now – think later) of other "policy"-led initiatives that failed to consider the greater complexity of working in the "community," this plan has been pushed forward without the organizational structures necessary to ensure links both with mainstream services and with (and therefore accountability to) the "community" (Transcultural Psychiatry Society UK, 2003). The hasty appointment of minority ethnic individuals believed to be "acceptable" to local ethnic communities appears to rest on the belief that "ethnic matching" and good intentions are sufficient to coax ethnic groups who are too shy, too ignorant or too hostile to the good sense of mainstream mental health services. The uncertain returns of "ethnic matching" have been dealt with elsewhere (Maitra, 2006b). Research that goes beyond user uptake and satisfaction repeatedly shows that more radical ideological overhauls are necessary (see below). Goodwill alone is scarcely adequate – coupled with power and naiveté; it is more likely to be dangerous.

Apart from a few notable attempts[8] to address the complexities of "cultural" work in mainstream British psychiatry, by and large services have confined themselves to easily identifiable and circumscribed areas, such as the provision of interpreting services for non-English speaking users (the need being seen as theirs rather than that of the service), and other "special needs" of minority groups (usually limited to a very small number of religious/dietary needs). Ethnic monitoring, despite endlessly problematic and multiplying categories, is believed to be necessary to ensure that organizations can audit equity of service provision. Health organizations rate themselves on criteria that revolve around "representation" (do "user" and employee statistics match ethnic population statistics?), and the relatively recent concept of "user satisfaction." While cultural psychiatry is slowly gathering force as an academic subdiscipline in Britain and elsewhere, little of this complexity appears to have entered organizational policies on "culturally competent practice."

Global markets – populations, professionals, and ideas

That the theoretical disciplines of psychology, psychiatry, the psychotherapies and mental health nursing are dominated by ideas arising from European, male, middle class society (usually summarized as "Eurocentric") is now an article of faith among the (racially) "aware" British public. However, the hegemonic control over the cultural color of ideas nurtured and promoted by Western academic institutions is faced with a number of challenges – from commercial interests, such as the pharmaceutical industry (Thomas et al., 2003; Lexchin & Light, 2006) and other potential funders of research (such as government bodies), from the culturally mixed pool that students and staff are drawn from, and from unpredictable global circuits of public interest and demand. The pathway from theory to practice is unlikely to be unidirectional. The two recent UK National Health Services (NHS) "initiatives" referred to above indicated that public opinion following a critical event may spawn policies (e.g., the *Delivering Racial Equality* plan following enquiries into the death of David Bennett) that by their very vagueness will trigger unpredictable changes in practice long before (or if ever) research is available to support it. So much for "evidence-based" practice.

What policy on "positive practice" initiatives and "community development workers" carefully avoids specifying is how ethnic "communities" are to be identified, by whom, and what qualifies the appointed community development worker to engage or represent any of these "communities?" Nevertheless, it seems clear that the ethnic composition of the workforce is neither culturally homogenous nor static. Thirty-one percent of UK entrants to medical school (BMA, 2001) and over a third of adult psychiatrists within the Royal College of Psychiatrists (admittedly only one of the influential disciplines in mental health) are from ethnic minority backgrounds (Decker, 2001). The recruitment crisis at consultant level in general adult psychiatry in England (Royal College of Psychiatrists, 2005) led to the recent drive to recruit doctors (Goldberg, 2003), nurses and social workers from low-income countries, and to an attempt to utilize the resources of refugee doctors already in Britain (Cohn et al., 2006; Desjarlais et al., 1995). A multicultural workforce such as this reflects, and reinforces, the influences of a culturally diverse population in major cities such as London. In other parts of the country that remain largely white, this workforce reflects the far-reaching impact of globalization. Tourism (both in the increasing access of Britons to foreign travel and the presence of non-white tourists in hitherto "white" communities), employment (and personal relationship) patterns that follow global markets, and an appetite for foreign goods and novel experiences fed by the media, all contribute to a heterogeneity of ideas – about satisfactions, and what constitutes deprivation. Can mental health practice help but be influenced, whether consciously or via largely unconscious mechanisms, by the cultural preferences of the individuals who form this motley workforce?

Early reports about both initiatives – the recruitment of senior overseas doctors and the utilization of refugee doctors – are carefully couched, and while they hint at power relationships (similar to those referred to in the opening vignette), almost nothing is said about cultural difference. In a recent qualitative study (Cohn *et al.*, 2006) refugee doctors spoke of their concerns about the role assigned to them – namely, to address the medical needs of their own ethnic group in Britain. They wondered whether working within their ethnic community might deny them the chance to make the most of their individual opportunities by "defining themselves as marginal. One (Doctor 8) explicitly said that working with the local community 'prevents me from going through'" (p. 76). George, Calthorpe and Khandelwal (2006) explored British trainees' responses to overseas consultant psychiatrists, a cohort distinguished from refugees by their status as seniors and the fact that they had been actively recruited from their countries of origin. Trainees were concerned about the consultants' capacities as trainers; others commented, "that some consultants recruited from overseas are granted the Membership far too readily, thus causing resentment in those who have worked hard to obtain the qualification" (George *et al.*, 2006, p. 230). These tensions are not mentioned by overseas consultants interviewed by Shah *et al.* (2006), who restrict their cautious reporting of initial difficulties to those located within their countries of origin and their families. While this may indeed be how they perceived their experiences, given the contradictions inherent within their positions as senior professionals and cultural novices within Britain, these doctors could not have spoken openly about professional difficulties and cultural tensions without threatening their professional credibility and their new positions. Both papers speak of the wealth of experience that these consultants bring, and that, "in general, it is only the form and not the content of postgraduate psychiatric training that tends to vary across countries." (George *et al.*, 2006, p. 230). While the success of Western medical training in non-Western countries is evident in the number of successful careers that have been built by immigrant doctors in the West, it cannot be assumed that the "cultural" content of *practice* is the same irrespective of the experiential backgrounds (personal and professional) of the individuals.

Despite ambitious government plans, the growing demand for social care and health services poses a real problem that is unlikely to be conclusively or easily met. Much has been written about a reversal of the "minority–majority" ethnic trends – attributed to falling birth rates of the indigenous European populations, the growth of resident "minority ethnic" populations, and the continuing influx of immigrants and refugees. Referring to US demographic predictions of this nature, Thernstrom (2002) argues that these are flawed, reifying quasiracial categories that suggest that these are more significant than other differences for the study of social phenomena, e.g., that the quasiracial category of "Hispanic" is more significant than, say, a religious category such as "Catholic." What these trends do suggest is that "cross-cultural" provisions of care are increasingly likely to be the rule, rather than the exception. This makes the examination of relationships between members of a culturally heterogeneous workforce, and the influence of a global flow of ideas on local institutions central to an understanding of emerging trends in theory and practice.

Cultural imports

Relatively little is known about the contribution of cultural beliefs to the interactions between non-Western practitioner and Western "patient." A fascinating study (Jadhav, unpublished data) of the relationships between South Asian trainee psychiatrists and their white British patients reveals that many of the latter saw these doctors in a more positive light in comparison with white British doctors. These South Asians were seen as friendly, "able to emote," sensitive to discrimination because of their own experiences, and more "holistic" than local British doctors because of the traditions of spirituality and complementary care in their culture of origin. British doctors were seen as belonging to the "upper" classes and unavailable (namely, choosing not to practice in the UK and migrating to Australia or the USA). Were these merely positive stereotypes of South Asian doctors, a category of service providers that is, after all, so familiar to the British public that their strange accents (also noted by the respondents, but not disparaged) had almost become part of the package of "otherness" that allowed psychiatric patients (a subgroup likely to be stigmatized) to construct a more benign version of medical authority?

This benign perception is especially unexpected in light of the beliefs that the South Asian psychiatrists held, particularly on matters that were relevant to diagnosis and patient management. Some doctors believed that their skills and medical resources were being misused by "the 'benefits' camp" (i.e., individuals they considered were exploiting the benefits of the welfare system). Others found local attributions and perceptions difficult to accept (e.g., that the loss of a pet, or dissatisfaction in a relationship with a boyfriend were significant psychological stressors). Distinctions between private disappointment and serious trauma, perceptions of personal/collective responsibility, assessments of what we are rightly entitled to – whether to sympathy or a (free) hospital bed, and what justifies access to public resources – are all judgments that are deeply influenced by one's personal and cultural history.

Clearly, these cultural systems had not been significantly touched despite many years of medical training, the psychiatric components of which would have relied exclusively on Western perceptions of individuals, relationships, and stresses. These doctors admitted to the researcher (also South Asian) that they would have liked the opportunity to discuss cultural issues, but were unable to declare this for fear of being thought incompetent at their jobs. Given this desire to conceal what they believed about their patients, what was it about their exchanges with their patients that permitted the latter to experience a quality of emotional engagement that was satisfyingly "holistic" ("spiritual," "complementary" as opposed to exclusively biomedical) and empathic (sensitive to "discriminations" due to social class and professional status)? Were they merely simulating empathy from a fear of losing their jobs, or were there satisfactions to "providing" (concern, compassion, hospital resources, medication) to a very particular other (white, British, vulnerable, and receptive, rather than the "superior" and disparaging stereotype of the colonial master filtered through collective history)? Would understanding these doctors' unconscious expectations of British/South Asian relationships improve the quality of the exchange between them? Should cultural training, were it available to psychiatric trainees, aim to convince them of the validity of other cultural viewpoints, or are there undiscovered riches in a degree of misunderstanding?

Other studies discuss the unpredictable direction of exchange when health beliefs intersect. Anderson (1987) found that differences in ideological structures between immigrant Indo-Canadian women and (Anglo-Canadian) health professionals in Canada prevented successful encounters. Based on ideologies about their roles as women these Indo-Canadian respondents considered their feelings of loneliness and depression to be "facts of life," rather than health problems. Health professionals' ideologies based on dominant beliefs about the roles of women in society and reflecting the rational individualism of Western capitalism, located these problems as being within the individual, stripped of her social context. This construction of social problems as health problems made their strategies to help their patients to "adjust" less than helpful.

Skultans (2006) describes the impact on newly independent Latvians of the influx of expensive Western medicines as part of a new ideology of economic liberalism. For Latvian women the individual focus and frame of illness that Western medicine emphasizes shifted the locus of responsibility for distress in problematic ways. Poverty and its effects were no longer seen in its historical and social embeddedness, but were re-described as personal failure. Their distress in the face of poverty was no longer a "natural" response to things beyond their control but "depression" (warranting expensive medication that they were unable to purchase). Skultans discusses the particular shape that Western liberal democracies and the "*psy* regimes" have given to ideas about the self, autonomy and choice. "Alien" value systems, implicit within imported medical technologies, have unpredictable effects. While South Asian negative perceptions of contemporary British culture appeared to transform itself into benign effects, Western liberal ideals translated in ways that did not enhance the lives of Latvians.

Global effects

The solutions, discussed above, to an ever-increasing demand for quick, high quality, and inexpensive health care for a British population told to expect nothing less, has significant effects on the health resources of distant countries. While providing welcome job opportunities for some individuals, they present serious dilemmas for others. Questions arise about the racism implicit in British policies that leave junior doctors who have qualified overseas effectively indentured to the NHS in a plight redolent of empire. Sudden change in immigration laws (Trewby *et al.*, 2006) has obliged another cohort of overseas doctors to return to their countries at great personal and financial cost. While the UK General Medical Council points out that no guarantees of employment are made to overseas applicants to the Professional and Linguistic Assessments Board examinations, these continue to be offered, and at considerable financial cost, tantalizing applicants in India, Africa, and other countries. The irony is that the basic medical qualifications these doctors have received are likely to have been greatly facilitated by subsidies from their own governments; limited career development, and economic prospects in their own countries prompt the choice to migrate West. To charges of exploitation, Western states have responded with contributions to developing countries and, with a somewhat curious logic, by "putting pressure on governments in developing countries to encourage them to place a greater emphasis on health" (BMA, 2006). Transfers of technology and personnel may merely be the bearable aspects of a widening global market that deals increasingly in human resources of another kind – whether in organs for transplant, or subjects for research. Iheanacho (2006) notes that the furore surrounding disastrous drug trials in Western countries may encourage the pharmaceutical industry to conduct these in developing countries, where Western research practices may mask important breaches of the rights of the poor or illiterate.[9] The following section discusses circumstances within some non-Western countries that are the recipients, or consumers, of health strategies devised in the West. This might explain to some degree the apparent passivity of individuals in the face of what may be newer forms of imperialism.

Mental health training and practice in low income countries

The continuing legacy of colonial psychiatry

The following case was presented at a family therapy workshop, held in a leading mental health institution in an Indian city.

A rejected admirer had subjected a young woman in rural India to a planned sexual assault. The threat of public dishonor to her and the family, the assailant's higher social status in the village, and a prevailing lack of confidence in the police and legal systems in this rural area prevented the young woman's family from pressing charges of rape. When her assailant made the young woman an offer of marriage, her family urged her to accept, promising no support if she was foolhardy enough to refuse this offer of an honorable solution. She had no choice but to comply, but her distrust and fear of her husband remained a major obstacle to any chance of a successful marital relationship. Thwarted in his expectations of love, and gratitude, the husband responded with increasing physical and emotional violence, leading eventually to his wife making several serious attempts at suicide.

The institution she was taken to offered the couple residential family therapy. Such resources are almost non-existent in India (as indeed they are in the UK!) and the treating team felt proud of being able to offer it. However, this largesse seemed to do little more than provoke an escalation in the husband's anxiety, ending in a brutal attack on his wife in the presence of professional staff. To the serious decline in her emotional state and the heightened risk of suicide, the team, horrified and apparently helpless, had proposed an increase in number, and dosage, of her antidepressant medications.

As therapists everywhere know, victims of socially sanctioned violence in any form may not be simply rescued by formulaic solutions, whether taken from women's movements ("empowerment"), mainstream psychiatry (antidepressants to treat depression triggered by trauma), or the psychological therapies.[10] The unspoken agreement among the therapists in this case *appeared* to be that patriarchal authority, as demonstrated in this man's unchallenged right to treat his wife as he chose, took precedence over any rights she might have had. Indeed, in seeking to "treat" her (with antidepressants) they had surrendered a great deal of the authority they might have assumed, though not without risk, to name the problem as social (and criminal).

Miyaji (2002) discusses the therapeutic paralysis engendered by a shared belief in a "cultural tradition" that has undeniably harmful consequences for some participants. Writing about attitudes to domestic violence in Japanese culture, she suggests that the clinical role obliges the therapist to shift between positions (and identities), moving to and from "traditional" and newer constructions of social roles and relative positions. What may get lost in this construction of tradition is the fact that traditions are rarely single, nor are they inevitably grounded in total consensus within a particular society. Indeed, the fact that traditions need to be taught, and constantly reinforced through repetition and ritual, suggests that they are vulnerable to change or to subversion by parallel and contradictory traditions. Therapists within a cultural system know, because of their own, even if partially successful, socialization into the system, of these internal subversions. Private discourses among women, among elders, and within families allow a wider variety of stances, alliances and "deals" to limit male exploitation, admittedly not always equally acceptable to all parties. It is these that need to be extended and developed *locally* in treatment strategies, creating a vital intermediate level of psychological reform.

The question here is whether Western schools of therapy, inevitably laden with culturally alien notions of good outcomes, are too distant from the repertoires of these clients. It seems clear, however, that there is strong interest in many non-Western countries in challenging old autocratic systems, and Western style therapies appear to offer a solution. However, what is likely to be lost to the reckoning by those who choose to train to become Western-style therapists is that what seem to be liberating new ideas, such as equality between the sexes and generations, may not be transposed easily to client groups that do not share the therapist's somewhat pro-Western ideals. Furthermore, what can not be discovered easily is what underlies the therapist's choice of a Western therapeutic tradition, and the degree of personal investment in distancing oneself from the admittedly negative aspects of own cultural communtiy. Kakar (1998) describes a therapeutic system that arises from within Indian cultural systems – that of the mystic/religious healer. Culturally knowledgeable, s/he has the option to broker solutions that address the problem in a manner congruent with the client's expectations, and simultaneously addresses allied problems at a number of symbolic and complex social levels. These solutions have little to do with the illness paradigm, or the linear analyses of causal factors and treatment strategy favored in dominant Western therapeutic models. To dismiss these as superstition laden, or unscientific, given their widespread popularity among all sections of the Indian public, merely begs the question – who are mental health strategies intended for? To the allied question of whether therapists do not have a duty to contribute to social change the response must surely be – "yes, but." What separates a "colonizing" mission to "civilize" the other from less problematic styles of change must be the degree of critical thinking brought to every stage of the project, along with a robust commitment to co-constructing solutions with those who wish for change.

The error, perhaps, in the case discussed above was the mistaken faith placed in Western therapeutic and logical premises. This legacy of a colonial mind-set persists in ex-colonized countries, and perpetuates the view of "native" (indigenous) culture as fixed, essentially backward, and so laden with immutable "traditions" that it could only be replaced by Western liberal humanitarian solutions. These perceptions are often kept in place by an earlier generation of Western trained "elite" psychiatrists. As Higginbotham and Marsella (1988) note, these "after-shocks" of colonialism in Southeast Asian centers undermine the confidence to develop local research and services.

It is not surprising that family therapy has achieved such popularity in India. Given the average Indian's discomfort with psychoanalytic ideas (perceived as overly preoccupied with sexual behavior and individual desires, and inadequately interested in social relationships), family therapy appears to promise the possibility of re-negotiating Indian cultural prohibitions. However, the uncritical acceptance of a therapeutic model premised on another culture's preoccupations cannot work beyond a certain point. Despite self-conscious anxieties about remaining in thrall to Western "superiority," the cultural embeddedness of the model remains unexamined. Rather like the Latvians Skultans describes (see above) these therapists seemed to see the failure of "cutting-edge" Western technology (antidepressants and residential family therapy) as personal failures, of themselves as therapists and of "Indian culture" itself. It is this inherited notion of one's cultural inferiority that afflicts the colonized individual, resulting in a failure to recognize locally occurring ethical systems that might offer solutions. Indeed, local cultural resources may only become recognizable after these have been identified by other (Western) eyes, and sanctified in print within academic Western journals.

The new imperialism of Western ideas

Mainstream British publications such as the *Psychiatric Bulletin* and *International Psychiatry* regularly publish accounts of mental health services in a wide range of non-Western countries, ranging from the affluent Middle East to economically disadvantaged nations in Africa and further afield. These papers demonstrate a range of positions with regard to the importance accorded to Western models (Burjorjee & Al-Adawi, 1992), including whether they argue for an approach that derives from local contexts and indigenous perceptions of mental health problems and needs.

Some writers from Bangladesh (Karim *et al.*, 2006) and Sri Lanka (Kuruppuarachchi & Rajakaruna, 1999) worry that cultural beliefs about illness causation (e.g., by supernatural influences) leads psychiatric patients to consult religious leaders and other practitioners of indigenous healing/medicine. These writers appear to share a belief in the efficacy of modern (i.e., Western) psychiatric treatments, and in the irrelevance of supernatural causation theories, which are considered to be the result of ignorance. They appear also to agree that local contexts and practices deny patients access to "proper," presumably universal, human rights. That significant numbers of British Asians who have access to Western psychiatry continue to consult traditional healers on visits to their countries of origin (Bhopal, 1986) suggests that more complex underlying meanings and motivations might lie behind these choices. Curiously, the finding that up to 80% of the patients with puerperal mental disorders attending a provincial general hospital in Sri Lanka (Kuruppuarachchi & Rajakaruna, 1999) also sought religious or traditional healing did not seem to prompt an enquiry into the evident pluralism[11] in health beliefs and help-seeking. Burjorjee and Al-Adawi (1992) appear as unquestioning about context when they proposed that the mental health needs of the population of Oman, with its distinctive geography of deserts and inaccessible mountainous terrains, and its nomadic Bedouin tribes, might be adequately served by young graduates briefly trained[12] to deliver psychiatric diagnosis, psychotropic drugs, and injections. There seems little question, again, in the minds of these writers that similar mental illnesses afflict populations, and respond to similar solutions, largely independent of local contexts and meanings.

Requests from low-income countries for training, and assistance in setting up "modern" mental health facilities, have prompted concern among some cultural psychiatrists. They argue for the need to ensure genuine partnerships between professionals in both centers if Western ideological hegemonies are not to be unwittingly promoted abroad (Royal College of Psychiatrists, 2001). When overseas training projects are described, there is often a disappointing lack of discussion of how much consideration has been given to ensure that a course translates effectively for a very different social and professional setting. For example, Dogra *et al.* (2005) describe the delivery of a course on child mental health in Varanasi, India, but make no mention of whether the course, considered useful in Leicester, UK, required any modification for a quite different set of Indian professionals. The fact that there appear to have been no cultural surprises for the British facilitators reminds one of a comment made by Chakraborty (1974, 1991), an important voice among the early transcultural psychiatrists, that Western observers seemed noticeably disinterested in material that did not support the universalistic assumptions of mainstream Western psychiatry.

Universals and counter arguments

Transcultural psychiatry

Beneduce and Martelli (2005) argue that the nature of its origins make conflict an unavoidable part of contemporary cultural psychiatry. The ethnocentric bias and racial stereotypes within contemporary psychiatry, Raimundo Oda *et al.* (2005) declare, originate within colonial ideas about the inferior brain development of colonized "natives," and the related vulnerability this produced to (Western) "civilization." This internal "fault" is made harder to explore by the many conflicting uses of the term "culture." From colonial misidentification of what was often political revolt as "cultural" tradition, or as defense of such tradition,[13] to the politicization of culture as in the current rhetoric of the clash between Islamic and Western civilizations, cultural difference appears "intractable" and problematic. Beneduce and Martelli make an interesting suggestion that a "historically founded ethnopsychiatry" may allow for the articulation of these elements, new trans-national identities, and the diversity of local worlds. In particular, it may permit a more effective challenge to the hegemony of Western psychiatry.

British "transcultural psychiatry" has focused on racism and oppression (Bains, 2005) within mental health services and the rights of minority ethnic groups. Some have gone as far as to advocate separate mental health services for them (Bhui & Sashidharan, 2003). Jadhav (2004) notes the steady growth in academic positions, courses, and journals dedicated to cultural psychiatry, and the irony of this being confined to Euro-American countries. Despite his optimism about the growth of the discipline, it would be premature to assume that academic orthodoxy, even when it includes "culture," is less hostile to its ideological premises being ques-tioned. There may well be patriarchs within this academic club, like those every-where, who are reluctant to question their own assumptions. Hsu (2004) writes with breathtaking dogmatism "While data are lacking, *those of us who have worked with different cultural groups will probably agree* that the problem of stigma is greater in non-Western than in Western cultures" (*italics mine*). And Jilek's[14] concern (1998) about the psychiatrist who "dismisses psychiatric diagnoses as Euro-American folk categories and discourages efforts at universal classification . . ., and even defines modern psychiatry as a culturally constructed Western folk system" suggests that some questions are still too "radical" for transcultural psychiatry.

Postcolonialism, multiculturalism and the future

> In order to understand the cultural conditions, and the rights, of migrant and minority populations we have to turn our minds to the colonial past, not because those are the countries of our "origins", but because the values of many so-called "Western" ideals of government and community are *themselves* derived from the colonial and post-colonial experience. (Bhabha, 1996, p. 209, italics in the original)

Current generations in Britain, as in other ex-colonial nations, may ask what they have to do with their nation's colonial past. They may point to the progress made in the West to provide a more secular, rational slant to human rights as evidence of how far these societies have come. Stuart Hall (1996), notes that "colonisation" was part of an essentially transnational and transcultural global process, and that decolonization "like colonisation itself, has marked the colonising societies as powerfully as it has the colonised . . ." For the ex-colonized, given the cultural upheaval that characterized the colonizing process decolonization could never provide a return to a pure set of uncontaminated origins. Neither party, it seems clear, emerges unchanged. What decolonization also reveals is the extent and significance of relationships between "diasporic" populations. Thus, while the center–periphery model of influence in which Western nations (central, grand, imperial) impinge on non-Western nations (peripheral, variants of the Western norm) may have seemed compelling earlier, it fails to address the complexity of directions and influences. Further, before we discuss which universally agreed system of values might underpin more open and receptive cultural exchange, a re-evaluation of basic concepts is essential. Bhabha (1996, p. 208) notes "The trouble with concepts like individualism, liberalism or secularism is that we understand them too well. These are ideas, and ideals that are increasingly complicit with a self-reflective claim to a culture of modernity whether it is held by the elites of the East and West, or the North and South." However, despite their having become "... instinctive to our sense of what civic society or a civic conscious-ness must be ..." it would be useful to remember that these ideas originated in parallel with the colonial enterprise.

Finally, McKenzie *et al.* (2004) comment on the resources hidden within the economic poverty of low income countries. The paucity of resources in many of these countries might suggest that there is little that psychiatry in developed countries can learn from poorer countries. However, this may be far from true.

Services in low income countries are often greatly under-resourced, under strain, and leave most people with mental health problems with no care. But there are examples of different ways to treat or prevent mental illness from which high income countries can learn. Some are born from the ingenuity of necessity, others from cultural knowledge. We do not aim to idealise low income countries, to demonise high technology and psychiatric care, or to offer the stereotype of cohesive traditional communities as a panacea, which could undermine the development of appropriate services. We simply present examples that challenge the orthodox, make us pause to think, and offer rational models for provision of care that high income countries may consider useful. (McKenzie *et al.*, 2004, p. 1138).

Conclusion

One of the rather unexpected ironies of globalization is that much of health care in many "First World" countries is provided by immigrant doctors from "Third World" countries, the vast majority of which are the ex-colonies of Britain and Europe. That medical training (and psychiatric training in particular) in these ex-colonies is deeply influenced by Western medicine, and its cultural matrix of individualism, positivism, and specific varieties of dualism, is scarcely surprising. There are, of course, many easily identifiable "imports" from non-Western cultures into the contemporary lives and health beliefs of Western societies. However, what is less obvious and unrecognized, is the degree to which immigrant doctors in the West continue to be influenced by their cultures of origin, and how and where these ideas leak into their practice.

The declining prestige and credibility of doctors in general, the re-definition of the boundaries of medical "professionalism" based on fear of blame, and various attacks on psychiatrists in particular, may explain why the profession appears to have little interest in further challenge. However, there has probably never been a better time to indulge that delight in the diversity of human experience that brought many of us into psychiatry. Given the trend of increasing diversity, and the disappearance of old certainties, alertness to multiculturalism and to history may provide important tools for the future.

It is hoped that concern about being seen as "radical" (or "political") will not dissuade doctors from lingering a little over these arguments, perhaps to ask whether any approach to emotional distress can legitimately overrule the system of meanings it is based upon. For immigrant doctors in Western countries it is perhaps an unavoidable part of development to undertake one's own "decolonization." Convictions of inferiority (sometimes unconscious), and the strategies we devise to manage or disguise them, interfere equally with understanding the plights of our patients, whether other immigrants or the native British. The dilemma posed by my colleague (in the first vignette) has stayed with me for this duration. While I believed his comment arose from a mixture of distress and disgust at the impact of their choices on the lives of our women patients, his locating the problem in a cultural undervaluing of shame (as an internal monitor) was too simple. The best face of gender relations in patriarchal societies, such as his and mine, was premised on a very particular take on public/private expressions of sexual modesty/desire. The expectation that one's own cultural solutions will make sense, let alone be accessible, to another culture is unforgivably naïve in a mental health professional. Only when the mental health disciplines have included cultural histories in how meaning is constructed will we begin to benefit from the riches of multiculturalism. What is necessary is an open curiosity about how cultural solutions to mental health dilemmas work, the specific contexts they were designed to serve, the costs they impose, and the alliances they need in order to work. When looking for new ideas about what mental health might mean in the twenty-first century, and how it might best be promoted, we might now look anywhere.

NOTES

(1) For example, as revealed in non-Western varieties of sexism (e.g., "forced marriage"), or patterns of distress (such as "somatization").

(2) A significant proportion of South Asian "trainees" had migrated with prior postgraduate qualifications in psychiatry from their countries of origin.

(3) The comment that one was "different," from the bulk of one's ethnic group kept one simultaneously grateful and puzzled by feelings of shame and resentment.

(4) The "aliens and alienists," respectively of Lipsedge and Littlewood's title. (1997).

(5) This sense of the *subaltern* was coined by the Marxist philosopher Antonio Gramsci, who also described as *cultural hegemony* the foundation for complex systems of domination by one group or class over a diverse culture through the medium of everyday practices and shared beliefs. In postcolonial theory the subaltern position refers to marginalized groups and the lower classes to describe a person rendered without agency by her/ his social status.

(6) For example, by problematizing women's freedom to express sexual choice.

(7) As evident in the Social Services' policy to place black and mixed race children with black carers (irrespective of cultural difference among "black" communities) in the belief that only black carers will be able to protect these children from the effects of racism.

(8) E.g., the Frantz Fanon Centre, Birmingham and Solihull Mental Health Trust; a training program run by University College London and Camden and Islington Mental-Health and Social Care Trust to help mental health professionals become more aware of cultural issues related to the treatment of Muslim inpatients.

(9) Such as ensuring "informed consent" by those unable to understand complex decision-making, or too much in need of the financial inducements offered.

(10) This is, of course, only at the most public level. Private discourse among women, and within families, allows a wider variety of stances, alliances and "deals", to limit male exploitation, though not always equally acceptable to all parties.

(11) The multiplicity of our own belief systems as researchers makes it, of course, perfectly possible that we might be pluralistic in our personal choices and rigidly linear in our academic endeavors. Clearly, the problem lies in the quality of medical training, and whether it can combine technical rigor with a more constructionist philosophical stance that allows for the realities of pluralism and competing systems.

(12) The trainers, the authors reassure readers, would be two senior psychiatrists, both "Maudsley trained."

(13) For example, the Indian Mutiny of 1857 was long described as an outbreak of violence motivated by religious feeling around a specific and relatively minor matter, rather than a nationalist uprising.

(14) He was writing as Chairman of the Transcultural Psychiatry section of the World Psychiatric Association.

REFERENCES

Anderson, J. M. (1987). Migration and health: perspectives on immigrant women. *Sociology of Health and Illness*, **9** (4), 410–438.

Bains, J. (2005). Race, culture and psychiatry: a history of transcultural psychiatry. *History of Psychiatry*, **16**(2), 139–154.

Beneduce, R. & Martelli, P. (2005). Politics of healing and politics of culture: Ethnopsychiatry, identities and migration. *Transcultural Psychiatry*, **42**, 367–393.

Bhabha, H. (1996). Unpacking my library … again. In *The Post-Colonial Question Common Skies, Divided Horizons*, ed. I. Chambers & L. Curti. London: Routledge.

Bhopal, R. S. (1986). The inter-relationship of folk, traditional and Western medicine within an Asian community in Britain. *Social Science and Medicine*, **22** (1), 99–105.

Bhui, K. & Sashidharan, S. P. (2003). Should there be separate psychiatric mental health services for ethnic minority groups? *British Journal of Psychiatry*, **182**, 10–12.

BMA (July 2001). The changing face of medicine: today's doctors. http://www.bma.org.uk/ap.nsf/Content/Changing+face+of+medicine+-+Today's+doctors.

BMA (2006). Feature – Flying doctors. *BMA*, 29 July, p. 13.

Burjorjee, R. & Al-Adawi, S. (1992). The Sultanate of Oman: an experiment in community care. *Psychiatric Bulletin*, **16**, 646–648.

Chakraborty, A. (1974). A challenge to transcultural psychiatry: whither transcultural psychiatry. *Transcultural Psychiatric Research Review*, **11**, 102–107.

Chakraborty A. (1991). Culture, colonialism and psychiatry. *Lancet*, **337**, 1204–7.

Cohn, S., Alenya, J., Murray, K., Bhugra, D., de Guzman, J., & Shmidt, U. (2006). Experiences and expectations of refugee doctors. *British Journal of Psychiatry*, **189**, 74–78.

Decker, K. (2001). Overseas doctors: Past and present. In *Racism in Medicine: An Agenda for Change*, ed. N. Coker. London: Kings Fund.

Desjarlais, R., Eisenberg, L., Good, B., & Kleinman, A (eds.) (1995). *World Mental Health Problems and Priorities in Low-Income Countries*. Oxford: Oxford University Press.

Department of Health (DoH) (2005). Delivering race equality in mental health care: An action plan for reform inside and outside services and the Government's response to the Independent inquiry into the death of David Bennett. London: DH. http://www.dh.gov.uk/PublicationsAndStatistics/Publications/PublicationsPolicyAndGuidance/PublicationsPolicyAndGuidanceArticle/fs/en?CONTENT_ID=4100773&chk=grJd1N.

Dogra, N., Frake, C., Bretherton, K., Dwivedi, K. N. & Sharma, I. (2005). Training CAMHS professionals in developing countries: An Indian case study. *Child and Adolescent Mental Health*, **10**, 74–79.

Fox, K. (2004). *Watching the English The Hidden Rules of English Behaviour*. London: Hodder and Stoughton Ltd.

George, S., Calthorpe, B., & Khandelwal, S. (2006). The International Fellowship Scheme for consultant psychiatrists: trainees' perspective. *Psychiatric Bulletin*, **30**, 229–231.

Goldberg, D. (2003). The NHS International Fellowship Scheme for Consultant Psychiatrists. *Newsletter of the Faculty of General and Community Psychiatry*, **6** (Spring), 5–6.

Hall, S. (1996). When was 'the post-colonial'? Thinking at the limit. In *The Post-Colonial Question Common Skies, Divided Horizons*, ed. I. Chambers & L. Curti. London: Routledge.

Higginbotham, N. & Marsella, A (1988). International consultation and the homogenization of psychiatry in Southeast Asia. *Social Science and Medicine*, **27**, 553–561.

Hsu, L. K. G. (2004). International psychiatry – an agenda for the way forward. *International Psychiatry*, **4**, 5–6.

Iheanacho, I. (2006). Drug trials-the dark side: this world. *British Medical Journal*, **332**, 1039.

Jadhav, S. (2004). How 'culture bound' is 'cultural psychiatry'? *International Psychiatry*, **4**, 6–7.

Jilek, W. G. (1998). Transcultural Psychiatry – Quo Vadis? *Transcultural Psychiatry Newsletter, January 1998*, xvi, 1. http://www.mentalhealth.com/newslet/tp9801.html.

Kakar, S. (1998). *Shamans, Mystics and Doctors: A Psychological Inquiry into India and its Healing Traditions*. New Delhi: Oxford University Press.

Karim, M. R., Shaheed, F., & Paul, S. (2006). Psychiatry in Bangladesh. *International Psychiatry*, **3**, 16–18.

Kuruppuarachchi, K. A. L. A. & Rajakaruna, R. R. (1999). Psychiatry in Sri Lanka. *Psychiatric Bulletin*, **23**, 686–688.

Lexchin, J. & Light, D. W. (2006). Commercial bias in medical journals: Commercial influence and the content of medical journals. *British Medical Journal*, **332**, 1444–1446.

Lipsedge, M. & Littlewood, R (1997). *Aliens and Alienists Ethnic Minorities and Psychiatry (3rd edn.)*. London: Routledge.

Maitra, B (2006a). Culture and the mental health of children. The 'cutting edge' of expertise. In *Critical Voices in Child and Adolescent Mental Health*, ed. S. Timimi & B. Maitra. London: Free Association Books.

Maitra, B. (2006b). The Many Cultures of Child Protection. In *Children in Family Context*, ed. L. Combrinck-Graham. New York: Guilford Publications.

McKenzie, K., Patel, V., & Araya, R. (2004). Learning from low income countries: mental health. *British Medical Journal*, **329**, 1138–1141.

Miyaji, N. T. (2002). Shifting identities and transcultural psychiatry. *Transcultural Psychiatry*, **39**, 173–195.

NHS Employers (2005). *Positive Action in the NHS*. London: NHS.

Raimundo Oda, A. M. G., Banzato, C. E. M., & Dalgalarrondo, P. (2005). Some origins of cross-cultural psychiatry. *History of Psychiatry*, **16**, 155–169.

Royal College of Psychiatrists (2001). Report of the overseas working group. Council report CR 93. London: Royal College of Psychiatrists.

Said, E. W. (1993). *Culture and Imperialism*. New York: Vintage Books.

Shah, M., Goswami, S., Singh, G., & Brown, R. (2006). Overseas consultant psychiatrists moving into the NHS: initial experience. *Psychiatric Bulletin*, **30**, 228–229.

Sinha, M. (1995). *Colonial Masculinity The 'Manly Englishman' and the 'Effeminate Bengali' in the Late Nineteenth Century*. New Delhi: Kali for Women.

Skultans, V. (2006). Psychiatry though the ethnographic lens. *International Journal of Social Psychiatry*, **52**, 73–83.

Thernstrom, S. (2002). The demography of racial and ethnic groups. In *Beyond the Color Line: New Perspectives on Race in America*, ed. A. Thernstrom & S. Thernstrom. Hoover Press.

Thomas, P., Bracken, P., Cutler, P., Hayward, R., May, R., & Yasmeen, S. (2003). Challenging the globalisation of biomedical psychiatry. *Journal of Public Mental Health*, **4**, 23–32.

Transcultural Psychiatry Society UK (2003). Response to: Inside Outside. Improving mental health services for Black and Minority Ethnic Communities in England (Summary). http://www.mind.org.uk/NR/rdonlyres/7ADC1B4D-1142-4BB5-81F2-6B82008F2341/1029/08TCPSInsideOutsideResponse1.doc.

Trewby, P., Williams, G., Williamson, P. *et al.* (2006). European doctors and change in UK policy. *British Medical Journal*, **332**, 913–914.

11

A new psychiatry for a new world: postcolonialism, postmodernism, and the integration of premodern thought into psychiatry

Ramotse Saunders, Amjad Hindi, and Ipsit Vahia

Introduction

In conceptualizing a new psychiatry for a new world, the authors found themselves having points of similarity as well as points of departure. They quickly realized that their differing viewpoints were influenced significantly by their backgrounds, their parent cultures, their adopted ones – in essence, their histories. This undoubtedly had an effect on the way this chapter was written. The aforementioned points of departure rendered a single chapter in a single voice an impossibility.

Instead, we are presenting three individually written essays. These essays contain as their organizing themes (in sequence) a postcolonial perspective, postmodern analysis, and an integration of premodern thoughts in contemporary psychiatry. It is our hope that these essays can, in conjunction, highlight some of the complexities and contradictions of psychiatry as it is faced with a "global" condition. This format is also intended to suggest that a "global vision" of psychiatry may only be possible if psychiatry is seen as a compendium of ideologies and philosophies which necessarily remain contradictory, but which may coexist within the context of multiple local discourses. Finally, we do not intend to provide a resolution to the many issues that prevail in the world of psychiatric thought, but to provide impetus to debate.

Part 1. Postcolonialism and psychiatry
Ramotse Saunders

The term "new world" itself presents a conundrum. What exactly is it and where might we situate it? For the purposes of this section, the "postcolonial new world"

Liberatory Psychiatry: Philosophy, Politics, and Mental Health, ed. Carl I. Cohen and Sami Timimi.
Published by Cambridge University Press. © Cambridge University Press.

refers to the portion of the world that emerged from colonialism altered to such an extent that there was discontinuity with its precolonial past. Clearly, the emergence of countries from colonialism occurred on a spectrum. Subsequent development has also occurred on a spectrum. The focus of this chapter will be those countries which emerged from colonialism significantly *damaged*, and in which development has continued to *lag*. However, use of these terms and their negative connotations are not a prelude to a rant. Rather they plead for a recognition that colonialism does not end on a given day of independence, that its imprint on a society is transformative, and that an emerging society must constantly grapple with these influences.

My identity (politics) requires some consideration. If we acknowledge that all positions have inherent biases, perhaps a simple disclosure can serve as starting point. I identify myself as a citizen of the postcolonial world. Such a designation is itself not singular. There are within the postcolonial diaspora, colonizer proxies, postcolonial subjects, and native speakers:

- *Colonizer proxy* – A colonizer proxy is a substitute for the original colonizer, invested in continuing the colonizer's agenda, preserving the status-quo, maintaining hierarchies. The colonizer proxy may be a citizen of the postcolony, but identifies more closely with the colonial "parent."
- *Postcolonial subject* (Spivak, 1999) – An individual who identifies as a citizen of the postcolony, but who has been so influenced/altered by the colonial experience (education, notions of self, migration, discrimination, history), that they are incapable of speaking in any voice but that of a cultural hybrid.
- *Native speaker* – Spivak's reading of *native informant* (Spivak, 1999) borrows the term from ethnographic studies and describes a plurality of interpretations including the (im)possible position of the native informant. Influenced by this, I have chosen the term native speaker to represent a third voice within the postcolonial diaspora, a voice that is dispossessed, that has the least political capital, and represents that residue of the citizenry least influenced by colonialism. Here the difference between *influenced* and *affected* is important. The native speaker has, doubtless, been affected by colonialism, but the assimilation of colonial impositions – the *influence* – is minimal (and ideally zero). The *native speaker* has taken upon himself or herself, a separate path of development, and justifiably claims a sense of belonging to the postcolony. This sense of belonging may not translate into ownership.

Inasmuch as all designations represent arbitrary distinctions (and foreclose upon the existence of a spectrum), they do provide useful organizing structures. Thus in the cloud of the postcolonial citizenry, I wish to identify these three as demonstrating separate agendas. Which one, or which combination, is most congruent with who I am will perhaps be revealed in a deconstruction of the text. It is possible also that, for the citizen of the postcolonial world, there is a constant switching between these positions.

Given that the postcolonial new world is a polynational, polydevelopmental grouping, an important question follows: What would lead to any cohesive view of what this new postcolonial world is, and so render this chapter writeable? Certainly, there are historical commonalities, and the number of colonizing powers was finite, but relying on such broad categories would render any analysis (with its contingent generalizations and lack of appreciation of the uniqueness of local narratives) to become a disguised repartitioning of the new world. In other words, a re-imposition of the colonialist project masquerading as an explanation. It is tempting to assume the rhetoric of oppressor and oppressed, but rather than mediating a discourse between poles, I shall attempt to approach this question from the perspective of the dyad. That is, the postcolony existing not as an entity unto itself, but as a stage in colony–colonizer entanglement. My position is not a prescription for a generic "New World." Nor is it a manifesto. Rather, it is a humble exposition of one aspect of the discourse.

Colonialism and psychiatry

The experience of colonialism is one of repetitive traumas: the abnegation of self, the distinction between primitive and civilized, those capable of self-governance, and those requiring supervision, the imposition of a foreign structure, and the control of labor. A notion derived from the concept of Caliban (Saunders, 2007) in subaltern studies (Roberto Fernandez, 1973–1974) is that the first step in this traumatization is the "caliban-ization" of the colonial subject. The reader will recall Shakespeare's Caliban in *The Tempest*, "a savage and deformed slave." Thus, the colonial subject is not rendered non-human (i.e., an animal, where anthropomorphization has clear limits), but *subhuman*, and this makes all subsequent impositions possible. The colonial master is invested with the permission, if not the moral obligation to embark on a process of humanization of this Caliban.

In this regard, what might be the impositions of medicine? Could its practitioners, while maintaining a professed concern with the provision of healthcare services, have reinforced colonialist categorizations? An answer to this question might begin with a reading of the history of medical experimentation on slaves (Washington, 2007) by physicians who have been lauded as medical pioneers. Similarly, texts on the conduct of medicine in the time of chattel slavery describe medical examinations for "soundness" (Fett, 2002) immediately prior to sale and give accounts of cost–benefit ratios – a parsimonious calculus – being used to determine when a slave should have access to a physician. Others give examples of enabling physician attitudes within the practice of slavery (Byrd & Clayton, 2000;

Schwartz, 2006). If the colonialist practice of medicine had a built-in doublethink, how might this be manifest, disguised, or sublimated in the postcolony?

Within medicine, the practice of psychiatry has been granted (or arrogates to itself) an additional imposition – that of madness (Foucault, 1988). The authority to designate individuals as mentally weak permits the *de facto* separation of the individual from reason and, in the case of the subhuman colonial subject, leads to a further caliban-ization.

The end of colonialism does not, in itself, dismantle these impositions. Rather, it is a redefinition of governance and the control of labor. The persistence of these impositions is assured by the existence of colonial proxies. As previously noted, this chapter considers the (colonizer/postcolony) and in that context, the colonial proxy requires additional consideration.

"Proxydom" is not a simple either-or condition. The proxy may come from the colonizer elite, or be a native-proxy, or some hybrid of these, and though proxies ultimately serve the colonialist project, it should not be assumed that they are equal or that all their actions are conscious. There exists a pecking order of distances from the colonizer ideal. Where medical elites find themselves in this order is likely closer to colonizer. Here, the question of the progeny of doublethink is partially answered. However, before all medicine is branded as imposition, the mitigating influence of self-reflection deserves mention. If medical élites have begun a process of analysis of their role, and this has occurred within the frame of individuation/independence – i.e., there is a societal project to differentiate from colonizer – then there may well be an absence or near-absence of proxydom. For psychiatry, this could translate into some restitution of the individual and a *transformed* range of impositions.

I say *transformed* and not reduced, because a project of nationalization and concomitant re-construction of local narrative may well lead to even harsher imposition of subhumanity on the individual "afflicted" with mental illness. The ability of local psychiatry to strip the individual of human characteristics remains problematic. Local psychiatry may be pernicious. In this case, a re-incorporation of psychiatry, as contemporarily practiced in colonizer countries could have a more benign consequence on individuals. But a measure of proxydom is restored as well. Postcolonial psychiatric practice is left to continually negotiate its place within the colony–colonizer dyad.

Legitimacy

The situation of medical elites is further complicated by the fact that the distance of postcolony from colonizer itself creates a hierarchical structure. Subsequent distances develop with the creation of local medical schools, the training of imported populations, and the eventual running of these institutions by locals. Questions about standards and competence arise the instant there is any separation from the north. There is the presumption of superior knowledge and clinical practice in the developed world. A quick perusal of a few developing countries' information on the US government's travel advisory website yields the following:

Medical facilities do not meet international standards and frequently lack medicines and supplies ... We strongly recommend you obtain comprehensive travel and medical insurance before traveling ... Care at public health facilities is significantly below U.S. standards ... Medical facilities are limited and medicines are sometimes unavailable ... Medical care is more limited than in the United States ...

There are also countries with favorable reports of healthcare in their cities but a rapid decline in more rural areas. On the colonizer side, some justification for this position may be found in the presence of superior facilities and equipment, advanced research, and higher standards of accountability. The consequence, though, is that postcolony medical élites are left striving for legitimacy. In the pursuit of this validation, a number of outcomes are likely. One is the persistent mimicry of current practice in the former colonizer/developed world. A consequential process is the confinement to cultural lag. The postcolony does not act *de novo*, but waits, observes, and adopts. Thus the cost of legitimacy is a perpetual self-imposed state of inferiority. In psychiatry these mechanisms translate into the uncritical adoption of nosological systems (e.g., DSM), educational systems (e.g., Problem-Based Learning), the dominance of particular standards of evidence (e.g., double-blind, randomized trials) and the directing of limited research resources to the kinds of research which will be published in the most prestigious journals – the portals of legitimacy. While these contribute to a common international language in which medical elites communicate and understand each other – and reinforcing notions of universality – there is a concomitant denial of other systems of knowledge. The counterbalance to an over-emphasis on legitimacy would appear to be an acknowledgment of *difference*, not inferiority, and a validation of local phenomenology. This is not to say that counteracting the impetus to legitimacy needs to validate unsafe care. Medical élites have the very real task of policing themselves and the local practice of medicine responsibly. It is important to recognize the potential problems such self-policing may face in extremely small societies with near-incestuous communities of physicians.

Systems of care

More muddled is the interaction between the medical training systems of developed and developing countries, the latter almost exclusively endowed with postcolony status. Physician undersupply in developed countries leads to a constant influx of physicians from developing countries (Torrey, 1973; Pearlin *et al.*, 1990; Sandhu, 2005). The similarity of medical systems in colonizer and postcolony tend to result in the vector of this migration being to the specific colonial sponsor or their most accessible proxies. Similarity of systems is but one of the reasons why this migration occurs. Other reasons relate to the aforementioned ideas of superiority/inferiority, and as such reveal notions of inadequacy in the postcolonial subject. In this regard, the concrete realities of economic benefits of migration cannot be ignored (Pearlin *et al.*, 1990; Rao *et al.*, 1998; Astor *et al.*, 2005; Shafqat & Zaidi 2007). A simultaneous process external to but derived from these migratory patterns is a refiguring of IMG roles within these developed nations (Rao, 2003). With rare exceptions, these international medical graduates are never treated equivalently and firmly occupy a second tier (Mick *et al.*, 2000; Weissman, 2001) in colonizer/developed nation healthcare systems, treating underserved populations and largely denied access to the most élite institutions. The consequences on the healthcare system of the postcolony are myriad. A large portion of these physicians never return to their home countries (Pearlin *et al.*, 1990). Thus, for psychiatry in the postcolony, this frequently results in understaffed facilities and treatment for the most severely mentally ill is limited solely to pharmacotherapeutic management. This point and its implicit suggestion that psychotherapy is necessary must, of course, be considered with the proviso that notions of psychotherapy are in themselves cultural impositions of colonizer healthcare systems.

A second scenario entails the return of these foreign-trained specialists into the local milieu. This may create problematic issues arising from application of their developed-country training to a population with a different narrative. Will their return lead to the pathologizing of local narrative, and the creation of disease where none existed previously? A second notion here is that much of their training may be irrelevant considering the environments in which they will be working. For example, in a non-Western society where there is less of a focus on individuation and an illness is experienced by an entire family, where enmeshment is considered the "norm," the practice of individual psychotherapy will be at the very least a difficult proposition, and one likely to generate more stresses than immediate solutions.

There is a potential for the ideas and practice that returning international medical graduates bring, especially in the context of psychiatry, to have transforming effects upon society, e.g., notions of personhood, mind, and the place of psychotherapy, the validity of imported psychiatric nosology, lifestyle normalization vs. postcolony mores. Certainly, the postcolony is not static and its culture is, through globalization, continually exposed to Western influence. Indeed, these psychiatrists are vectors of globalization. If this society becomes increasingly

Westernized, then the ideas of Western psychiatry may present an easier fit with what it is becoming. For example, the effects that increase inclusion of individuals, are likely to be beneficial to the most ostracized in society.

It also necessitates that the postcolony consider whether the contrasting conceptualizations of this process as colonial re-imposition vs. assimilation of knowledge via globalization are really distinct processes, and if so, whether they are occurring simultaneously. These systems of care issues generate compromises. The ultimate accounting of these compromises would seem to lie in comparing the benefits across the dyad. If the colonizer is benefiting more than postcolony, then, it would appear that the traditional vectors of exploitation are in operation, and the relationship requires reassessment and renegotiation.

The postcolonial subject in the developed world

The medical migrants discussed above are but one part of a larger population of postcolonial subjects who find themselves as residents inside the former colonizers. Thus far the analysis has focused on their effects on the postcolony. But these displaced postcolonial subjects are also agents of dialectical interaction (between postcolony and colonizer). Indeed, they may function as *postcolony* proxies. Whether they perform the latter function, and whether it is intended, is influenced by the complicated position of the migrant cum *immigrant*, never fully belonging to the adopted home but complicit in the abandonment of the original home (Schmiedeck, 1978).[1] The immigrant physician may assume within herself the position of a native speaker (Spivak 1999), and attempt to speak for "her people" while enacting the behaviors of a postcolonial subject. Or by an imposition, the colonizer may label the immigrant physician a native speaker. And this labeling, in its imposition-differentiation of self and other, is a repetition of the very machinations of colonialism. Might this be a Caliban-physician? Following the imposition, with what voice does this individual speak?

Consider another scenario, where a migrant physician, initially a postcolonial subject, becomes so inured of colonizer culture, so assimilated as to take on the persona of a colonial proxy, i.e., the migrant physician becomes an immigrant physician and this immigrant physician dissolves into the adopted culture. It would be an over-simplification to explain such transformation as a hapless immigrant succumbing to overwhelming forces. The prerogatives of legitimacy and mimicry discussed previously, also apply.

Likewise, the tiering of health care in the developed world also applies (Blanco *et al.*, 1999). The immigrant physician, in spite of all the assimilation she can muster, may be confined to the treatment of immigrant populations. Add to this mélange, the fact that the treated immigrant populations may come from many places. Will they be treated hierarchically? Universalistically? Ahistorically? Aculturally? The migrant cum immigrant cum colonizer proxy scenario has a multitude of potential outcomes. The caution is that this individual can easily become a doublethink double-agent.

In the above paragraphs, the term *physician* has been used, but when we substitute for this *psychiatrist*, these considerations assume special significance. A brief digression to the templates of *culture* (and its empiricist progeny – *cultural competence*) may provide further elucidation of the problem. Cultural competence is clearly preferable to cultural incompetence, but its assertion of a teachable, quantifiable ability to treat another precludes an acknowledgment of complex distances and differences which do not vanish in the presence of a few learned techniques. If cultural competence is assumed in the graduate of a residency training program, or in the board-certified psychiatrist, then what is the outcome of a colonizer proxy who is considered culturally competent treating immigrant populations? How does she perceive those immigrant populations – i.e., "her people" – and others who are immigrants but not "her people" who are given as her charges to diagnose and treat. Psychiatric diagnoses are often stigmatizing, pejorative, and most importantly, enduring. There is significant potential for misrepresentation of immigrant patients, postcolonial subjects and native speakers alike, thereby making careful consideration of disguised agendas necessary, and demanding the continual questioning of claims of cultural competence.

As previously, when there was a measure of self-disclosure, the above considerations beg the questions: What voice or voices have I assumed in the practice of psychiatry? What voice am I assuming in writing this? Am I culturally competent to expound views on a new psychiatry for a new world? Am I misrepresenting "my people"? Is there any alternative but for the migrant/immigrant physician to constantly ask these questions, and what damage might their repetition wreak upon the self?

Consequences of entanglement

The constant tension in the (colonizer/postcolony) dyad often engenders a discussion of what position should be taken by the postcolony and its citizenry (postcolonial subjects and native speakers). There are those who advocate active opposition to any manifestations of the colonialist project, the perspective here polemicized in its most extreme by Fanon (1966, 1967). Others believe that maintaining a critique without active opposition is sufficient. The internalization of this critique by the body politic ultimately may result in transformation by making "ruptures" possible, i.e., theory as revolution (Foucault, 1989).

In this regard, I believe there must be consideration of size, the vector of globalization, and the influence of capital. It is likely that larger, more powerful economies with more pervasive media dominate how influence is manifested in our present economy. The summation of these elements reveals a power relationship with postcolony on the receiving end. As assimilation proceeds, how does the discourse change? Is the increasingly Westernized postcolony less likely to mount any sort of critical (far less self-critical) examination of globalization and its discontents? If the lessons of history are to be instructive, then the postcolony will not actualize liberation without active resistance. Psychiatry is but a small part of the meta-narrative of globalization, but these principles would appear to apply similarly. However, by virtue of its smallness, a fair counter-argument to the rhetoric of resistance is that the loudest yell of this minority will amount to little more than a voice in the wilderness. Perhaps, the best that can be realistically envisioned is the maintenance of criticism.

Conclusion

As stated earlier, I intended to take a jaunt along one path of the discourse on the status of psychiatry in the new world. In assuming a postcolonial perspective, it has joined a dialogue that is still being written. While identity politics – my ownership of my difference, my history, my fundamental position – makes neutrality impossible (and undesirable), it is my hope that this text has escaped the rhetoric of the oppressed and managed to discuss, instead, the position of the entangled subaltern.

Part II. Towards a new psychiatry for a new world
Amjad Hindi

Introduction

I dream of the intellectual destroyer of evidence and universalities, the one who, in the inertias and constraints of the present, locates and marks the weak points, the openings, the lines of force, who incessantly displaces himself, doesn't know exactly where he is heading nor what he'll think tomorrow because he is too attentive to the present . . . (Foucault, 1989)

From the outset, two sets of political relations privileged themselves in this work, and displaced my attempts to begin it with a traditional scientific statement. Essentially, the two relations led to rethinking the identity of the author in psychiatry. The first was a *production* type of relation – namely producing a text, accompanied by a string of questions about the meaning of authorship, authority and originality. The second relation – one of *power* – emerged from the series of values and biases that preceded my proposed knowledge of this essay and unveiled my biographical core. In both orders, one faces a set of related questions of: Who speaks psychiatry and in which voice? Or, who is at the least entitled to theorize it in the present? I present this polemic as a necessary introduction to the analysis I use in this essay to comment on the relation between world psychiatry and postmodern critique.

Postmodernism is an intellectual school that still remains today not easily defined. The difficulty in asserting a definition probably lies in postmodernism's defiance of universal or traditional description and its attempt to stay away as much as possible from generalized deductive reasoning. Nonetheless, I think it is fair to say that postmodernism is seen as representing a break with modernism, which is an intellectual movement that began in the eighteenth century and continued into the late twentieth century, roughly corresponding to the period between the French revolution and the dominance of global capitalism. Modernists are adherents of the Enlightenment position which holds that the progress and advancement of the humankind depends on rational and scientific thought (Thomas & Bracken, 2004). Postmodernism, on the other hand, sees in the Enlightenment a rigid ideal-ism and a collection of absolute arguments that may have been very popular in the past, but no longer seems applicable to the conditions of our present time. On the historical level, postmodernism refers to the new globalization and information age, and the associated breakdown of cultural, linguistic, and national identities. On a theoretical level, it challenges grand theories or "narratives" of history and science that seek to explain wide swathes of the world, and it questions guarantors of truth such as science and religion, and whether absolute reason and rationality lead to progress and improvement. Moreover, postmodernism emphasizes that these grand narratives and science in general, far from being value neutral, have built-in biases and assumptions that reflect Western culture and socio-political structures.

The aspirations of this book, placed nakedly in its title, are of psychiatric liberation and socio-political change. That is what I tried to press this essay to embrace from its instance of conception. Yet, I don't claim that this stated value is all that can be said, since, through careful reading any text opens up disseminated assumptions and re-representation hitherto unknown to the author. In this sense, any written text becomes the sole property of the analytic reader who releases the work to its multitude of different meanings, not that of the author. This essay revolves around unfolding this representative meaning to the best of my limits as an author, while leaving the reader to add to it what she or he finds fit.

Postmodern psychiatry and the position of local authorship

Any serious reading of politics in psychiatry will encounter three assumptions
(1) That "the personal is political", i.e., what people emotionally experience as thought and feeling, regardless of psychopathology or normalcy, is grounded

in the socio-political structures they come across in their daily lives. These structures are universally common to any society, and include things like poverty and economic standards, type of government, size of the population and so forth. It is important to point out that while modernism holds that these variables affect the individual in a universal and predictable manner (e.g., the psychological effects of low socioeconomic status are almost the same across the world), postmodernism asserts that these structures assume a discursive function. Thus, "discourse" is considered to be a way of thought and behavior that is institutionalized by the powers specific to each society, and that affects all the individuals living it. In essence, a discourse produces the social boundaries that limit what can be defined as "real." For example, the discourse on sexuality in certain places governs the language and vocabulary allowed to describe sex, which can in turn prevent polygamy or homosexuality from being seen as real as mainstream sexuality. In social sciences, the way a discourse shapes the reality of people is termed "institutional power."

(2) The second assumption holds that, similar to the way a discourse shapes the personal, people can fight back and empower themselves by narrating their own stories in response to the institutions they live in. To clarify this, consider how people feel empowered by psychotherapy. They learn how to re-tell the same story of their lives, albeit with empowering insights they learn from psychotherapeutic language. By adopting words that reflect their own power, people learn how to shape their reality as much as the way a discourse does. This corresponding *local* knowledge leads postmodernism to say that the meaning of socio-political structures can only be understood by the people living under them, and that universal conclusions regarding their effects on the individual are dubious. Further, this form of personal power does not respond well to quantitative scientific enquiry and can only be represented through narratives and stories.

(3) The third and final assumption states that any critique wishing to grapple with, or re-read the relation between psychiatry and politics can only be meaningful through what I call a *local narrative of psychiatry*, which I will come to explain at a later point in this essay.

This "focus on the political" as *method* does not merely follow postmodern ethos; rather, the postmodern argument holds that it should precede all endeavors to theorize psychiatry, elucidate its societal function, and critique its current form. Undoubtedly, many modern psychiatrists adopt the position that deems such efforts to revive the political origins of science as subversive and too subjective, leading psychiatry to lose its standing as a legitimate science. They distance themselves from politics in the name of a value-free science. However, as Adorno (Adorno & Crook, 1994) points out, their stance can be deemed as tantamount to the *most political statement of all.*

Psychiatry's history has been dominated by a majority of Western writers who, in the service of scientific legitimacy and objectivity, believed they should be answering only to abstract scientific calculations, and should divorce themselves from hermeneutics and any imbedded politics. The necessity of "scientific legitimacy" led psychiatrists to deny the existence of roles that were clearly more political than medical, and were delegated by societal structures wishing to suppress social deviance and aiming at conforming human behavior. While psychiatrists still claim their field to be strictly medical, their continued denial only serves at sharpening, in some instances, the obvious political content of their work, especially by some stakeholders who often find it difficult to tell psychiatry apart from legal institutions. This "history of objectivity" has effectively meant abandoning problems one may encounter in the transparency of psychiatric language and turning a blind eye to advances in philosophy, linguistics and the rest of humanities. Even recently, with the increased ascendance of *Culture Theory*, modern psychiatry refocused it as *Cross-Cultural Psychiatry*. Within this framework, the *social* has been viewed typically – *à la* Durkheim's and Comte's nineteenth-century sociological theories – as a set of *objective facts* that obey natural laws (Ingleby, 1980). Thus, the socio-political are merely summed up as a set of quantifiable variables to be used in psychiatric research and DSM cultural formulations. With a few exceptions, for example, the work of Arthur Kleinman (1988), cross-cultural psychiatry has not adequately incorporated the theoretical views accepted by most other fields of the humanities in which culture is understood as a work-in-progress or a process operating reciprocally at two levels: the level of discursive knowledge/institutional power and that of situated local knowledge/personal power (Jenkins & Barrett, 2004).

One could say that this has had an exclusionary effect on service users (patients), who, despite benefiting from psychiatric healing, found at times their stories morphed into something that meant less than what they hoped for. Postmodern psychiatry advocates a new reading of psychiatric ethics aimed at exactly retrieving this political potential, this personal form of power, hoping to re-insert the stories and narratives that fade away in an apolitical and rational psychiatry. That is, postmodern psychiatry aims to help the service-users adopt the political language that empowers them, as much as providing the necessary clinical care they need. To illustrate this point, consider the movement towards having user-led publications that complement the science of psychiatry; for example, see *City Voices* published in New York (http://www.newyorkcityvoices.org).

To say then that a new psychiatry – or rather postmodern psychiatry – is a *local social praxis*, is to acknowledge the necessary contextuality of any discourse, and acknowledge that psychiatric authorship is located in a whole web of related discourses: psychiatric, medical, political, humanitarian, cultural studies, linguistics, and others. This transformation unlocks modern psychiatry's reliance on the special authority and expertise of its authors; for example, consider the function of the DSM as a way of asserting the complex and exclusive technicality of psychiatric texts. In contrast, postmodern psychiatry opens the space for the other: the patient, the non-Western form of psychiatry, the non-professional, and invites them to become local psychiatric authors. Additionally, postmodern psychiatry calls on psychiatrists to search their textbooks and journals for the lines of politics and power just as they would for scientific facts and opinions; and to examine, critique, and supplement all the incumbent universalities and statements, rather than simply accept them in the name of professionalism and scientific orthodoxy.

Situating postpsychiatry in the world

The question of method

This essay starts from understanding the condition of psychiatry in the world as being *already* postmodern. Therefore, before pushing the argument any further, I will present the kinds of theoretical assumptions and tools of analysis that I intend to use and attempt to answer the questions of method. The most pressing seems to be whether the interpretive systems of "postmodern theory" are operational at the level of non-Western knowledge: that is, can one prevent postmodern critique from becoming the latest venture of the West theorizing the "other" (Said, 2004)? And if a postmodern condition indeed exists outside traditional Western thinking, how can it be applied to world psychiatry?

Given that almost all scientific works on world psychiatry assume a modernist perspective, below I shall answer why I think a postmodern condition applies to the rest of the world, with respect to psychiatry or other studies.

(1) Often what prevents thinking of the non-West as postmodern is the biased assumption of the existence of a *"cultural lag,"* in which the state of non-Western society is said to lag in adopting sociological technologies that of the West, and then to be determined by this technological status (Smith & Marx 1994). Similarly, it is assumed that International Medical Graduates psychiatrists trained in the United States return to their native country and practice a form of psychiatry that is frozen in the era of their residencies, e.g., 1970s or 1980s. You can see how the proposed cultural-lag can deny the non-West any possibility of an independent history – modern or post – as if it could not possibly experience *simultaneously* with the West a postmodern condition. This concept is further explained in this chapter's essay on postcolonialism and the world.

(2) Consider postmodern theory's opposition to the notion of *linearity* on psychiatry's history. As per modern ideology, and based on the way the West's history was deemed to be progressive and gradual, world psychiatry could not witness, or leapfrog to a postmodern condition or postpsychiatry, *before* it had fully lived both the successes and the failures of modernity. This demonstrates a form of neocolonialism where the "*other*" is understood through Western eyes. It seems true that the inclusion of a postpsychiatric critique is easiest in communities where there is an already established modernist psychiatric tradition as opposed to a premodern one. However, this does not necessarily mean that this modern form of psychiatry cannot rapidly accelerate or, to use a postmodern term, rupture into a condition where postpsychiatric practice is possible. On the other hand, this rupture with the modern form of psychiatry need not be a society-wide phenomenon in which all psychiatrists need to practice postpsychiatry. Rather, it is hoped that similar to other fields of social science, it will lead to a ripple-effect that leads to a new psychiatry in a new world.

(3) Finally, a number of other observations have been conducive to a postmodern perspective: (a) the fact that I write this essay as a non-Western person; (b) the way postmodern critique has been received in other fields of humanities in non-Western areas; and (c) multiple social phenomena that indicated the appearance of a postmodern condition in the world, of which I shall lay emphasis on two, globalism and the World Wide Web.

Psychiatry, Globalism and the internet

In my native city of Damascus Syria, the horizon is plugged with satellite dishes through which people tune in daily to the latest techniques of becoming consumers of the global economy. Little time is left for them to pursue other ways of "*becoming*," e.g., critical or sceptical of their everyday conditions. Similarly, in Globalism, under a capitalistic umbrella, psychiatry sells its Western expertise and clinical appraisal to people who are shaped daily and increasingly as clients. Thus, the Delphic reminder "know thyself" (Gnothi Seauton) is mutated into "know what to buy", and people adopt a language of self-understanding, or a "technology of the self" (Foucault, 1990), that is presented to them through advertisements and simulations of reality. Perhaps under this rubric we may soon start watching reality shows in which psychotherapy is simulated. The point here is not whether Globalism according to the modernist ethos is morally good or bad, since it is in my view both and neither. Rather, this brings forth a condition in which psychiatry is constantly under the structure of being a commodity, presented and calculated as an efficient worth-the-while buy; its technologies are at once repressing at the institutional level and empowering on the personal one, complicating any attempt to argue for one possibility over the other.

I invoke Globalism in problematizing a new psychiatry for two reasons: (1) to declare the futility of ignoring a post-modern *global* condition that engulfs medicine, psychiatry and science in general; and (2) to reject the assumption held by many psychiatrists that this requires an even stronger case for a positivistic psychiatry. The strategy of universal psychiatrists is expressed here mainly as a process of eliminating any "market competitor" to its theory of mental suffering. It becomes a commodity that casts traditional pre-modernist meanings and beliefs into oblivion, guaranteeing a full reign for a bio-reductive psychiatry that treats people with hi-tech psychopharmacologies. Though, it is true that premodern notions of psychiatry may be at times harmful, it does not automatically mean that modern psychiatry offers marked advances over it. (This is further explained in this chapter's accompanying essay on premodernism.) I will assign import to this last observation since it constitutes a rupture point in people's experience, and a new limit in their history in which acts of alienation and silencing will be achieved in the name of universal objectivity, human rights and world health.

The other phenomenon I wish to emphasize is the impact of the Internet's *informatics culture* on psychiatry. Across all academic disciplines, the World Wide Web is the topic of daily discussion in which people tend to view it as having either a positive or a negative effect on their field (a modernistic perspective), while missing the point that it leads to both conclusions. To the extent that it impacts on psychiatry, one can claim that the web has transformed the knowledge/power equations and the control over speech, writing and reading. It presents itself as a self-regulating system, or an archive of knowledge, that is slowly making its medium the primary source of meaning in the world. Thus, more and more, the traditional institutions of family, tribe, and custom are no longer seen as the main containers of psychiatric experience.

Postpsychiatry

In *Postpsychiatry: A New Direction for Mental Health* and their other writings (Bracken & Thomas, 2001, 2005; also see their chapter in this volume), Patrick Bracken and Philip Thomas located postmodern psychiatry in the social practice of hermeneutics that privileged ethics over technology, and Heideggerian ontology of contextual meanings over the Jasperian phenomenology of psychopathology. Similarly, in the United States Bradley Lewis (2000; also see his chapter in this volume) has advanced a postmodern *rewriting* of modernist psychiatry, in which modernity's "quest for objective truth" becomes Lyotard's (1984) *crisis in representation*. Its "faith-in-method" becomes *incredulity toward metanarratives*, and the modern goals of progress and emancipation become those of struggle and compromise. These seminal works opened the space for theorizing psychiatry along postmodern lines, and re-inserted the *power* relations back into the fabric of its science. It is important here to invoke the position of the authorship (the relation of production) called for in the beginning of the essay, and state that this essay merely attempts at an extension to a debate already ongoing. It deals with the question of context in situating postpsychiatry in the world, along with the problematizing of universalities vs. locality when psychiatry faces a post-modern condition.

The question of temporality between modern and postpsychiatry

Postpsychiatry is a *moment* in the history of psychiatry. It is continuous with the modern version, yet separated by a transformation in each other's method. In other words, postpsychiatry denies any categorical cessation from modern psy-chiatry, insisting that a psychiatrist can be *both*. Postpsychiatry simultaneously affirms and rejects modern psychiatry, or what Agger (1998a, b) calls "Continuous and Discontinuous Relationship". To say it simply, postpsychiatry does not gen-erally reject the use of medications and other current treatments to relieve suffer-ing, nor does it attempt to deny the existence of mental illness as defined over the past century. What it radically opposes is the modernist view that the accumu-lation of *facts by scientific progress and research*, when set apart from hidden values and politics, will solve any dilemma. To stress this further, the meaning of the prefix "post-" does not make postpsychiatry a chronologically later (more advanced) stage of evolution that supersedes modernity, nor is it the newest phase of progress capable of effacing, and replacing the theory and technique of its predecessor. Rather, postpsychiatry springs from the depth of universal-psychiatry's fracture lines, from the gaps and discontinuities of positivism, from the crisis in representation in its grand narrative (Agger, 1998a, b). Similar problematization can be found in the work of Thomas Kuhn (1996) who, despite being unrelated to postmodern thought, stressed the non-cumulative nature of scientific work, its historicity, and its governing paradigm.

The above needs to be said to address the critique that postpsychiatry is attempting to *de-legitimize* modern psychiatry, or more interestingly, that post-psychiatry is *not* psychiatry. Again, consider postpsychiatry to equal a politico-contextual modern psychiatry, where the line that separates each attitude (modernist or post-) is constantly open to interpretation and dialogue, never defined or fixed to eternity. Postpsychiatry is an addendum to psychiatry "as we know it," which unwraps its values and power for examination, and supplements it with a local political critique, or a *local narrative* (cf. Derrida, 1978; 1981).

A problematization of the local narrative in world psychiatry

There are currently two ways of understanding psychiatry and psychiatric conditions in the world. The first is the idea that mental illness is the same around the globe and that a competent psychiatrist can treat any patient anywhere when helped by translation. This is what I call "Global Psychiatry." The other perspective contends that psychiatrists need to develop sensitive *cultural* competence prior to every venture into a different area of the world. This is known as "Cross-Cultural Psychiatry." The difference between the two conceptualizations lies in how each considers the question of interpreting signs and symptoms, and whether the emphasis is more on similarity or difference. I shall pause for a moment to highlight each attitude and move then to post-modern narratives.

In *Global Psychiatry* the assumption is the universality of human experience based on the similarity in genetic structures and resemblances in brain anatomy across the world. Backed by an identical attitude in general medicine and surgery that exalts efficiency and cost-analysis, Global Psychiatry actively marginalizes the meaning of political or mental "difference" as inconsequential and propounds a unified social change in all of its host communities. Western concepts dominate its vision of world health. It is a model that is rife with assumptions (about the meaning of family, the individual, human rights, etc.), but nonetheless, it meshes well the aspirations of a global capitalistic economy. Here, psychiatry can be an effective tool in instilling the values of modernity and the meaning of "normal" functionality, so prevalent in DSM and ICD criteria that define and categorize mental illness, and consequently, fostering a slow merging of all world communities with that of the West.

On the other hand, *Cross-Cultural Psychiatry* assumes that mental and political differences exist between communities, but falls short of fully realizing its meaning. Although there is increasingly a "new" form of cross-cultural psychiatry – the work of Arthur Kleinman(1988) is an example – in which difference is fully appreciated, for the most part it remains true that cross-cultural psychiatry assumes that difference happens only in the context rather than the form of mental illness, and thus tries to study it as a quantifiable number of reduced variables that may contain different contents, but that ultimately leads to a similar categorical form (i.e., a type of syndrome or a constellation of signs). Here, the way of reducing and abbreviating culture into a tangible corpus remains somewhat archaic and ill defined, in the sense that it follows classical ideas of philology and anthropology that have been revised appreciably, if not discarded altogether.

In essence, cross-cultural psychiatry deals with the West as a fully understood monolithic unity. For example, the culture of a 30-year-old homeless man from the Netherlands can conceivably be lumped together with that of an American single mother from the Midwest. On the other hand, it gazes at the rest of the world as "*The Other*" that needs to be understood and studied, and around whom the idea of cultural competence is woven. The other becomes everyone and everything else, a blank paper that can be inscribed with the knowledge of the West. If global psychiatry seeks to emancipate the other, cross-cultural psychiatry seeks to understand the other. Yet the latter model theorizes identity as stable and unified, as opposed to the postmodernist view of the subject as provisional and contingent. Cross-cultural psychiatry conceptualizes "the social real" as that which harmonizes with the traditional understanding of the culture at hand (invariably using variables such as race and gender in a static and simplified way), while the latter holds that identity is formed both by discourse and personal narrative. One possible consequence of the cross-cultural perspective is to enhance the legitimacy of the local psychiatric academics who, in concert with renowned international cultural psychiatrists, command the discourse on cross-cultural psychiatry. Sadly, this process ensures a reproduction of timeless monolithic cultures that are prone to structuralist assumptions and stereotypes (e.g., the Indian caste system, Japanese feudal animisms and Arab tribal structures), and serves as an instrument that freezes and supports all the local institutions and symbols of domination in the non-West. Paradoxically, cross-cultural psychiatry in many ways recreates the otherness in other cultures.

The final act of situating local narratives in the non-Western world

I shall define a "*local narrative*" as any conceptual model of psychiatric knowledge that holds two main functions:

(1) Stresses the differences and the non-linearity that set its working theory apart from any artificially synthesized "grand-narratives" of psychiatry, be it universal (e.g., a global state of consumerism, the commoditization of humanity) or cross-cultural (hegemonic cultural monoliths).

(2) Employs the interpretive stories and narrations of local people in the interest of mobilizing their personal power. In this, the "*locals*" are seen as best equipped to negotiate and compromise, if need be, the idea of psychiatry and its political aspiration. The authorship of such narrative is best left to a multidiscipline (scientific, academic, folklorist, mythical, etc.) collection of authors. In this model, psychiatrists are seen mainly as contributors, not as final-sayers, who help service users both medically and politically. The latter happens by assisting the users to verbalize their stories and clearing the way for them to lead the discussion.

In being user led, a local narrative contains the methods in which the users argue for their lives, and interpret their own stories. These methods shall not only reflect their subjectivity, but also the discoursed reality they inherited in their local structures. This idea of *the real* as being both reified by institutional discourse and subjectified at the level of the individual becomes important when considering the problematic of "psychiatric insight." A pitfall that modernity is the belief that people can reach a stage in which full emancipation/insight is possible; where their interpretive stories are true and valid, never acknowledging an element of falsity; and if such an effort is not feasible (due to mental illness and anosognosia), then the determinacy of *Meaning* should revert to the expert person of a psychiatrist.

The response to the modernity framework involves two levels. First, the philosophical understanding of "meaning" (in both epistemology and ontology) is no longer as transparent and holy as once thought. There is indeed a constant deferral of it in every act of understanding, and the only measure that protects us from engaging in infinite discussions (Agger 1998a, b) is our potential human capacity to act *as if* we have pinned down meaning after exhausting ourselves with enquiry. However, while modern psychiatry continues to assume the potential existence of a fully valid and rational "*Real*," postpsychiatry stresses that truth is a constructed social phenomenon and that *dialogue* is what helps us find a temporary anchor point to act *as if* we have fixed meaning.

Second, the risk of falsity of certain local psychiatric narratives is plausible. For example, some locations may revert to premodernity altogether, while others may further the local institutional power structures, leading to what I term as the *detached* local narrative, as in Voodoo. However, I am more swayed to the argument that allowing people to be at once both true and false is a far better method than the alternative of a "policed" global psychiatry. It can be such because postpsychiatry can promote "reflective examination" as a technique used by the locals to constantly examine the line that separates the personal construction of mental illness, from the prefabricated discourse by dominant institutions. A local psychiatric narrative calls on its constituents to inspect their specific conditions of repression and domination, while empowering people with techniques of the self that help people make different statements about themselves using psychiatric terms, linguistic constructions and insights (e.g., I feel depressed or traumatized by my daily living conditions).

I shall end with a reiteration for the need for a certain brand of dialogue, one that sees the reader of this text as a coauthor who instils his or her own meaning on it and reconstruct one's differences into its content. The reader is also invited to examine my values and to marry this essay with the positional context I write from. Thus, I close with a bit of irony derived from the theme of Barthes' *The Death of the Author* (Barthes, 1977): My disappearance as the expert subject of this work is juxtaposed with my affirmed identity as a Syrian-born resident psychiatrist writing in the United States.

Part III. Premodernism, modernism and psychiatry
Ipsit Vahia

Premodernism and medicine

In attempting to think about psychiatry as an emancipatory tool for the new world (here used synonymously with the "developing world"), it is essential to examine the system of psychiatric practice in the developing world. As a discipline, psychiatry has always been a modernist tool. Furthermore, it remains a "Western" ideology. Early Kraepelinian and Freudian theory attempted to provide "scientific" explanations for what had until then been largely perplexing phenomena explained by a myriad of animistic or metaphysical hypotheses.

Ideology predominating in large parts of Asia (India, China, Japan, the Middle East), Africa, and South America tended to be more premodern, and was based on principles of totality, unity, and purpose. It celebrated continuity and community and tended to believe in human lifespan as part of a larger narrative determined by either a "cosmic law" or deified entities. Principles of pantheism and panpsychism were commonly observed in these belief systems (Gier, 2000). In these societies, mental illness was conceptualized and described within this context. Prior to the birth of psychiatry, treatment of mental illness was done by "traditional healing" that consisted of a mixture of religion, mysticism, and rational healing (explanation of illness in the context of moral values, e.g., illness explained as a "divine" punishment for social "misdeeds" and therefore treated by performing penance for such acts believed to be the reason for the illness). Their treatment methods included rituals, use of somatic treatments, and herb-based medications that had to be inhaled, ingested, or massaged to the head, hair, or skin.

The impact of psychiatry on premodern thought is a topic that has not received much attention, largely because modernist thought largely dismisses premodern notions. There is nothing in the medical or psychiatric literature specifically addressing this topic. (A search by this author on the National Library of Medicine's PubMed online database yielded no citations.) Yet, it is impossible to neglect the fact that premodern concepts continue to provide the most prevalent explanations for mental illness in large parts of the world. If psychiatry is truly to serve an emancipatory function, it must acknowledge this ancient way of thinking and its impact on populations. Psychiatry remains an alien concept to large numbers of the world's population that live in rural Asia, Africa, or South America. In attempting to discuss how psychiatry may need to adapt itself to better understand this way of thought, I will largely restrict myself to discussion of psychiatry in India and use it as an example to illustrate some of the conflicts between premodern thought and modern psychiatry.

The conflict between psychiatry and premodernism

Early psychiatric concepts based on Freudian or Jungian theory were found to be of little value in the developing world when applied in their original theoretical forms. Dreams have a symbolic significance in premodern cultures and are believed to be means of communication with metaphysical entities of religious/cultural significance. Also, symptoms suggestive of mental illness were believed to be a consequence of retribution from gods or spirits for wrong deeds done by the individual. An example of the resistance to analytical principles can be found in the Indian culture where the concept of "Karma" or a "cosmic" cycle of action and reaction of individuals is considered the driving force or the principle behind problems encountered by individuals, i.e., a person would be rewarded for good deeds/behavior and punished for misdeeds. Hence, mental illness was believed to be a form of punishment. Based on this principle, activities such as repentance and penance were thought to be the major factors that could alleviate psychic distress.

Therefore, it was not surprising that practitioners of psychoanalysis-based psychiatry found considerable resistance to their Western-based views of mental illness and the mind (Astor *et al.*, 2005). Such a theory, because it largely denied the agency of god, was received with skepticism. Moreover, it was also ineffective for most people because they were unable to comply with many of the basic methods such as interpretation of dreams and free association. In cultures where doctors were classically exalted as persons of higher learning, psychodynamic interpretation of transference, and subsequent development of insight were found to be largely impossible, since therapy came to be seen as discourse (Barthes, 1977). The influence of colonialism is discussed in greater depth elsewhere in this chapter, but it is important to mention here that anticolonial sentiments in largely premodern societies such as India led to much stagnation in the professional and intellectual realms of psychiatry. Astor and colleagues (Astor *et al.*, 2005) describe this phenomenon as it relates to the world of psychoanalysis and also attribute it to the largely racist tones used by early British analysts in precolonial India. The authors show how British analysts created a discourse where the Indian psyche was described as infantile, native and submissive and in need of the enlightened parent represented by the colonizers (Astor *et al.*, 2005). In the aftermath of a political and intellectual climate of this nature, postcolonial rejection of analysis and psychiatry should hardly be surprising.

The biological narrative

Historically, the practice of psychiatry changed dramatically with the advent of medications in the mid twentieth century. The massive paradigm shift that followed – labeled by Cohen (1993) using the term "Biomedicalization" – led to significant changes in the way psychiatry was practiced throughout the world. In the developing world it had the unfortunate, albeit temporary, effect of eliminating any dialog between premodern thought and the contemporary discipline of psychiatry (Foss, 2002). Over the next 40 years, the narrative of biological paradigm has expanded relentlessly. It is important to acknowledge that biomedicalization did make psychiatry and mental health accessible to a larger population.

Medications' ability to assist in the management of acute behavioral disturbance served to revolutionize the practice of psychiatry in both the developed and in much of the developing world. However, this also provided grounds for the assumption that treatment implies causation. While some symptoms can be traced to a direct causative cycle that is reversed or interrupted by medication, in reality the chain of causation is very complex. The incorrectness of this view has become increasingly clear as the search for the "locus of causation" has intensified. Kenneth Kendler (2005), one of the pre-eminent researchers into the genetics of mental illness describes how mental illness can only be accurately formulated using a multidimensional model, and that there is no "locus of causation." Critique of the reductionistic view exists in Western literature dating back to the 1970s. Alexander Luria (1971), a prominent neuroscientist said "The idea that the fundamental processes of psychological life are of a universal ahistorical nature and must be viewed either as a category of the soul or as a natural function of the brain, independent of socio-historical conditions turned out during the course of our investigations to be incorrect."

In the developing world, psychiatry seems to have largely succumbed to the biological narrative. Phillips and colleagues (2003) have suggested that the development of psychiatric nosology and the Fifth Edition of the *Diagnostic and Statistical Manual* (DSM-V) will be based increasingly on biological evidence. Since DSM V is destined to become the international standard for classification of psychiatric illness, this will serve to lend further credence to the notion of universality of psychiatric illness. The American Psychoanalytic Association has recently published the *Psychoanalytic Diagnostic Manual* (PDM Task Force 2006) to serve as "a complement to the DSM" and provide a more narrative-based framework within which to diagnose, label, and conceptualize mental illness. While this is a commendable exercise, it supports the notion stated earlier, that psychiatry tends to neglect the premodern world view.

The marginalizing of premodern thought

An important question to address is why there has been no concerted movement to promote assimilation of some features of premodern thought into contemporary psychiatric thinking. A precedent for this may be found in the historical correspondence between Freud and Girindrashekhar Bose, the founder of the Indian Psychoanalytic Association. They corresponded for 17 years and, by published accounts, enjoyed a warm regard for each other. However, their relationship seems to be marked by a strong mutual ambivalence. Freud tended to disagree with some of Bose's views on theoretical aspects of psychoanalysis, which may have been influenced by Bose's experience working among people in India, with a premodern mindset. Bose's theories, especially on castration anxiety and repression, spoke of concepts like projective identification before their description in the Western literature (Bose 1921; Astor *et al.*, 2005). His theory was strongly influenced by Hindu philosophy, whereas Freud's views involved direct and vociferous questioning of religion (Astor *et al.*, 2005). For example, in his book, *Concept of Repression* (Bose, 1921), Bose describes the theory of the opposite wish, which bears similarity to the philosophical concept of karma (Astor *et al.*, 2005). He states that every wish gives rise to an opposite repressed wish. He uses this to suggest sophisticated ideas of primary feminity and repressed wishes in males to be female. In his correspondence with Freud, he applies this to castration anxiety, and attributes castration anxiety to this wish. He also makes a note of how this wish to be female is unearthed more easily in Indian patients. However, Freud disagreed with Bose and stood by his theories, based on phallic monism (Astor *et al.*, 2005).

Freud seems to have appreciated communication with Bose, and the influence of psychoanalytic thinking in India. Nevertheless, he did not seem to have ever granted him true collegial autonomy (Astor *et al.*, 2005). This rejection of a non-universal approach to analysis seems to have permeated into subsequent theories and the changing paradigms of psychiatry.

In the recent decades, within psychiatry, psychoanalytic thinking has been marginalized by the biological approach to mental illness, and the impact of the environment acting on a biological substrate has been stressed. Thus, one may argue that psychiatry should have been able to assimilate the notion that local environments can impact on both the clinical manifestations and biopsychosocial management of mental illness. If this notion was fully accepted and implemented, then psychiatry would evolve locally rather than globally. Yet this has not happened, and one must ask why? Part of the answer may be found in the economics of worldwide healthcare and the major role that economic concerns have played in shaping models of healthcare delivery and systems of care. In many parts of the developing world, with patent laws coming into force only recently, there is often cutthroat competition among manufacturers of generic medications. The result is a phenomenon where the pharmaceutical industry promotes the prescriber rather than the prescription (Roy, 2004). In addition, developing nations are being seen increasingly as viable populations in which to test new medications, without due consideration for regulation and the ethics of such practices (Gulhati, 2004). There has been a lack of meaningful dialog regarding the impact of such a medication-focused approach on the development of psychiatry in areas where it is often culturally alien.

There is another interesting pattern that has emerged recently. Rural psychiatry in the developing world tends to deal with primarily acute behavioral disturbances. This tends to be the commonest site of interface between psychiatry and premodern thought, but owing to the fact that rural psychiatry operates more along the lines of the medical model, it has not been a tool for influencing society or change in thought. On the other hand, urban psychiatrists who, in clinical practice, tend to encounter issues borne from high-stress lifestyles, related to work and economic demands, have increasingly been finding techniques such as psychoanalysis useful (Astor *et al.*, 2005). This counter-intuitive revival of psychoanalysis in developing world urban environments may provide a breeding ground for new ideas about psychiatry that take premodern ideas into account, although presently this does not seem to be occurring.

There is a small body of literature that describes modification of classic analytical principles to facilitate their application in premodern societies. N. S. Vahia and colleagues (1966, 1973) in the 1960s and 1970s describe techniques based on the classical Hindu philosophical texts of Patanjali, who is considered the founder of yoga. Treatments described in their work include regulated breathing to promote relaxation and the use of meditation as a means of stress relief. These treatments would today be considered part of the spectrum of cognitive behavioral therapies. However, this literature predates Aaron Beck's initial work. The need for this type of work came from the fact that psychoanalytic principles could not be used in treating persons who had a distinctly premodern worldview. This is one of the few examples of a truly assimilative model of psychiatry.

As psychiatry marches towards an even more evidence-based DSM-V era, it is important for the field to remember that it can and must be a much broader social tool than simply a means of treating an illness. The "biomedicalization", although effective for dealing with one aspect of mental illness, tends to ignore external and intra-psychic environments. For psychiatry to succeed as an emancipatory tool, it must understand and assimilate local thought. It is heartening that critiques of psychiatry have identified this need.

Constructive postmodernism

Postmodern thinking and its role in critique of psychiatry have been written about extensively elsewhere in this volume, and more specifically with respect to the developing world, in the second section of this chapter. Such a critique frequently employs deconstructionist theory (Gier, 2000). This involves rejection of not only a modern worldview, but any worldview whatsoever. For the premodern world, thought and existence have been defined solely by a worldview. Eastern cultures have an extremely complex notion of existence that describes the current state as a minor part of a much greater cosmic cycle, and the agency of existence is the soul, rather than the body and the mind. It is easy to see why a deconstructed narrative would lead to insurmountable conflict within such schools of thought, and foster further alienation. It raises the question of whether a postmodern approach is a legitimate approach in such societies. On the other hand, it is hardly practical to suggest a return to an entirely premodern scheme of thought. In addition to the considerable obstacles to implementing such a way of thought and practice, this would mean rejecting many of the contributions of scientific and modern thought, such as technology and universality.

Gier (2000) has used an attractive term "constructive postmodernism" in describing a way of thought that attempts to imbibe the more relevant and influential tenets of premodern thought with modernism. While modernism talks about the transition of reason from mythos to logos, and deconstruction calls for the elimination of reason, Gier describes "constructive postmodernism" as a transition from logos as analytic reason to logos as a synthetic, esthetic, and dynamic reason. Constructive postmodernism attempts to keep intact the modern principles of autonomy and cosmology, but also acknowledges that reason is shaped by culture and values. There is evidence that, throughout the world, the value of premodern/holistic techniques for alleviation of stress is increasingly being recognized. Techniques such as yoga and meditation are now considered lifestyle choices to promote "health." Multiple studies (Nespor, 1994; Walter & Rey, 1999; Krisanaprakornkit *et al.*, 2006) have demonstrated the value of such techniques as adjunctive modalities in the treatment of mental illness.

The academic institution of psychiatry has chosen largely to ignore the value of these "alternative" treatments and has focused its energies and resources on the construction of treatment systems and guidelines that rely on "scientific" proof of their effectiveness in rigorously controlled testing environments. In doing so, psychiatry has attempted to ally itself more closely with the larger establishment of allopathic medicine while minimizing the element of subjectivity in psychiatric illness. This approach is delineated in the American Psychiatric Association's Practice Guidelines (2004), which make no mention of alternative treatments or even psychoanalysis. Were psychiatry to recognize the observable subjective value of including such decidedly premodern techniques, it would provide one example of the field acknowledging the importance of an individual's experience of mental illness, in addition to the biological phenomena that may be responsible for it.

Premodern thinking emphasizes the importance of an individual's subjective inner world. In the developing world, entire systems of traditional medicine (e.g., Ayurveda in India, Unani medicine in Pakistan and the Middle East, Shamanism in North America, ancient Chinese medicine) were founded on holistic principles that sought to modify a persons subjective experience of their illness and frame physical and mental illness in a broader context of society and/or religion. The value of these traditional systems has been largely neglected by psychiatry, but the fact that they remain immensely popular is testimony to their value to the population in this part of the world. Angermeyer and colleagues (2005) reported in a comparative study in different regions of Eastern Europe, that in places with less developed mental health systems, there tended to be a greater reliance on "traditional alternative" treatment methods. While psychiatry questions the actual scientific value of such practice, it would do well to acknowledge some of the principles that make it relevant even today.

Application of Constructive Postmodernism would mean a psychiatry system that expands the scope of its own teaching, and that acknowledges and incorporates local (traditional) systems of care. Such practice would imply collegial rather than adversarial outlook toward other systems of care, and a recognition of the principles that have allowed such practices to remain popular despite the lack of standard empirical evidence. Psychiatry would enrich itself by accepting an external paradigm of health and illness. Such practice would allow psychiatry to be perceived as an expanded local narrative, and as a friendly rather than authoritarian tool for change, while preserving its more modernist aspects.

Several writers have proposed closer collaboration with traditional systems of healthcare as an effective way of doing outreach, especially in more rural parts of the developing world where it may improve accessibility to, and quality of, healthcare (Shaikh & Hatcher, 2005). There are three ways to view this collaboration: (a) that empirical evidence for the utility of traditional methods to improve mental well-being has been, and will continue to be, documented, and consequently they may complement and/or add to the impact of validated Western techniques; (b) that the traditional methods may be viewed as inherent to the culture and that Western techniques will not be countenanced or ever attain effectiveness without the concomitant use of traditional methods; (c) as a combination of (a) and (b). If psychiatry could assimilate such notions, it would emerge as both a medical and social science that bridges the chasm between science and faith, premodernist ideas and modern practice, as well as a scientific discipline that also serves as an emancipatory tool.

Chapter conclusion

Our reckoning of a new psychiatry for a new world began with three perspectives, which we admit are not exhaustive of the possible perspectives. This tripartite discussion was not intended to be a *de novo* synthesis of the debate, but has involved traversing some uncharted territory.

In our initial trajectories the voices with which we were speaking seemed clear and defined our viewpoints on the matter, but, governed by a discourse that is auto-generative of its own critique, the question morphed into what constituencies our voices represented. For example, have we been seduced into the position of colonizer proxies, or did we manage in our mutterings to represent the views of the most disenfranchised? Have we imposed yet another grand narrative, or did we highlight difference in a critique of power and psychiatry? Is an acknowledgment of local historical traditions an answer or a tool, and if so, whom does it serve?

In each of these essays, binary opposites of local vs. global, legitimacy vs. marginality, difference vs. common ground, and cultural reductionism vs. complexity, have emerged. Perhaps, one intersecting point of agreement lies in our own origins in nations of the developing world along with a shared ideal of a liberatory psychiatry. Whether this leads to a manifestation of new world reactionism or whether we elucidate a bona fide discursive position remains a question. We cannot be divorced from our otherness.

In conclusion, it is the authors' position that a fully globalized unified psychiatry is impossible and that a utopian dream of homogeneity is easily transformed into hegemony. *Vive la différence*!

NOTE

(1) The literature has described differing processes of emigration and immigration from a developmental and cultural perspective, but here I have attempted to introduce in the postcolonial the additional notions of political relinquishment, reaction, interacion, and metamorphosis.

REFERENCES

Adorno, T. & Crook, S. (1994). *Adorno*. London: Routledge.

Agger, B. (1998a). From Derrida to difference theory. In *Critical Social Theory: An Introduction*, ed. B. Agger. Boulder: Westview Press, pp. 56–77.

Agger, B. (1998b). Theorizing postmodernity. In *Critical Social Theory: An Introduction*. Boulder: Westview Press, pp. 34–55.

American Psychiatric Association (2004). *Practice Guidelines for the Treatment of Psychiatric Disorders*. Arlington, VA: American Psychiatric Publishing.

Angermeyer, M. C., Breier, P. *et al.* (2005). Public attitudes toward psychiatric treatment. An international comparison. *Social Psychiatry and Psychiatric Epidemiology*, **40**(11), 855–864.

Astor, A., Akhtar, T., Matallana, M. A. *et al.* (2005). Physician migration: views from professionals in Colombia, Nigeria, India, Pakistan and the Philippines. *Social Science Medicine* **61**(12), 2492–2500.

Barthes, R. (1977). The death of the author. In *Image, Music, Text*. New York: Hill and Wang, pp. 142–148.

Blanco, C., Carvalho, C., & Olfson, M. (1999). Practice patterns of international and U.S. medical graduate psychiatrists. *American Journal of Psychiatry*, **156**(3), 445–450.

Bose, G. (1921). *Concept of Repression*. Calcutta: Sri Gouranga Press.

Bracken, P. & Thomas, P. (2001). Postpsychiatry: a new direction for mental health. *British Medical Journal*, **322**, 724–727.

Bracken, P. & Thomas, P. (2005). *Postpsychiatry: Mental Health in a Postmodern World*. New York: Oxford University Press.

Byrd, M. W. & Clayton, L. A. (2000). *An American Health Dilemma: A Medical History of African Americans and the Problem of Race – Beginnings to 1900*. London: Routledge.

Cohen, C. I. (1993). The biomedicalization of psychiatry: a critical overview. *Community Mental Health Journal*, **29**(6), 509–522.

Derrida, J. (1978). *Of Grammatology*. Baltimore: Johns Hopkins University Press.

Derrida, J. (1981). *Dissemination*. Chicago: University of Chicago Press.

Fanon, F. (1966). *The Wretched of the Earth*. New York: Grove Press.

Fanon, F. (1967). *Black Skin White Masks*. New York: Grove Press.

Fett, S. M. (2002). *Working Cures: Healing, Health, and Power on Southern Slave Plantations*. Chapel Hill, NC: University of North Carolina Press.

Force, P. T. (2006). *Psychodynamic Diagnostic Manual*. Silver Spring, MD: Alliance of Psychoanalytic Organizations.

Foss, L. (2002). *The End of Modern Medicine: Biomedical Science under a Microscope*. Albany, NY: SUNY Press.

Foucault, M. (1988). *Madness and Civilization: A History of Insanity in the Age of Reason*. New York: Vintage Books.

Foucault, M. (1989). The end of the monarchy of sex. *Foucault Live: Interviews, 1961–1984*.

Foucault, M. (1990). *The History of Sexuality*. New York: Vintage Books.

Gier, N. F. (2000). Chapter 2. *Spiritual Titanism: Indian, Chinese, and Western Perspectives* Albany, NY: SUNY Press.

Gulhati, C. (2004). Needed: closer scrutiny of clinical trials. *Indian Journal of Medical Ethics*, **12**(1), accessed at www.issuesinmedicalethics.org/1220065html.

Ingleby, D. (1980). Understanding "mental illness". *Critical Psychiatry: The Politics of Mental Health*, ed. D. Ingleby. New York: Pantheon Books, pp. 28–29.

Jenkins, J. H. & Barrett, R. J. (2004). Introduction. In *Schizophrenia, Culture, and Subjectivity*, ed. J. H. Jenkins & R. J. Barrett. New York: Cambridge University Press, pp. 4–5.

Kendler, K. (2005). Toward a philosophical structure for psychiatry. *American Journal of Psychiatry*, **162**(3), 433–440.

Kleinman, A. (1988). *Rethinking Psychiatry: From Cultural Category to Personal Experience*. New York: Free Press.

Krisanaprakornkit, T., Krisanaprakornkit, W. *et al.* (2006). Meditation therapy for anxiety disorders. *Cochrane Database Systems Review*, (1), CD004998.

Kuhn, T. S. (1996). *The Structure of Scientific Revolutions*. Chicago: University of Chicago Press.

Lewis, B. (2000). Psychiatry and postmodern theory. *Journal of Medical Humanities*, **21**(2), 71–84.

Luria, A. (1971). Toward the problem of the historical nature of psychological processes. *International Journal of Psychology*, **6**, 259–272.

Lyotard, J. F. (1984). *The Postmodern Condition: A Report on Knowledge*. Minnesota: University of Minnesota Press.

Mick, S. S., Lee, S., & Wodchis, W. P. (2000). Variations in geographical distribution of foreign and domestically trained physicians in the United States: "safety nets" or "surplus exacerbation"? *Social Science and Medicine*, **50**, 185–202.

Nespor, K. (1994). [Use of yoga in psychiatry]. *Cas Lek Cesk*, **133**(10), 295–297.

Pearlin, L. I., Mullan, J. T., *et al.* (1990). Caregiving and the stress process: an overview of concepts and their measures. *Gerontologist*, **30**(5), 583–594.

Phillips, K. A., First, M. B. & Pincus H. A., eds. (2003). *Advancing DSM: Dilemmas in Psychiatric Diagnosis*. Washington DC: American Psychiatric Association.

Rao, N. R. (2003). Psychiatric workforce: Past legacies, current dilemmas, and future prospects. *Academic Psychiatry*, **27**(4), 238–240.

Rao, N. R., Meinzer, A., Manley, M., & Chagwedera, I. (1998). International medical students' career choice, attitudes toward psychiatry, and emigration to the United States: examples from India and Zimbabwe. *Academic Psychiatry*, **22**, 117–126.

Roberto Fernandez, R. (1973–1974). Caliban: Notes towards a discussion of culture in our America. *The Massachusetts Review*, **XV**.

Roy, N. (2004). Who rules the great Indian drug bazaar? *Indian Journal of Medical Ethics*, **12**(1), 2–3.

Said, E. (2004). *Orientalism*. New York: Vintage Books.

Sandhu, D. P. (2005). Current dilemmas in overseas doctors' training. *Postgraduate Medical Journal*, **81**(952), 79–82.

Saunders, P. (2007). *Alienation and Repatriation. Translating Identity in Caribbean Literature*. Lexington Books.

Schmiedeck, R. A. (1978). The foreign medical graduate and the nature of emigration. *Psychiatric Opinion*, **15**(3), 38–40.

Schwartz, M. J. (2006). *Birthing a Slave: Motherhood and Medicine in the Antebellum South*. Cambridge, MA: Harvard University Press.

Shafqat, S. & Zaidi, A. K. M. (2007). Pakistani physicians and the repatriation equation. *New England Journal of Medicine*, **356**(5), 442–443.

Shaikh, B. & Hatcher, J. (2005). Complementary and alternative medicine in Pakistan: prospects and limitations. *Evidence Based Complementary Alternative Medicine*, **2**(2), 139–142.

Smith, M. R. & Marx, L., eds. (1994). *Does Technology Drive History? The Dilemma of Technological Determinism*. Boston: MIT Press.

Spivak, G. C. (1999). *A Critique of Postcolonial Reason: Toward a History of the Vanishing Present*. Cambridge, MA: Harvard University Press.

Thomas, P. & Bracken, P. (2004). Political psychiatry in practice. *Advances in Psychiatric Treatment*, **10**, 361–370.

Torrey, F. (1973). Cheap labor from poor nations. *American Journal of Psychiatry*, **130**(4), 428–434.

Vahia N. S., D. D., Jeste, D. V., Ravindranath, S., Kapoor, S. N., & Ardhapurkar, I. (1973). Psychophysiologic therapy based on the concepts of Patanjali. A new approach to the treatment of neurotic and psychosomatic disorders. *American Journal of Psychotherapy*, **27**(4), 557–565.

Vahia N. S., V. S., Doongaji, D. R. (1966). Some ancient Indian concepts in the treatment of psychiatric disorders. *British Journal of Psychiatry*, **112**(492), 1089–1096.

Walter, G. & Rey, J. M. (1999). The relevance of herbal treatments for psychiatric practice. *Australia and New Zealand Journal of Psychiatry*, **33**(4), 482–489; discussion 490–493.

Washington, H. A. (2007). *Medical Apartheid: The Dark History of Medical Experimentation on Black Americans from Colonial Times to the Present*. New York: Doubleday.

Weissman, J. (2001). Residents' preferences and preparation for caring for underserved populations. *Journal of Urban Health: Bulletin of the New York Academy of Medicine*, **78**(3), 535–549.

12

Neoliberalism and biopsychiatry: a marriage of convenience

Joanna Moncrieff

Introduction

Since the end of the 1970s there has been a change in the nature and activity of institutional psychiatry. Neuroscience research, which aims to uncover the biological origins of psychiatric disorders, has burgeoned and flourished, gaining a high degree of credibility outside psychiatry as well as within (Cohen, 1993). In addition, psychiatry is no longer confined within the walls of an asylum, ministering to the severely disturbed, but now plies its wares to a widening proportion of the population. Use of psychiatric drugs has risen dramatically. In the UK, for example, prescriptions for antidepressants rose by 235% in the 10 years up to 2002 (National Institute for Clinical Excellence, 2004). In the USA 11% of women and 5% of men now take an antidepressant drug (Stagnitti, 2005). A larger proportion of the general population are now willing to identify themselves as needing psychiatric help and psychiatry has become a more confident and biologically inclined profession.

These developments in psychiatry parallel profound social and economic changes, referred to here as "neoliberalism," that have occurred to varying degrees throughout the world. The question I shall address in this chapter is whether these two developments are related. Does a newly invigorated biologically oriented psychiatry help to create the social and cultural milieu favoured by neoliberal policies? Have those policies in turn helped a certain view of psychiatry to become hegemonic?

Psychiatry and economics

Psychiatry has always had an intimate relationship with economics. The modern institution of psychiatry emerged at the beginning of the industrial revolution and can be seen as a response to the "massive reorganisation of an entire society along market principles" which undermined traditional ways of caring for the sick and

Liberatory Psychiatry: Philosophy, Politics, and Mental Health, ed. Carl I. Cohen and Sami Timimi.
Published by Cambridge University Press. © Cambridge University Press.

non-productive (Scull, 1993). The new system of wage labor required a commitment to work and the problematization of idleness. The insane threatened the order and discipline necessary to foster the work ethic and urge people into the labor market and so the state funded a segregational response to madness in the form of the public asylums (Foucault, 1965; Scull, 1993).

The characterization of psychiatry as an institution of "social control" by social scientists and other theorists is also a comment on its political and economic relations. According to this view, psychiatry is a means of medicalizing difficult social problems, previously often referred to as "deviance," in order to make them amenable to a technical, in this case a medical, solution. In this way, the problems and proposed solutions appear to be uncontentious and evade democratic debate (Conrad, 1992). The particular problems that psychiatry can be thought of as managing are twofold. First, it deals with disturbing behavior, which, for various reasons, is difficult to deal with in the criminal justice system. Second, it helps to police non-engagement in the workforce which is not obviously attributable to physical sickness.

For thinkers on the political right such as libertarian psychiatrist and anti-psychiatrist, Thomas Szasz, psychiatry is a tool of bureaucratic, leftist state-centered regimes, as epitomized by the former communist states, where it was commonly suggested that psychiatry was used to medicalize political dissent. In a truly "liberal" regime with a minimal state, such social problems would be ignored unless they met criteria for the application of criminal sanctions (Szasz, 1994). Thinkers on the left have emphasized how the medicalization of deviance serves the interests of the political status quo in capitalist countries too, but the nature of the specific relation between psychiatry and capitalism has been little elaborated, with some exceptions (Cohen, 1993; Lewis, 2003). This chapter attempts to take this analysis further in the context of the increased virulence of capitalism unleashed by the neoliberal "reforms" of the last few decades. In particular, I will look at the coincidence between the ideology of neoliberalism and the recently popularized psychiatric notion of the "chemical imbalance."

Capitalist economics in the twentieth century

Although neoliberalism has been thoroughly dissected by critical economists and social scientists, under many different names including "late capitalism," "late modernity," "multinational capitalism" and others, it is useful to highlight some of its main features in order to appreciate how modern psychiatric ideas and practices relate to the new world order that it represents. The economic and social trends that are referred to here as neoliberalism date from around 1980. They represent a departure from policies of the preceding period, which was dominated by the rise of the welfare state.

From the beginning of the twentieth century, governments in the developed world were starting to assume responsibility for a widening array of social problems. The dominant Liberal ideology of the nineteenth century, with its emphasis on the minimal state and free trade, started to be replaced by an acceptance of the desirability of state provision and planning. State-funded education and social insurance programs for health and welfare were introduced and in psychiatry the state promoted a more strongly medicalized approach (Unsworth, 1987). This change in political ideology is usually attributed to the increasing power of organized labor, expressed in the Trade Union movement and political parties such as the British Labour Party, and to the linked development of universal suffrage. Parallel with these developments in the West, the Russian revolution brought into being a state which eschewed capitalism entirely and organized itself on the principles of Marxist socialism. The Soviet Union, based on the power of the organized working class and later on the bureaucracy of the Communist Party, undertook planned economic development and wealth redistribution under state control.

After the world recession of the 1930s and the Second World War, the arguments against unrestrained free market capitalism seemed to have won out. The horrors of the depression, the rise of fascism and the war led European electorates to vote in parties that supported the creation of the Welfare State and Keynesian economic policies that prioritized full employment and the alleviation of poverty. Economically, this involved state investment in and protection of national industries via subsidies and trade barriers and the nationalization of key industries in some countries. State provision and funding of health, welfare, and education services were extended. Such policies required that the state maintain tight controls over finance and investment. The state became, in effect, more responsive than it had previously been to the needs of labor in its historic task of regulating and balancing competing interests. For these reasons the period is sometimes referred to as one of state "corporatism," referring to the way in which the state incorporates the interests of both capital and labor.

Throughout the 1950s and 1960s the developed world prospered, with rapid economic growth accompanied by near full employment. Then came a period of economic turmoil in the 1970s, whose origins are still debated. Whatever its causes, it was associated with a decline in profitability, inflation, and industrial unrest (Garland, 2001).

The economics of neoliberalism

The "neoliberal revolution" started as a reaction to the turmoil of the 1970s and was ushered in by Margaret Thatcher in the UK and Ronald Reagan in the USA. It was backed and inspired by international financial institutions such as the IMF and the World Bank, by financial markets, and by multinational corporations, who all perceived themselves to be threatened by inflation and the rising power of labour in the developed world (Newton, 2004). It consisted of a "decisive turn away from the interventionism of the period since 1945" (Newton, 2004, p. 130) and a turn towards the "liberalization" of trade, financial transactions, business, and industry. This was accompanied by a massive transfer of resources from public to private ownership through the sale of nationalized industries and contracting out of services previously provided by the public sector.

The first part of the neoliberal period was characterized by "monetarist" economic policies. These involved increasing interest rates and reducing government spending in order to reduce inflation by engineering recession and producing high unemployment. Although government spending was subsequently increased again, especially spending on defense in the USA, partly as a consequence of the disastrous consequences of monetarism, unemployment has remained high in many parts of the developed world (Fig. 12.1). It is also certainly much higher than official statistics present. In Europe, many more people became classified as "inactive," such as those on incapacity benefits, who might in other circumstances be part of the labor market (Glynn, 2006). Unemployment can be seen as a structural feature of neoliberal economies that acts as a significant depressor of wages, conditions, and Trade Union power.

Trade liberalization and deregulation of foreign financial investment have lead to increased volume of trade and what has been termed the "financialization" of modern economics. This refers to the process by which the mobility and importance of financial capital produces intense pressure to increase short-term

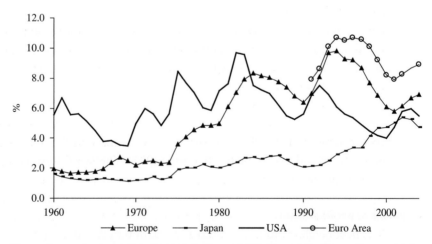

Fig. 12.1.   Unemployment rates, 1960–2004. Data from OECD (reproduced from Glynn, 2006).

profitability and to prioritize this over other activities such as investment in research and development. Domestic financial transactions were also liberalized, including removal of restrictions on credit. This facilitated a demand-led consumer boom fueled by debt especially in the UK and USA, in which consumption is temporarily decoupled from income (Glynn, 2006). In the developed world, the process was accelerated by the Structural Adjustment Programmes imposed on countries by the IMF designed to facilitate debt repayments in return for neoliberal market deregulation, privatization, and welfare and wage cuts (Newton, 2004).

Multinational corporations, including the pharmaceutical companies, have been major beneficiaries of the neoliberal policies that they helped to formulate and promote through institutions like the European and US Round Tables of Industrialists, the International Chamber of Commerce and the Council for International Business. Trade liberalization helped them find new markets for their goods, when demand in the West was reaching saturation. Reduced barriers to investment helped create outlets for over-accumulated capital (Arrighi, 2005). Opening up of investment opportunities in Asia and the developing world provided sources of cheaper labor and benefits in terms of downward pressure on wages and conditions in Western countries. Newton has described the expansion of the multinationals as "one of the most striking features of the world economy during the last decades of the 20th century" (Newton, 2004, p. 159). After the decline of profits in the 1970s, the profitability of multinational corporations has soared since the 1980s. The 200 leading firms profits rose by 362% from 1983 to 1999 (Glynn, 2006; Newton, 2004).

At the other end of the scale, the neoliberal economic revolution has changed the nature of the labor market. As well as chronic unemployment, there has been a transfer of manual employment from relatively well-paid unionized jobs to lower paid, often temporary or part-time jobs with little job security or benefits. This has been accompanied by increased work intensity and poorer working conditions, including less control over how and where work is done. Trade Union membership has declined and ghettos of long-term unemployment have developed especially in inner cities (Glynn, 2006).

The increased inequality that has accompanied neoliberalism has been well documented. There has been increased disparity of wealth both within and between nations since 1980 and the disparity is more visible than ever before due to the spread of the media (Bauman, 1997). The wealth gap has opened up mainly between the richest sections of society and the rest. In the USA real wages for the top 10% of wage earners grew 27% compared with an average growth of 10.2%. Most of the increase in the wages of the top 10% occurred amongst the top 5%, and about two-thirds in the top 1%. Wages for the bottom 10% did not grow at all in real terms (Glynn, 2006). In most OECD countries and the USA wages at

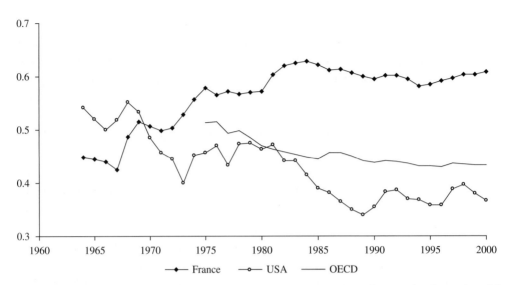

Fig. 12.2.   Minimum wages – ratio of average pay, 1964–2000. Data from OECD (reproduced from Glynn, 2006).

the bottom have declined comparatively (Fig. 12.2, Glynn, 2006, p. 119). The decline in the value of welfare entitlements such as benefits and state pensions have also increased poverty, and Western countries that undertook the strongest neo-liberal changes such as UK and New Zealand saw the greatest growth of poverty between 1980 and 2000 (Glynn, 2006). As well as increased inequality, there has been an increase of absolute poverty in many poorer nations.

In developed countries, increasing inequalities partly reflect the changing nature of the welfare state as governments increasingly identify the interests of capital with the interests of the nation, and no longer attempt to reflect and promote the interests of labor (Abraham & Lewis, 2002; Lasch & Urry, 1987). In liberalizing countries, welfare entitlements have declined despite growing levels of government expenditure. Pensions and benefits have lost value compared to other earnings. State provision, for example, the British NHS, has been scaled down by piecemeal privatization and contracting out services. The rhetoric of "risk" has shifted the burden of responsibility for welfare and health from the state to the individual (Higgs, 1998).

To summarize, neoliberal policies of deregulation and privatization have unleashed the pursuit of profit from the fetters imposed by welfare capitalism and reflect the waning power of labor in relation to capital (Glynn, 2006). Volumes of trade and commercial activity have exploded, demanding ever-growing levels of consumption. The level of exploitation of labor has also grown through the depression of wages, deregulation of working conditions and privatization of the public sector. Neoliberal policies therefore demand increased and highly visible consumption, but also entail the polarization of wealth, power, opportunity, and life experience. They have enriched the already wealthy, empowered multinational corporations and impoverished a significant proportion of the population in both developed and developing countries.

Ideology of neoliberalism

Neoliberal economic policies have been accompanied by an evolving cultural and moral ethos, which is best summed up by a change from broad acceptance of collective virtues such as equality and solidarity to the individual and intertwined values of competition and consumerism. This change was facilitated by the achievements of the preceding period of welfare capitalism. The alleviation of poverty increased equality, weakened social class ties, the significance of gender roles and the nuclear family and fostered individuality, thus producing the conditions necessary for a mass consumer society (Lasch & Urry, 1987). Paradoxically, the possibility of mass consumption encouraged individuals and households to differentiate themselves from each other thus eroding the commitment to equality that had supported the development of consumer society in the first place (Higgs & Gilleard, 2006).

Consumerism is the idea that buying things is a good in itself, independent of their use value. It is rarely promoted blatantly, but it suffuses society through the increasing intrusion of advertising that helps to "universalise the values of the market place" (Newton, 2004, p. 162). The constant message about the benefits of choice and the commercialization of more and more aspects of life also help to make consumerism seem a normal and desirable state. Its pervasiveness can be seen in the way that people are increasingly defined and define themselves through what they buy rather than through what they do. The fact that shopping has become a leisure pursuit and the most popular by recent polls, rather than a means to an end is the cultural expression of consumerism.

Consumerism is closely related to competition because consumerism depends on aspiration and is antithetical to equality. Advertisements and brand labels play on people's desire to acquire greater social status than others. As economist Clive Hamilton points out "the pursuit of wealth is inherently competitive" (Hamilton, 2003, p. 42). The idea of the virtue of competition is used explicitly to justify neoliberal policies. Trade and investment liberalization and privatization of state enterprises are justified on grounds that competition will increase growth and reduce prices for consumers. The depressing effect of competition on workers wages and conditions is presented as a necessary and inevitable byproduct. Being competitive is also presented as an individual virtue and something that should be encouraged throughout the workplace and in other arenas. People who are prepared to push their way to the top are lauded and those who don't wish to are derided. A London underground advertisement for a job agency of a few years ago suggested that anyone who wanted a job for life was contemptible.

Parallel with the modern orgy of consumption in Western nations has been a growing trend towards authoritarian social policies and more pervasive systems of regulation. Society has become obsessed increasingly with law and order, increasingly retributive in its inclinations and more amenable to the idea of public surveillance (Garland, 2001). Rates of imprisonment have increased steadily in most Western countries. In the USA 1.3% of the male population and almost 5% of the black male population are now in prison (Bureau of Justice, 2005). Sentences have got longer and harsher (Garland, 2001). Forced labor in chain gangs has been reintroduced in some southern United States and the death penalty has been extended. Procedural safeguards have been reduced such as the abolition of the "right to silence" and the reduction of jury trials in the UK and antiterrorist legislation passed in the wake of 9/11 allows suspects to be held without trial. Other UK legislation in recent years has introduced child curfews, antisocial behavioral orders, known as "ASBOs," and "parenting orders." Trade Union activities have been curbed radically, along with rights of protest by the Criminal Justice Bill, 1999. There has also been a burgeoning of crime control and prevention measures including CCTV cameras, community policing, and neighborhood watch. Despite the effects of the European human rights legislation in the opposite direction, overall citizens of the UK are subject to more controls on their liberty and less legal protection from wrongful accusation and punishment than they were a few decades ago.

Neoliberalism and psychiatry

The chemical imbalance model

Although psychiatry has always embraced many different theories of human behavior, as a medical specialty, the premise that mental disorders are the result of abnormal biology of some sort has generally predominated.[1] In recent decades this idea has taken the form that psychiatric disorders are due to "chemical imbalances." This "chemical imbalance" theory suggests that psychiatric disorders are caused by abnormalities of neurotransmitter chemicals in the brain (chemicals that are involved in transmission of nerve signals) and that abnormalities of different neurotransmitters cause different psychiatric disorders. What is remarkable about this current theory is its widespread popularity. The combined efforts of the pharmaceutical industry and the psychiatric profession have established the idea as if it were fact among the general population.

I do not have space here to review all the evidence for chemical imbalance models of psychiatric disorders. Elsewhere, others and myself have pointed out that there is very little evidence that there is a link between serotonin (a neuro-transmitter) and depression and that what evidence that exists is contradictory and inconsistent. Leading psychopharmacologists acknowledge that this is the case (Lacasse & Leo, 2005; Moncrieff & Cohen, 2006). The theory that schizophrenia is caused by over-activity of dopamine, another neurotransmitter, was formulated in the 1960s. It was first thought to be supported by evidence of increased dopamine receptors in the brain, until later it was found that this was due to the effects of long-term ingestion of dopamine blocking neuroleptic drugs (Valenstein, 1988). There is no direct evidence that there is any abnormality of overall dopamine concentration in the brains of people with schizophrenia on postmortem. The only tenuous evidence for any dopamine abnormality comes from a motley collection of studies using various indirect measures of dopamine activity levels (Moncrieff, 2006). Some, though not all, of these studies have found an indication of slightly raised dopamine activity levels in people with acute psychosis, rather than schizophrenia *per se*. However, dopamine is known to be raised in many situations, including acute stress, and it may be something non-specific like increased stress or arousal that explains these findings rather than a specific link with psychosis or schizophrenia.

Despite the tenuous nature of the evidence, the chemical imbalance notion of psychiatric disorders is promoted widely by the psychiatric profession and by pharmaceutical advertising, as illustrated by the quotations in Table 12.1. This publicity has been successful in persuading people in the mental health field and the general public that psychiatric disorders are known to be caused by abnormal-ities in brain chemicals. Even when psychiatrists admit that there is no conclusive evidence for this supposition, they still maintain that the idea of the chemical imbalance is a "reasonable shorthand for expressing that this is a chemically or brain based problem and that medications help to normalise function" (Meek, 2006, p. 754).

In questioning the notion that psychiatric disorders can be attributed to bio-logical dysfunction, I am not denying that mental events are likely to be accom-panied by biological changes. Like ordinary mental and physical activity, psychiatric disturbance will be mirrored in the brain. However, unlike neuro-logical disorders, there is no evidence as yet that there are discrete and specific anatomical or functional defects associated with the vast majority of what we label as mental illness.

This chapter suggests there are political reasons that may explain why the chemical imbalance model has been so successful despite the lack of supporting evidence. My argument is that the chemical imbalance idea of psychiatric prob-lems facilitates the neoliberal project and that features of neoliberalism in turn strengthen the chemical imbalance theory and biopsychiatry more generally. The

Table 12.1. Examples of promotion of the chemical imbalance model of emotional distress by psychiatric institutions and the pharmaceutical industry

Source	Quotation
British Royal College of Psychiatrists (Royal College of Psychiatrists, 2006)	"two … neurotransmitters (serotonin and noradrenalin) are particularly affected" in depression and "we think that antidepressants work by increasing the activity of certain chemicals in our brains called neurotransmitters."
American Psychiatric Association (American Psychiatric Association, 2005)	"antidepressants may be prescribed to correct imbalances in the levels of chemicals in the brain."
British Royal College of Psychiatrists (Royal College of Psychiatrists, 2004)	Psychosis and schizophrenia involve "an imbalance in brain chemistry"
American Psychiatric Association (American Psychiatric Association, 1996)	Antipsychotic medications "help bring biochemical imbalances closer to normal."
An early advertisement for Prozac quoted by Eliot Valenstein (Valenstein, 1988) (p. 181).	"like arthritis or diabetes, depression is a physical illness."
A leaflet produced in 1996 by the consortium called "America's Pharmaceutical Research Companies" quoted by Eliot Valenstein (Valenstein, 1988) (p. 182)	"Today scientists know that many people suffering from mental illnesses have imbalances in the way their brains metabolise certain chemicals called neurotransmitters. Too much or too little of these chemicals may result in depression, anxiety or other emotional or physical disorders. This knowledge has allowed pharmaceutical company researchers to develop medicines that can alter the way in which the brain produces, stores and releases neurotransmitter chemicals, thereby alleviating the symptoms of some mental illnesses."
Pfizer's website suggested (Pfizer, 2006)	"No one knows the exact causes of schizophrenia …. Imbalances of certain chemicals in the brain are thought to lead to symptoms of the illness. Medicine plays a key role in balancing these chemicals."
Eli Lilly (Eli Lilly, 2006)	"a growing amount of evidence supports the view that people with depression have an imbalance of the brain's neurotransmitters … many scientists believe that an imbalance in serotonin may be an important factor in the development and severity of depression."

pharmaceutical industry has played a key role in these processes by disseminating the theory of the chemical imbalance in a way that could probably never have been achieved by psychiatry alone.

The pharmaceutical industry

Although the biological model of psychiatric distress has dominated mainstream psychiatry for much of its history (Scull, 1994), until recently, it was generally restricted to people with severe psychiatric problems. The psychiatric profession lacked the capacity and maybe the will to spread the model much wider. The activities of the pharmaceutical industry from the early 1990s have changed this situation dramatically. The industry mounted and funded huge promotional campaigns that have greatly expanded the application of the idea of the chemical imbalance. The United Kingdom Defeat Depression Campaign, run by the Royal College of Psychiatrists and General Practitioners but part funded by Eli Lilly (makers of Prozac), is a good example, and typical of other national depression campaigns. The campaign message was that depression was an under-recognized problem and it sought to persuade GPs that they should diagnose more people as depressed and prescribe more antidepressants. The campaign literature suggested that 5% of the population suffer from depression at any one time and that around 20% of GP attenders have symptoms of depression, with half of these needing treatment (Paykel & Priest, 1992). As a result of this campaign and more general marketing, use of antidepressants soared. Many more people came to see their problems as resulting from a medical disease, a chemical imbalance, that drugs could help correct. People came to view themselves as "neurochemical selves," as Nikolas Rose has recently put it (Rose, 2004).

In the United States drug companies have launched other disease awareness campaigns. In some of these, such as the "Social Anxiety Disorder" campaign mounted by SmithKline, the companies concerned took a minor diagnostic category from the American Psychiatric Association's Diagnostic and Statistical Manual (DSM), and set out to present it as a real and uncontested entity, to demonstrate how prevalent it was and that it required treatment. The fact that the meaning of the condition is uncertain, and that the DSM was formed by professional haggling over the validity of disorders (Kirk & Kutchins, 1997), is unknown to most of the audience. The latest diagnoses being invented and popularized are "compulsive buying disorder" and "intermittent explosive disorder." Research on both these "conditions" has been funded by a number of drug companies. Companies have also funded campaigns to extend the diagnosis and drug treatment of childhood behavioral problems, such as those diagnosed as attention deficit hyperactivity disorder (ADHD), and have successfully medicalized psychiatric disorders that were previously not thought to be amenable to drug treatment such as post-traumatic stress disorder, bulimia, and substance misuse. The success of their activities can be measured by the co-operation of the academic psychiatric community as well as the response of the media and the wider population. Drug company-funded research on "intermittent explosive disorder" was conducted at Harvard University and published by a Harvard-based professor (Kessler *et al.*, 2006). Research on "compulsive buying disorder" is being conducted at Stanford University. There is no hint in the medical literature that these conditions might be controversial. A published paper entitled "The psychopharmacology of compulsive buying" (Bullock & Koran, 2003) illustrates the extent of penetration of a biochemical conception of these areas. The general media report the results of this research, often not realizing or reporting that it was conceived and funded by drug companies.

The pharmaceutical industry has been phenomenally successful in the period of neoliberalism. Since the early 1980s its profitability relative to other commercial sectors has risen substantially (*Public Citizen*, 2002). By 2001, US pharmaceutical firms' profits averaged 18.5% of revenue compared with 2.2% for the rest of the Fortune 500 companies (Fig. 12.3). It has become increasingly influential too. It conducts or funds a substantial proportion of drug research. It provides much medical journal funding through advertising and supplements and it donates funding to medical associations such as the American Psychiatric Association. Governments in the United States and New Zealand brought in legislation in the 1990s allowing direct to consumer advertising of drugs. In other countries drug companies are allowed to conduct disease awareness campaigns aimed at the general public. The industry provides funding to sympathetic

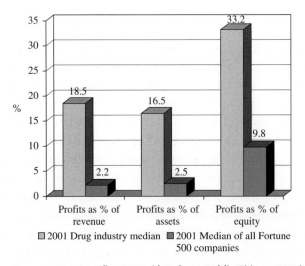

Fig. 12.3.   Drug company profits, 2001 (data from *Public Citizen*, 2002).

patient and carer groups and it provides an increasing proportion of drug regulatory agency fees, such as the US Food and Drug Administration. This reduces the independence of these agencies and increasing numbers of drug withdrawals, suggests that the drug regulation process has become less effective as a result (Abraham & Davis, 2005). In the United States the pharmaceutical industry has a large number of political lobbyists and makes substantial contributions to political party funds, mostly the Republicans. In the UK, the industry is also increasingly influential over government policy (National Institute for Mental Health England (NIMHE) and Association of British Pharmaceutical Industry (APBI) Partnership, 2002) and there is little evidence of consideration of the possible conflicts between public interests and commercial ones. Although public concern was such that a House of Commons Select Committee was recently set up to investigate the undue influence of the pharmaceutical industry, and issued a report which was very critical of its actions and government collusion, the report has not resulted in any policy initiative (House of Commons Health Committee, 2005).

The increasing power of the pharmaceutical industry illustrates the changing balance between labor and capital that has been achieved by neoliberal policies. The industry can be seen as a beneficiary of neoliberal policies that have made governments more responsive to the interests of multinational corporations (Abraham & Lewis, 2002). Its activities can also be seen as part of the driving force behind neoliberalism, both in its aggressive campaigns to forge new markets, and in its increasing influence on political life, which sets a precedent for continuing transfer of authority from governments to the corporations (Hamilton, 2003).

Consumerism, competition, and the chemical imbalance model

The chemical imbalance model of human distress is a perfect companion to the ideology of consumerism and helps the neoliberal project in various ways. Consumerism necessarily involves aspiration, and the precondition of aspiration is dissatisfaction. Marketing campaigns set out first to "create a dissatisfaction in the market place," in order to persuade consumers that they need the company's product (Pharmaceutical Marketing, 2000). Economist Clive Hamilton has described "a permanent state of unfulfilled desire" as being the "essential state for consumers in modern capitalism" (Hamilton, 2003, p. 87).

The idea that there is an ideal chemical balance, which has no foundation in science, suggests that there is an ideal state of neurochemical balance against which everyone can be measured and can measure him- or herself. Thus it plants the seeds of doubt in people's minds. Are our brains perfectly chemically balanced? Do we not need some fine-tuning to reach a state of ideal mental functioning? Maybe we are missing out on something if we do not try the effects of Prozac? Just as the pervasive advertising of goods makes people feel discontent with their material possessions, the promotion of the chemical imbalance idea has made people discontent with themselves. People are encouraged to aspire to be something different from their current self, in their emotional lives as well as in their material lives. Difficulties, imperfection, mundanity should not be tolerated. We should all expect to lead permanently exciting, successful, and perfectly "balanced" lives. If we don't, we are encouraged to feel that we have settled for second best and will somehow be unfulfilled. Individual consumption, whether of prescribed drugs, alternative medicines, or therapy, is presented as the means of achieving this ideal state. However, as for material acquisitions, the act of consumption does not dispel the dissatisfaction, but confirms the need to consume more. "No amount of acquisitions and exciting sensations is ever likely to bring satisfaction" says Bauman (Bauman, 1997, p. 40). The taking of medication only confirms feelings of inadequacy and anxiety; leading people to feel they need more drugs each time they experience further difficulties or anxieties. As Hamilton notes, the effects of consumerism are to "reinforce the insidious sense that something is missing, to create the conditions for serial disappointment, yet to sustain hope that more of what has so far failed will ultimately succeed" (Hamilton, 2003, p. 89).

In this way, discontent is transformed into a commercial opportunity – it is commodified. It has been categorized into different types. You may now have depression, social anxiety disorder, PTSD, etc. or a combination of these and others. And it has been "reified," that is, as situations come to be seen as mental disorders they are characterized independently of the history of the individual sufferer and his or her social context. And, where levels of distress are inadequate to present a commercial opportunity, they can be inflated by careful advertising. Human distress can now be marketed in its various new forms along with a purchasable and profitable "solution." The fact that the solution never satisfies means that the cycle of consumption is perpetuated and escalated, in a vain attempt to chase the elusive ideal emotional state.

It is for the real losers of neoliberalism that the medicalization of discontent is most significant and most prevalent. Rising inequality, falling social mobility (Glynn, 2006), and the public parade of wealth presented by the media's obsession with celebrity, mean that expectations are pushed up at the same time as the chance of achieving relative social progress falls. This gives rise to a widening gulf between expectations and reality, especially for the poor (Monbiot, 2006). The modern epidemic of psychological disorders in children and adults in Western nations is concentrated among the poor. It is a clear instance of the medicalization of political discontent. But this situation is not overtly coercive. This view has not been imposed on people by direct force. People themselves have come to see their problems as individual problems, emanating from their brain chemistry. Usually, no one demands that they seek medical help, there simply appears to be no other obvious way to conceive of their problems or any other source of help.

As well as medicalizing discontent, the pathological self-dissatisfaction suggested by the idea that our behavior and problems are due to a brain disorder helps to produce a state of mind that accepts the changing nature of working life wrought by neoliberal policies. Feelings of anxiety and personal inadequacy make people vulnerable. People are more susceptible to the promotion of the value of competition and to the increasing demands and declining conditions and security of modern day work. Therefore, keeping people in a perpetual state of anxiety and self-doubt is useful in communities in which access to well paid work has been destroyed and low-paid "flexible" work and unemployment are the only alternatives. Self-doubt is a state of mind that is compatible with a placid and unchallenging workforce and undermines people's abilities to see problems and their solutions in collective terms. People are more likely to locate the source of their troubles in themselves, and see their doctor, than to look at their working environment and see the Trade Union.

The fact that large numbers of people have been persuaded to "recode their moods and their ills in terms of the functioning of their brain chemicals" (Rose, 2004, p. 28) means that society as a whole is increasingly deaf to social and political critique. Instead of highlighting the destructive effects of unemployment and low wage labor, we diagnose people as depressed and sign them off sick. Instead of recognizing the difficulties of imposing a certain sort of schooling on naturally lively boys, we pathologize the individual children and try and drug them into conformity (Timimi, 2005). Instead of acknowledging the potentially devastating effects of international conflicts, we tell people they have Post Traumatic Stress Disorder (PTSD) and prescribe them pills to mollify their anger (Summerfield, 2001). This is not to imply that social action can eliminate madness and distress. They are part of the human condition. But medicalizing them obstructs a political response to the social consequences of life in neoliberal societies. As psychiatrist Bradley Lewis has put it: "If we plug human suffering, misery and sadness into the calculus of bioscience, there is no need to make changes in the social order, instead, we only need to jumpstart some neurotransmitters" (Lewis, 2003, p. 56).

Because it blends well with the prevailing cultural value of consumerism, the medicalization of discontent is difficult to challenge, which is why conditions as absurd as "compulsive shopping" can become respected academic pursuits. It therefore constitutes a particularly effective form of social control, helping to obscure the consequences of neoliberalism and suppress possible resistance to them.

Authoritarian psychiatry

Social scientists have suggested that the apparently contradictory correlation of liberalizing economic polices with authoritarian social policies results from the need to control the victims of neoliberal policies and assuage the fear of the rich and the middle classes (Garland, 2001). Poverty has been transformed from a social problem to individual failure and the consequences of failure have been intensified, as have the rewards of success. To sustain mass demand, the "seductive" message of the benefits of lavish consumption must be transmitted "in every direction and addressed indiscriminately to those who will listen" (Bauman, 1997, p. 40). This creates an incentive to criminal behavior among those who cannot legitimately afford such commodities. The urban underclass, or the "outcasts of a thriving society of seduced consumers," frequently resort to theft and consumption of drugs "the poor man's (and illegal) substitutes for the rich man's (and legal) tools of consumer ecstasy" (Bauman, 1997, p. 61). Whereas welfare politics defined poverty as a collective problem requiring a political solution in the form of welfare, neoliberal societies have redefined the problem as an individual problem of crim-inality, requiring a punitive response. In Bauman's words "The prisons now fully and truly deputise for the fading welfare institutions" (Bauman, 1997, p. 41).

Psychiatry was founded on the incarceration of the severely disturbed, and neo-liberal capitalism has expanded its coercive function along with, and alongside, the prison system. The chemical imbalance model promotes a coercive as well as a consumerist response to disturbance through its suggestion that there is such a thing as a "normal" brain. The idea of the "normal" abolishes the tolerance of difference and diversity. Instead of accepting that human beings have an infinite variety of propensities and abilities, the idea suggests that people who don't conform to some theoretical ideal state need to be chemically corrected.

In the UK, the use of the Mental Health Act has increased dramatically since the 1980s, both in absolute terms, and relative to non-compulsory admissions (Fig. 12.4) (Wall et al., 1999). Several additions were made to the legislation during the 1990s that allowed patients discharged from hospital to be kept under closer surveillance and control than before. A supervision register was introduced for patients thought to present risks of aggression, self-harm or self-neglect and a "supervised discharge" order was created to enable restrictions to be placed on people at discharge including the requirement to take medication and accept professional supervision. Proposals to reform the Mental Health Act have focused on facilitating further compulsory community treatment, as well as incarceration of people with personality disorders who are not thought to be treatable. The government, at one stage, proposed scrapping the exclusion clause for people with drug and alcohol problems, possibly demonstrating within government a desire for the psychiatric establishment to undertake the policing of public drunkenness and homelessness.

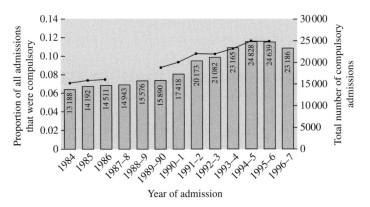

Fig. 12.4.   Admissions to psychiatric hospital under Mental Health Act 1983, 1984–1997 (data from Wall *et al.*, 1999).

The proposals have been justified by rhetoric of increasing access to care and *treatment*. In particular it is sometimes stated by those who advocate increasing controls over psychiatric patients that new psychiatric drugs have made the treatment of mental disorder much more effective and less problematic than it used to be (Rethink *et al.*, 2006).[2] Thus, the idea that mental disorder is due to a potentially identifiable biological abnormality that needs correcting and if possible annihilating, is the rationale for a policy of increasing incarceration of the mentally disturbed and disturbing.

Bauman writes of how the materialistic values of society, coupled with increasing inequality, produce an inevitable pull towards crime (Bauman, 1997). But there is also an inevitable impetus to madness. A society that is increasingly socially fragmented and divided, where the gulf between success and failure seems so large, where the only option open to many is highly demanding and low paid work, where the only cheap and simple route to carelessness is through drugs, is likely to make people particularly vulnerable to mental disintegration in its many forms. It has long been known that urban life and social deprivation are associated with high levels of mental disorder. Neoliberal economic policies are likely to further increase their pathogenic effects. By medicalizing these effects, psychiatry helps to obscure their political origin. It is also being used to provide a punitive response to these consequences of neoliberal policies.

Conclusions

Since the 1980s there has been a radical shift in economic and social policy away from state intervention in the market to facilitate redistribution of wealth, towards the unleashing of untrammelled market forces. It has involved the transfer of power from labor to capital, which has resulted in increased inequality. The philosophy associated with these policies extols the virtues of consumerism and competition. However, there is also a trend towards increasingly authoritarian policies and harsh punishments for those who challenge the system or fail to meet its demands. Psychiatry as an institution of social control, as it was conceived of by social critics of the 1960s and 1970s, is well placed to aid and abet the neoliberal agenda. The chemical imbalance model of mental disorder has allowed discontent to be medicalized, and this has been achieved on an unprecedented scale by the activities of an increasingly unfettered multinational pharmaceutical industry. This mode of medicalization allows emotional distress to be commodified and marketed, which is perfectly consistent with the ideology of consumerism. The promotion of a narrowly biological model of mental disorder also allows the introduction of increasing controls over psychiatric patients in the name of increasing access to medical treatment.

But just as welfare capitalism sowed the seeds of its demise, neoliberalism appears to breed its own resistance. A political challenge to the liberalizing policies of the French government has been witnessed in student protests and industrial unrest. In South America, Hugo Chavez in Venezuala and more lately Evo Morales in Bolivia have defied the international neoliberal community by nationalizing industries, redistributing wealth and creating state-funded health and education programs. The international anticapitalist movement has managed to turn meetings of the World Trade Organization and G7/G8[3] summits into siege-like affairs, conducted behind armored defences. Some of the most radical neoliberal policies, such as the Multilateral Agreement on Investment, proposed by organizations of leading multinational corporations, were defeated by the reluctance of national governments, showing that, in Newton's words "globalisation was not inevitable, and that not just its own flaws, but politics, could impose a limit on how far it could go" (Newton, 2004, p. 172).

Despite its concurrence with some neoliberal ideals and its lack of economic analysis, postmodernism, in its rejection of the certainties and structures of modernism, opened up spaces for the expression of numerous points of view, including many that were previously unheard. Some authors have talked of a transformation from passive to active citizenship, encouraged by the erosion of the certainties of the welfare state (Abraham & Lewis, 2002). New social movements have arisen, including numerous "consumer" groups. These politically active, "reflexive" groups have been at the forefront of monitoring and criticizing the activities and influence of multinational companies and government bodies as well as challenging the privilege and authority of professionals. Health service consumer groups supported the introduction of a Medicines Information Bill into the United Kingdom parliament in the 1990s, which would have established public access to information on safety and efficacy of drugs. The Bill was defeated after the drug companies threatened to withdraw their business form the UK (Abraham & Lewis, 2002). However, consumer pressure did finally persuade drug companies to publish figures for suicidal behavior in antidepressant trials in 2006 (GlaxoSmithKline, 2006). Within the medical profession and the wider public as well, there has been mounting concern about the influence of the pharmaceutical industry, with numerous books now charting its influence and misdemeanors.

Earlier critics focused on the coercive nature of psychiatry. This aspect has been strengthened over recent years, in line with increasingly authoritarian policies in other areas of social life. But the most significant development in psychiatry has been the willing co-option of a large proportion of the population to the idea that they are mentally imperfect and require treatment, usually in the form of drugs. Modern-day psychiatry has therefore become a focus of consumerist aspiration and in the process has turned people's discontent away from society and into themselves. The social catastrophe produced by neoliberal policies has been washed away and forgotten in the language of individual distress. In this sense biopsychiatry acts to support the whole neoliberal project, by redirecting potential disaffection and opposition. The relation between psychiatry and economics is thus more entangled than ever. The waning of neoliberal hegemony may therefore be a potential opportunity at which to develop an alternative vision of psychiatry.

NOTES

(1) The influence of psychoanalysis in the USA in the twentieth century is an important exception, but it was incorporated by the medical establishment in a way that never fundamentally challenged a biomedical perspective.

(2) This is despite the fact that research does not demonstrate that the new drugs are more effective than the older ones, and it is becoming increasingly apparent that their side effects are just as severe, albeit, different.

(3) G7/G8 stands for Group of 7 or 8 leading industrial nations.

REFERENCES

Abraham, J. & Davis, C. (2005). A comparative analysis of drug safety withdrawals in the UK and the US (1971–1992): implications for current regulatory thinking and policy. *Social Science and Medicine*, **61**, 881–892.

Abraham, J. & Lewis, G. (2002). Citizenship, medical expertise and the capitalist regulatory state in Europe. *Sociology*, **36**, 67–88.

American Psychiatric Association (1996). Schizophrenia. Pamphlet.

American Psychiatric Association (2005). Let's talk facts about depression. Pamphlet.

Arrighi, G. (2005). Hegemony unravelling- 1. *New Left Review*, March–April, 23–80.

Bauman, Z. (1997). *Postmodernity and its Discontents*. Cambridge: Polity Press.

Bullock, K. & Koran, L. (2003). Psychopharmacology of compulsive buying. *Drugs Today (Barc.)*, **39**, 695–700.

Bureau of Justice 2005, *Statistics, June 2004*. Washington, DC: Bureau of Justice.

Cohen, C. I. (1993). The biomedicalization of psychiatry: a critical overview. *Community Mental Health Journal*, **29** (6), 509–521.

Conrad, P. (1992). Medicalisation and social control. *Annual Review of Sociology*, **18**, 209–232.

Eli Lilly (2006). Eli Lilly website. 6-2-2006. Eli Lilly. Ref Type: Electronic Citation.

Foucault, M. (1965). *Madness and Civilisation*. New York: Random House Inc.

Garland, D. (2001). *The Culture of Control*. Oxford: Oxford University Press.

GlaxoSmithKline (2006). Important prescribing information. Letter to healthcare professionals. GlaxoSmithKline. 2006. Electronic Citation.

Glynn, A. (2006). *Capitalism Unleashed*. Oxford: Oxford University Press.

Hamilton, C. (2003). *Growth Fetish*. Crow's Nest Australia: Allen & Unwin.

Higgs, P. (1998). Risk, governmentality and the reconceptualisation of citizenship. In *Modernity, Medicine and Health*, ed. G. Scambler & P. Higgs. London: Routledge.

Higgs, P. & Gilleard, C. (2006). Departing the margins. Social class and later life in a second modernity. *Journal of Sociology*, **42**, 219–241.

House of Commons Health Committee (2005). *The Influence of the Pharmaceutical Industry*. London: Stationery Office Ltd.

Kessler, R. C., Coccaro, E. F., Fava, M., Jaeger, S., Jin, R., & Walters, E. (2006). The prevalence and correlates of DSM-IV intermittent explosive disorder in the National Comorbidity Survey Replication. *Archives of General Psychiatry*, **63**, (6), 669–678.

Kirk, H. & Kutchins, S. A. (1997). *Making Us Crazy*. New York: Free Press.

Lacasse, J. R. & Leo, J. (2005). Serotonin and depression: a disconnect between the advertisements and the scientific literature, *PLoS.Medicine*, **2**, (12), e392.

Lasch, S. & Urry, J. (1987). *The End of Organised Capitalism*. Madison: University of Wisconsin Press.

Lewis, B. E. (2003). Prozac and the post-human politics of cyborgs. *Journal of Medical Humanities*, **24**, (1/2), 49–63.

Meek, C. (2006). SSRI. *Canadian Medical Association Journal News*, **174**[6], 754.

Monbiot, G. (2006). We are making our children ill with unrealistic expectations. *Guardian*, 27–6–2006. Manchester.

Moncrieff, J. (2006). The dopamine hypothesis of schizophrenia and psychosis: where does the evidence stand now? *in press*.

Moncrieff, J. & Cohen, D. (2006). Do antidepressants cure or create abnormal brain states? *PLoS.Medicine*, **3**, (7), e240.

National Institute for Clinical Excellence (2004). *Depression: Management of Depression in Primary and Secondary Care. Clinical Practice Guideline Number 23*. London: National Institute for Clinical Excellence.

National Institute for Mental Health England (NIMHE) and Association of British Pharmaceutical Industry (APBI) Partnership (2002). *Meeting of Minds.*

Newton, S. (2004). *The Global Economy 1944–2000.* London: Arnold.

Paykel, E. S. & Priest, R. G. (1992). Recognition and management of depression in general practice: consensus statement, *British Medical Journal,* **305**, (6863), 1198–1202.

Pfizer (2006). Pfizer website. 6–2–2006. Pfizer. Ref Type: Electronic Citation.

Pharmaceutical Marketing (2000). Practical Guides: Medical education parts I and II. Pharmaceutical Marketing.

Public Citizen (2002). *America's Other Drug Problem: A Briefing Book on the Prescription Drug Debate.* Public Citizen.

Rethink, Sane, & Zito Trust (2006). *Behind Closed Doors.* Rethink.

Rose, N. (2004). Becoming neurochemical selves. In *Biotechnology, Commerce and Civil Society.* ed., N. Stehr. New Brunswick, NJ: Transaction Publishers. pp. 89–128.

Royal College of Psychiatrists. (2004). *Mental health and growing up.* Pamphlet

Royal College of Psychiatrists. (2006). *Antidepressants.* Pamphlet

Scull, A. (1993). *The Most Solitary of Afflictions.* New Haven.

Scull, A. (1994). Somatic treatments and the historiography of psychiatry. *History of Psychiatry,* **5**, 1–12.

Stagnitti, M. (2005). *Antidepressant Use in the US Civilian Non-Institutionalised Population, 2002. Statistical Brief #77.* Rockville, MD: Medical Expenditure Panel Agency for Healthcare Research and Quality.

Summerfield, D. (2001). The invention of post-traumatic stress disorder and the social usefulness of a psychiatric category, *British Medical Journal,* **322**, (7278), 95–98.

Szasz, T. (1994). *Cruel Compassion. Psychiatric Control of Society's Unwanted.* New York: John Wiley & Sons.

Timimi, S. (2005). *Naughty Boys. Antisocial Behaviour, ADHD and the Role of Culture.* London: Palgrave Macmillan.

Unsworth, C. (1987). *The Politics of Mental Health Legislation.* Oxford: Oxford University Press.

Valenstein, E. (1988). *Blaming the Brain.* New York: Free Press.

Wall, S., Hotopf, M., Wessely, S., & Churchill, R. (1999). Trends in the use of the Mental Health Act: England, 1984–96. *British Medical Journal,* **318**, (7197), 1520–1521.

13

Psychoanalysis and social change: the Latin American experience

Astrid Rusquellas

Introduction: Freud, Marx and progressive psychoanalytic theory

Throughout the twentieth century, Leftist psychoanalysts and psychoanalytically inclined Marxists have tried to achieve some sort of a synthesis between psychoanalysis and Marxism. Thus, through the years the confusing term of "Freudo-Marxism" has popped up periodically. The reality is that no authors ever recognized themselves as a participant in a Freudo-Marxist current. As Alejandro Vainer put it, "Freudo-Marxism never existed."

In Latin America, when someone is accused of being a Freudo-Marxist, he or she is seen as somebody who is theoretically sloppy; who establishes a cross of little theoretical and clinical consistency between Marxism and psychoanalysis. Supposedly, in that mélange, patients get poorly psychoanalyzed and badly politicized. From that point of view, a Freudo-Marxist is somebody that you would not want to introduce as your associate to your colleagues in the intellectual and scientific fields. Freudo-Marxist is a name that was utilized to disqualify Marxist psychoanalysts.

Leon Rozitchner is a philosopher who has contributed brilliant insights to the problem of articulating psychoanalysis and Marxism. In his classic work, *Freud and the Problem of Power*, Rozitchner analyzes the internalization of power in the formation of subjectivity according to Freud and Marx:

When Freud finds that the fortress with which Power contains us is not outside, but imprisoning us from inside ourselves, installed in the domain so called "interior", organizing with its apparatus of domination, our own psychic apparatus, is he not showing us the ways for an analysis of the problem of domination and an analysis of Power that necessarily has to involve the subject as a locus where this resides and debates with itself? Freud opens the paths and attempts, in a way perhaps precarious, but at the same time precise, to render the historical determination in subjectivity. He shows the manner in which history is present articulating and organizing the psychic apparatus where society has internalized itself to the point in which the

Liberatory Psychiatry: Philosophy, Politics, and Mental Health, ed. Carl I. Cohen and Sami Timimi. Published by Cambridge University Press. © Cambridge University Press.

subject is congruently integrated inside the re-production of the system that produced it. This psychic apparatus is nothing but the extreme pole of the projection and internalization of social structure in the subjective sphere. (Rozitchner, 1982, p. 14)

When we talk about the liberatory goals of psychiatry and we mention Pinel we need to understand that Foucault among others has pointed out to another movement implicit in traditional psychiatry and that is the adaptational effect of psychiatry and psychotherapy. Rozitchner contends that:

In reality this "liberalization" is inscribed in the discovery of a technique more important, effective, and subtle than chains; a technique that is going to characterize on the other hand, the development of all other institutions and which will be linked with the discovery of subjectivity as the locus of implantation of exterior domination . . . Freud understood this and was critical of the classical image of liberatory psychiatry; he understood this external domination and showed that within the subjective field persist the categories present in the repressive social order as descriptive categories of its comprehension and functioning. Many of the explanations that Freud develops are based in models of the repressive social institutions that had been internalized: the police, the military, religion, economy, and the family. All that we see in action outside permits the theoretical construction of a subjective organization inside, which determines us as a replica of the social organization. Freud shows us a psychology, which he includes in the historical sciences. In other words he constitutes the individual as a locus where the sense of history is verified and debated and without which behavior becomes insignificant. (Rozitchner, 1982, p. 23)

From the very beginning of psychoanalysis, there was a significant group of Freud's disciples who explored the radical potential of psychoanalytic theory. They endeavored in their theoretical writings and clinical practice, to offer an alternative to the prevailing interpretation of Freud as conservative. In fact, they thought that in Freud's work there were elements of a radical, political and sexual philosophy, which could undermine the established culture.

I will mention here the teachings of Marie Langer, who happened to be my training analyst, because she belonged both to the old world of European Freudian Left, and to the newer Psychoanalytic Left in Latin America. She was a leader of a psychoanalytic movement committed to social change that took place in Latin America in the 1960s, 1970s, and 1980s. At the end of this chapter we will refer to the present contributions of this movement in Argentina, where psychoanalysts have helped, within the specificity of their discipline, the struggles of workers occupying more than 600 factories.

When Marie Langer was asked (in an interview reproduced in her autobiography, *From Vienna to Managua*) about what would be scientifically valid today from Freud's and psychoanalytic theory, she answered

What remains still valid today are the main theoretical concepts of Freud, such as the unconscious, infantile sexuality, repression and latent motivation; in other words, the unconscious as a formal–abstract object of investigation. Also valid are the theoretical–technical concepts of transference and counter-transference. When we enter into the ideological sphere (such as Totem and Taboo, which delves into the past, or Civilization and Its Discontents, which analyzes the present and the future), we find that Freud's discourse deliberately omits the relations of production, in other words the social context. He derives our "discontent" from the repression of our libidinous and aggressive impulses, a repression imposed upon us by society. (Langer, 1989, p. 136).

Moreover, classic Freudian theory ignores the discontent caused by ideology. Langer explains:

Ideological distortions appear with most clarity in relation to the concept of reality. When Freud says that the ego should submit itself to reality, along with submission to the id and the superego, we ask ourselves, which reality and what concept of reality he is referring to. If we don't have another relevant scientific body of knowledge as an instrument (like dialectical materialism) in order to analyze reality, then we cannot increase the patient's ego capacity to recognize it. Reality does not exist independently of a social historical process. (Langer, 1989, p. 139)

Langer points somewhat ironically to the fact that, although Freud has been criticized for the paradox that when he speaks about reality, he limits his discourse to its manifest aspect. The paradox is that this came precisely from somebody who knew how to see beyond the appearances of things (the meaning of latent motivation, the unconscious). Moreover, Langer observes that while Freud never understood people as products of history, he, nevertheless, provided the best explanations of the psyche as a product of history. For example, in *Group Psychology and the Analysis of the Ego* he points out that, "In individual psychic life, the Other always appears effectively as model, object, assistant or adversary; and as such, individual psychology is at the same time and from the start social psychology in a board but fully justified sense" (Freud, 1921).

There are elements of the social world throughout Freud's work. Freud's discoveries arise out of a bi-personal situation in which the establishment of transference (the analyst analizand-link) is fundamental. A third is always present in this relationship in the discourse of the analizand. As in early infancy, the father is soon included in the previously mother–child relationship. In resolving the oedipal complex, the child introjects society through the establishment of the superego. Although Freud does not omit the social level when he analyzes relations, he does omit it at the historical level when he tries to apply the Oedipal triangle, based upon the model appropriate to the primitive horde. He explains how a male child upon introjecting the paternal prohibition of incest also introjects society. However, Freud makes no effort to explain how people in turn act back on society. Langer notes that Freud never explicitly speaks of ideology, although he refers to it implicitly in its broadest sense when he says that it is very difficult to change humans because their superegos do not in fact correspond to their fathers but to their forefathers.

Finally, another common criticism of Freud is that he concentrates entirely on the first years of life and invalidates other factors, which clearly take place later. A Marxist, for example, would mention work. However, in all fairness, Freud doesn't ignore it. Describing neurosis, he says that a present-day trauma causes the adult to return to the point of infantile fixation, the result of a stage of depravation, frustration or over-gratification. For Freud, there exists a dialectic interrelation between infancy and adulthood.

Because of these limitations in classical Freudian theory, a variety of Leftist theorists attempted to extract what they perceived as the radical elements in Freudian theory that could be used to promote and explain revolutionary change. Wilhem Reich was among the first to attempt at a synthesis of Freud and Marx. He termed his theory and practice, "SexPol." The kind of practice manifest in Sexpol has not been studied sufficiently. It is a surprisingly modern idea to liberate the political potential of areas that have always been considered apolitical, such as sexuality and the family.

Sexpol became a victim of the intellectual, social, and political climate in which it arose. It originated in Vienna in the 1920s, organized by the Viennese Psychoanalytic Society with the help of the Social Democrat Municipality. The Communists also cooperated in the creation of family centers dedicated to family planning and sex education. Reich devoted himself to his work with zeal. Although today it is recognized among social scientists that the family often acts as an ideological tool and reproduces the subjects that the state needs, in the 1920s, Reich was the first and only one to say it. A sexually repressed and frustrated mother is easily converted into a conservative entity, submissive to men and dominating and repressive with children. Langer states that,

These were the mothers who reproduced the subjects prone to obedience with more or less sublimated homosexuality, which led them to submission and admiration to the Fuhrer. (Langer, 1989, p. 156)

Together with Jung, Adler, and Stekel, Reich adhered to the Freudian ideas with a critical attitude. Together with Ferenczy, Otto Rank, and Fenichel, he criticized Freud from the point of view of a radical perspective that tried to reconcile Marxism with psychoanalysis. While he was still a medical student, he was accepted as a member of the Vienna Psychoanalytic Society in 1920. He developed his technical innovations as a head of the technical seminar of the Vienna Psychoanalytic Society from 1922 to 1930. In those years he acquired a reputation as a brilliant and innovative therapist. Through systematic case studies, he developed the essentials of his own psychological system based on the theory of orgasm, the theory of character, and the technique of character analysis.

In 1927 Reich presented his first theory of orgasm in the monograph titled *Die Funktion des Orgasmus*, which was dedicated to Sigmund Freud. He reasserted Freud's concept of actual neurosis and made it the centerpiece of his systematic pathology. Initially, Freud had explained the dynamics of the actual neurosis in "economic terms" in which the actual/neurotic symptom was nourished by undischarged libido. Reich embraced the aspects of Freud's scientism – e.g., blocks, cathexes and displacements – that were later abandoned by Freud. What later critics considered a naïve set of metaphors derived from thermodynamic theory was for Reich what he found most akin to his thought. He coined the term "sex economy" suggesting a synthesis of Freud and Marx to describe the science of biopsychic energy.

The Christian establishment states that, although orgasm can be an important pleasure, human beings can do without it. Orgasm becomes important for the survival of the species. However, Reich believed that true orgasms, that resulted in the complete release of dammed up libido, were fundamental for human mental health. Therefore, the clinics that he later founded and directed called SexPol, considered full orgasmic enjoyment as the means and goal of therapy.

A second prong of Reich's psychological system was his theory of character. He conceived his idea of character in trying to deal with the obstacle and critical problem of resistance. Character structure was for him the way the patient's general personal style interfered with analytic progress, rather than one or two conscious or unconscious defenses. He then coined the term of character resistance and character neurosis. In reality, his theory of character was a theory of the ego with character being a kind of armor or rigid outer shell that protected the individual from painful reality at the same time limiting his ability to experience life fully. His most famous work *Character Analysis* consists of articles written from 1928–1933 and could be characterized as Reich's systematic attack on the Ego.

The main contrast between Freud and Reich's theory can be located in Freud's fondness for the ego, and Reich's great hostility for it. Reich's theory of personality can be described as a structure with three layers. The deepest level was the person's social and sexual spontaneous joy along with the pleasures of work and the capacity for love. In our society, sex is repressed and the second layer becomes dominant. This second layer can be equated with the Freudian unconscious and expressions of sadism, envy, greed, etc. This second layer is in turn kept in check by the third layer, the "characterological superstructure." This is the artificial mask of self-control, insincere politeness, and artificial sociability. Reich considered that, ultimately, character itself was the illness; and a very noxious one, because it was an illness in disguise.

Reich was especially critical of Freud's *Civilization and Its Discontents*. The main theme of *Civilization and Its Discontents* was derived from the hydraulic theory of psychic energy. That is, the energy that made civilization possible was subtracted from direct erotic experience.

Reich suggested that, just as Marxism represented a critique of bourgeois economics brought forth by the contradictions within capitalism itself, psychoanalysis was a critique of bourgeois morality, which in dialectical fashion arose from the contradictions inherent in sexual repression.

Marx recognized the existence of a gap between the economic structure and the ideological superstructure including politics. That is, groups did not always behave in accordance to their economic interests. Marx terms this false consciousness. Reich explored how ideology developed at the individual level. For Reich, ideology became internalized or anchored in the character structure of the individual. He thought that it was this psychological fact that traditional Marxism had neglected. Values, ideas, moral commands, and religious beliefs reflected economic and historic elements, but were not just pertaining to the intellect, they actually get submerged in the very structure of personality. Because of the weight of ideology, people not only thought differently but also became different. Because ideology was internalized psychologically, it was possible to understand how political activities could fail to be the reflection of economic reality.

When a society is changing rapidly, because ideology was anchored in the very structure of personality, it can supersede the actual economic interests of a group or a class. For example, German masses voting for and supporting Nazism. Reich showed how, and in which locus, this process develops.

He considered that family was the locus of character formation through child-rearing practices. Of course, the family was itself a product of historical and economic determinants. He anticipated the later work of Eric Fromm in pointing out that the triumph of Nazism in Germany could not be understood just because of Hitler's personality or for the trickery of the German Bourgeoisie. Nazism, as well as any significant political movement, was rooted in the psychology of the German people.

He explained the psychological grounds of Nazism as an ambivalent relationship to authority peculiar to the German lower middle classes who simultaneously desired strong authority and opposed it. He pointed out that this psychological trait was the result of being trapped between the rich capitalist and the militant proletariat. Character structure was a result of the manner in which the family handled infantile and adolescent sexuality. In the lower middle class of Germany the economic structures of the small business or small farm coincided in that the workers were members of a family under the authority of the father. These features of fathers with the double authority of their paternity and economic power have been the subject of literature and filmography. For example, in the Italian film, *Padre Padrone* (father boss), the father–farm owner, is also a despotic boss. This double authority, and his constant presence, creates the conditions for much greater control of the father over the children than the father of the proletarian family in which children "disappear" in the factory at 12 or 13 years. Reich thought that it was precisely the fears, and sexual repression, characteristic of the lower middle class, which made possible the authoritarian personality from which Nazism nourished itself.

In summary, for Reich, repression existed not for the sake of civilization, morality, or religion, and neither did it exist for the sake of culture as Freud proposed, but simply in order to create the character structure necessary for the preservation of an authoritarian social regime. Reichian theory has directly or indirectly affected many of the Leftist Freudians up to the present day. Elements of Reich are found in Fromm, Marcuse, Lacan, Deleuze, and Guattari.

Application of psychoanalysis to progressive social change: early European attempts

Reich proposed lifting the financial barriers to psychoanalysis in the capitalist world. The SexPol outpatient clinics of Vienna and Berlin began a process that had the potential to affect profound changes in psychoanalysis, removing it from cloistered offices and projecting it into the lively world of the streets, apartment blocks, bars, and factories. In addition to Reich, who had the distinction of being thrown out of both the psychoanalytic society and the Communist Party because of his radical views, Otto Fenichel and Bernfeldt made serious attempts to reconcile Marxism and psychoanalysis. Fenichel more quietly pushed for the construction of a Marxist psychoanalysis within the International Psychoanalytic Association.

During the 1920s and 1930s there were other important if less well-known examples of applied psychoanalysis committed to social change in Europe. For example, the 1920s Experimental Children's home in the Soviet Union directed by psychoanalyst Vera Yanitskaya a.k.a. Vera Schmit.

Her husband Otto was the founding member Soviet Psychoanalytic Society and a prominent official in the Bolshevik government. Vera Schmit, a lay analyst who had no medical degree, recognized the profound implications of the Freud's child sexuality theory in education. In the Experimental Children's home, there were no punishments, and praise and blame were always directed to the action and not to the child.

In 1923, Sabina Spillrein developed family and children's clinics under the theoretical postulates of both psychoanalysis and Marxism. She was also active in the Moscow Institute of Psychoanalysis and headed the Department of Child Psychology at the University of Moscow. An important contributor to psychoanalytic theory according to Freud, she had been the analyst of young Jean Piaget and Alexander Luria, to whom she was also a respected mentor.

Application of psychoanalysis to progressive social change: recent examples in Latin America

In 1982, after the Sandinista victory, Silvia Berman, M.D. and Marie Langer, M.D. organized the Mental Health Workers Internationalist Teams that were to establish the teaching and delivery of mental health services in Nicaragua. In the words of Marie Langer, "We were 12 specialists, psychologists and medical doctors with psychoanalytical training, most of which were Argentinian and Mexican."

The Internationalist Teams took turns and flew to Nicaragua from Mexico during the years 1981–1985. They met with the Department of Mental Health to discuss cooperation with the School of Medicine at Leon, where there were two psychiatrists who treated their patients with drugs and never listened to what they had to say, as well as two Sandinista psychologists, and one female social worker. When the psychiatrists complained about the long lists of patients, the team suggested group therapy. One young psychologist was going to start doing group therapy and the team asked him which theoretical approach he had selected. He answered, as though it was taken for granted, "The Marxist approach, of course, because we know how relations of production are reflected in the psyche . . . " Langer then notes, "At that point it became clear to us that we had to start teaching seriously the basic elements of psychoanalysis and group therapy."

The team made compiled a sort of Ten Commandments, a list of concepts and principles that would become the core of their first lectures in psychoanalysis:

(1) We must be able to listen, to question and to assimilate the meaning of catharsis. (2) The unconscious exists; this is easily proved through the interpretation of slips, dreams and fantasies. Everything which appears illogical in us has a meaning. (3) Hence our attitude and actions are over-determined. Our ideology is in part unconscious. (4) We are a sum of conflicts. We are apprehensive of changes, which awaken our basic fears. Every symptom has a primary and secondary benefit. (5) We are a sum of contradictions. Even the mother who loves her baby hates it at the same time (Winnicott). (6) The history and sexuality of our childhood are important because they are repeated – generally without our realizing it. (7) Transference relationships are important, because we repeat them. (8) Counter-transference is important; nobody is neutral. The practice of psychotherapy is a political task. (9) The sequences of complementary events explain why one person becomes ill in a particular traumatic situation and another does not. (10) We are all wonderful, but also mad; we are heroes but also cowards (how to cope with fear?); we are loving but at the same time perverse. Feelings of guilt have to be diminished, as they don't help but paralyze. (Langer, 1989, p. 215)

Among other tasks the Internationalist Teams supervised group and individual therapy; taught psychoprophylaxis and prevention; taught rudiments of family therapy to pediatricians; taught medical psychology to medical students; started plans of sexual education; and started Balint groups with doctors and nurses in the Ministry of Health. (Michael and Enid Balint were psychoanalysts who started seminars for general practitioners in London in the 1950s. In essence, Balint group members listened to the presenting doctor's story and then discussed the case, trying to concentrate on the doctor and patient relationship, with particular attention to the feelings aroused in them by the patient.)

In addition, the Internationalist Teams taught psychopathology in the Psychiatric Hospital of Managua, where they were responsible for part of the training for future psychiatrists. They imparted the teaching of a different, and to them unknown, form of psychotherapy to social workers and behavioral psychologists. Various approaches were used including assessments of the relationship between the individual and the family based on psychoanalytic theory, the analysis of relationships within the family based systemic theory, and the role of the family in society as defined in terms of the Marxist theory. The success of the teams was achieved with the help of other internationalist workers such as psychoanalysts from France, Switzerland, Israel, and Austria.

Another Latin American example of a successful movement in the direction of articulating a psychoanalysis committed to social change is exemplified by the international encounters of Marxist psychology and psychoanalysis that took place in La Havana, Cuba in 1986, 1988, 1990, 1992, 1994, 1996, 1998, 2000, and 2003. Psychoanalysts of all countries in Latin America which professed their commitment to social change and a few psychoanalysts from France, Switzerland, Italy, and Austria met in Havana every 2 years. Marie Langer and Juan Carlos Volnovich from Argentina were originally responsible for the initial organizing steps. Eventually, the organization of the encounters was the responsibility of an International Committee composed by Cuban psychologists and by psychoanalysts from Mexico, Brazil, Argentina, and Europe, and was sponsored by the University of Havana and by the Society of Cuban Psychologists.

I was part of two of these encounters in 1986 and 1990, and I have maintained contact with the main presenters and continue to follow the proceedings of all other meetings. It would be impossible to cover in this chapter even the minimal summary of the contributions and agreements reached by the different currents in Latin American psychoanalysis and Cuban psychology. For now, I will refer the reader to some of the extensive literature on the subject. I acknowledge that written texts will convey only part of the marvelous, exhilarating feeling of exchanging ideas and thinking together with the community of therapists committed to social change under the blue skies of Cuba.

In the words of Juan Carlos Volnovich after the 6th Latin American encounter of Psychoanalysis and Marxist Psychology in Cuba:

It is not an "alternative clinic," the one that spoke at this encounter. We are not trying to inaugurate another pole of power in the disputed psychoanalytic market. We are not hoping to find a technocratic clinic updated in a rush so that it would be able to compete in the saturated psychoanalytic universe. We aspire to replace a decadent psychoanalysis by an innovative and, if you want, troublesome orthodox psychoanalysis. Far from any demagogic proposal, we vindicate a clinic so orthodox (if by orthodoxy one understands the psychoanalytic legitimacy that supports it) as hidden or covert. It is to that clinic and that psychoanalysis to which we convoke. It is "our psychoanalysis" that is emerging from these encounters. The newness of the psychoanalysis that these encounters invoke is already built. It inhabits hospitals, offices, schools, and mass media in Latin America. It is not necessary to invent it. What is necessary and would be extremely novel is that the multiplicity of its discourse would become legitimate before our own eyes and the eyes of others. (Volnovich, 2003)

Psychoanalysis committed to social change in Argentina

The Argentinian Psychoanalytical Association, APA, was officially founded in December of 1942. Of the six signatures of the foundation document, two: Enrique Pichon-Rivière and Marie Langer, were Marxists. Initially, the APA and its members devoted themselves to clinical and theoretical issues primarily in the sphere of the intrapsychic conflict. However, Marie Langer, Emilio Rodrigue, Pichon-Rivière, and others became progressively more interested in the articulation between psychoanalysis and social issues.

From the beginning, the Argentinian APA, which was one of the largest and powerful analytic institutions in the world during the 1940s and 1950s, did not follow the orthodoxy of Sigmund and Anna Freud, but the heresy of Melanie Klein. Still the Argentinian APA was a powerful member of the International Psychoanalytic Association (IPA) and received through the years the visits of prominent psychoanalysts like Hanna Seagal and Heinz Hartman. Many European psychoanalysts such as Angel Garma and Heinrich Racker, who had come to Argentina because of the triumph of fascism and its persecutions, enriched the ranks of Argentinian psychoanalysts.

Marie Langer, who was part of the founding group, had been born in Vienna in 1910. There she graduated as a medical doctor and was analyzed by one of Freud's inner circle, Richard Sterba. As Nazism advanced, she emigrated to Spain with her husband and joined the International Brigades as surgeon and anesthesiologist, respectively. After the defeat of the Republic, she had to go into yet another exile and reached Argentina in 1942.

Eventually Pichon-Rivière founded the School of Social Psychology and Marie Langer and younger members became more and more involved in Leftist politics within the Argentinian Federation of Psychiatry. In the psychoanalytic field they emphasized the weight and importance of social issues in psychoanalytic theory.

As the time passed, an important current developed in the APA, which presented significant ideological and theoretical differences from the more conservative official line. It was constituted by training analysts such as Marie Langer, Emilio Rodrigue, and others, and younger analysts and candidates. Ultimately in the International Psychoanalytic Conference of Vienna in 1971, the Argentine delegation was unable to present a unified document for the APA. Marie Langer and the other dissidents introduced their own document titled *Psychoanalysis and/ or Revolution*. On their return to Argentina, Marie Langer and the group of dissidents broke with the APA and founded Platform Psychoanalytic Association.

Their break with the APA and the creation of Platform must be understood in the social and political climate of the 1960s and early 1970s in Argentina. These years were marked by the succession of elected governments being toppled by military coups. The military juntas responded to the popular struggle for democracy, and trade union-led fights for better living conditions, with progressively massive and bloody repressions.

The book by Enrique Carpintero and Alejandro Vainer *Las Huellas de la Memoria* (*The Tracks of Memory*), which deals with the history psychoanalysis and mental health in Argentina, states that the general strike that started in Córdoba in 1969 (called Cordobazo) with mobilization of students and workers that paralyzed the country was a milestone which marked a before and after in Argentinean Mental Health. In 1970 the Argentinian Federation of Psychiatrists elected a Marxist president Dr. Gervasio Paz with the considerable support of psychoanalysts/psychiatrists, who identified themselves as committed to social change.

In those years General Menéndez, attempting to justify and explain the assassinations and disappearances of psychoanalysts, psychologists, and psychiatrists stated that "the analytic couch was the crib of the subversion." In other words, the military of the 1970s accused psychoanalysts of politicizing their patients and society. In reality, it was the other way around, during the late 1960s and 1970s, the patients (the people) wound up politicizing and teaching political reality to the professionals of mental health. This social awareness resulted in professional activities that felt increasingly threatening to the military establishment.

In 1976 the government of María Estela Martínez de Perón (nicknamed Isabel) was toppled by the military junta presided by General Videla inaugurating the bloodiest repression of Argentinian history. More than 300 mental health professionals were either assassinated or disappeared; trade unions became illegal and during the years 1976–1982 more than 40 000 people were assassinated or disappeared. The book *Huellas de la Memoria*, dedicates a whole section in the second volume, just to mention the names of the numerous psychoanalysts and other mental health professionals who "disappeared" in the 1970s.

Psychoanalysis was pronounced by the military, as a subversive profession and the state universities fired all professors with a background in psychoanalysis. Because of the exclusion of psychoanalysis from public education higher curriculum, psychoanalytic institutions remained very active and private study groups flourished. People were afraid to talk and the climate of oppression created by the regime transformed psychotherapy into a very special experience, which in as far as one was expected to say whatever came to mind, was in total contrast with the predominant climate in society.

The military attempt to abolish psychoanalysis backfired and it gave psychoanalysis a heroic aura, leading to an identification with the Freud of the days of his so-called "splendid isolation."

During the years of the military dictatorship, 1976–1982, the Lacanian interpretation of psychoanalysis became very popular for a number of reasons, not the least of which was the fact that its hermeneutic character made it more impervious to military repression.

There is ample evidence that psychoanalytic psychotherapy helped families and children of the disappeared or tortured and had an important role in maintaining a degree of mental health in the political resistance and the society at large. In the exile communities in Mexico, Brazil, other Latin American countries, and Europe the analysts were involved in active professional solidarity with the recent arrivals who had suffered torture, loss of dear ones, or other considerable trauma. Group and individual therapy, was administered as the free contribution of the professionals committed to social change and an enormous body of clinical and theoretical materials were created and exchanged during that period.

Marie Langer exemplifies the application of Kleinian concepts to better understand how certain political militants were able to withstand torture. This is a smaller illustration of the extremely active and creative, theoretical and clinical original work of those years:

Political militancy, like any other impassioned activity, is nurtured on feelings which arise from the paranoid–schizoid and depressive positions. Or, in simple terms, along with the desire and the goal of repairing social injustices and achieving a more just society – reparation, depressive position – there exists a schism somewhat unavoidably dualistic, yet effective, whereby compañeros are idealized and enemies are loathed. With respect to the latter, you could speak in a certain sense of feelings arising from the paranoid–schizoid position. But in borderline situations, as in torture, I suppose one can only resist it by carrying those feelings to the extreme. This dreadful reality, is obviously conducive to the enemy-torturer being experienced as the embodiment of evil, and "the cause", as the salvation of humanity. Those who carry out repression also know that the strength of the torture is derived from this conviction; that's why there is usually a "bad" torturer and a "good" interrogator. If the prisoner begins to believe in the interrogator's "good faith", he becomes confused, breaks down, and confesses. Kleininan concepts, which are so focused upon the internal world and apparently so little connected to social reality, can nevertheless be used to interpret socio-political phenomena. (Langer, 1989 p. 150)

As the filmmaker Naomi Klein in her documentary *The Take* has put it "Argentina was not the typical third world country with its chronically marginalized important sections of the population, but has become impoverished by 10 years of following 'the model' prescribed by the Internationally Monetary Fund." Joseph Stiglitz, Nobel Laureate in Economics, former Chief Economist of the World Bank, one of the most influential economic thinkers of the last 20 years wrote *Globalization and its Discontents* denouncing the disastrous effects of the IMF policies of which he himself had helped create and implement.

At the beginning of the twentieth century Argentina was one of the most prosperous nations in the world. This economic prosperity was the substructure of the cultural, artistic, and scientific production that rendered two Nobel Peace Prizes and three Nobel Medical Prizes. In the 1940s Argentina's European identified intelligentsia and its educated middle and working classes produced a predominant center of psychoanalytic practice. The whole popular culture was permeated by psychoanalytic ideas. Because of the disastrous results of the neoliberal policies recommended by the International Monetary Fund, thousands of factories and business and an important portion of the industry of Argentina, collapsed. The result was that from the year 2000 until the present there are about 600 factories occupied by workers.

In November of 2003, there were 262 factories in Argentina occupied by the workers. They had been abandoned by their owners during 2001 to 2003. At the present time there are more than 600 occupied factories. More than half of them were legally covered under the umbrella of Cooperative Law, a respected institution that originated in the last 20 years of the nineteenth century. Because the owners of the factories were in many cases indebted to state banks, some were in the process of being nationalized by the state.

In 2001, Argentinian psychoanalysts found themselves working under a complete economic collapse that had to be understood in the context of the triumph of neoliberalism. As Juan Carlos Volnovich, M.D. put it,

The reality that we psychoanalysts are forced to grapple with, is how to help our patients recover the ability to construct internal systems of representations of reality, that re-establish the right to think and to structure projects ... that do not reduce human beings, marginalized by the system to their pure biological essence ... [To] a great extent the debate regarding the possibility of challenging hegemonic ideology, revolve around the right of the subject to transgress superego mandates and reformulate the social contract according to specific historical circumstances ... Psychoanalysts have been forced to struggle with the paradoxes of ego and superego phenomena within the context of a history of extreme situations including economic crisis and political repression ... As psychoanalysts we need to help our patients recover a reality, based on an ability to construct ... (Volnovich, 2002, p. 88)

The psychoanalysts who are helping workers within the occupied factories categorized their activities as help to produce self and to produce reality. Some of the techniques are not original or new. Group techniques, family techniques and occasionally one-to-one techniques, come from the past 40 or 50 years. What is completely new is the context. That is, the movement, the workers' collective inviting the psychoanalyst to provide his or her help in the occupied factory. Applied psychoanalytic techniques are used in remarkably creative ways to foster the process of development of new relationships between the workers. A new horizontal structure is emerging; now workers no longer relate to a boss that tells them what to do; they have to relate to each other.

Social sources of superego and humans' original helplessness predisposes individuals to remain subordinate in relationship to power. Power promotes consensus by encouraging us to identify our desire with lethal representations it offers: "destroy yourself," "exterminate the others," "kill off insignificant ones that don't matter." The military dictatorship in Argentina caused massive social trauma and subsequent democratic regimes have not dealt with its sequelae.

Workers in occupied factories need to open a new way to deal with those aspects of the superego that direct unconscious behaviors in relation to power and authority, that need to be brought to consciousness. Juan Carlos Volnovich stated:

A surplus of innovative energy is generated by the system's own contradictions. That energy resists the tenacious hold power has, by creating an opening for new possibilities. The psychoanalytic situation entails two possibilities for re-enforcing unconscious and semiconscious complicity with power or for questioning it: (1) By means of the transference, it can reinforce submission to power. (2) Conversely it can also help to deconstruct myths. (Volnovich, 2002, p. 90)

Psychoanalysis can help to create new meaning, to re-signify such myths, so as to dismantle the subjects relationship to power. Psychoanalysis can help to construct an alternative system of representations that recovers the right to think more critically and to feel more authentically. Psychoanalysis can help in reconciliation of the subject with his/her passions. Volnovich argues:

From a theoretical perspective we are thinking of the fundamental importance of the effort made to open a bridge between the subject and his/her deadly identification with power, so that something akin to desire can circulate within that space. Psychoanalysis has an important role to play in this process: if there is an "other" who can listen and also desire, if there is an other who invites the subject to speak, then something of the violence that destroys us, something of the destructive compulsion can give way to an elaboration that can become transformative action in the social domain . . . The mere fact that resistance and struggle exists, opens a space for the human screams that when they are listened to, become language. (Volnovich, 2002, p. 89)

Juan Carlos Volnovich describes his experience with women in the community and factories occupied by women. He states, the methodology adopted by the self-convoked assemblies and by the workers' cooperatives that take the direction of bankrupt factories, carries the mark of feminism and of the women's movement, "This is an example of a clear transference of the technology and the political praxis of the women's movement, which is significantly influencing the anti-capitalist praxis" (Volnovich, 2002, p. 90).

   This author tells us in summary that this transference of political praxis from the women's movement translates itself in the occupied factories by: (1) the horizontal model that replaces the vertical hierarchy in the conception and conducting of political and entrepreneurial projects; (2) the heterogeneity of the different people that comprise the working movement and the body of assemblies, which is one of the non-negotiable slogans of the women's movement; (3) critical attitude towards the theory of representation; (4) the autonomy of "auto-gestion". In the words of a woman worker of Grissinopoli/New Hope, "What we did two months ago, is exactly like giving birth . . . To occupy a factory is a political act, and without knowing, we were involved in a political act . . . When the owners/bosses left, the base remained. The workers, which are the most important part of the factory, remained . . . If we have to establish an alliance, the only possible alliance is with the other worker's of the recovered factories, with the self-convoked assemblies and with the task forces of workers that have taken responsibility for the factories. It's not the case of becoming a boss. The point is to become responsible so that the future, your future, would depend on the work that you yourself initiate."

   Volnovich places the experience of the women in the occupied factories in the context of what he terms the three discourses. The discourse of suffering, the discourse of resistance, and the discourse of struggle:

The discourse of suffering is concerned with the endless economic and cultural anguish imposed by contemporary global capitalism. This discourse defines the parameters that measure subjective pain, internal schism, and the daily devastation suffered by the majority of Argentines in the present period. This discourse provides a lens through which to view how men, women, adolescents, and children are damaged by social exclusion (unemployment, homelessness, hunger, and so forth) and how the inequitable distribution of material goods is reflected symbolically in the culture's representations of power privilege, status, and identity . . . Whereas the discourse of suffering addresses the experience of pain and trauma, the discourse of resistance highlights the innovative strategies that people have developed to deal with the devastating policies imposed by corporate capitalism. (Volnovich, 2002, p. 90)

Volnovich and the other authors of the book about psychoanalysts working within the occupied factories described in detail the different strategies that people have found for survival and resistance. Thus, they describe the pot-banging demonstrations that forced the government of De la Rua to resign, which led ultimately to the elections of 2003. They also describe the strategies for demonstrations of the unemployed (piqueteros) who cut roads and maintained a continuous presence near the government palaces of the capital and the provinces. They acknowledge the originality and creativity of people that, without the leadership of political parties, create and reconstruct social links emphasizing solidarity and building networks of urban organizations such as the neighborhood assemblies.

Volnovich states that:

The discourse of struggle calls for a construction and re-construction of the social bonds and emphasizes the urban webs based on creative solidarity ... Just as women in the feminist movement learn that the struggle against the most damaging effects of patriarchy cannot be waged without addressing the most harmful effects of capitalism, in Argentina since the "corralito" and triumphant globalization people are becoming conscious of the many converging factors responsible for our oppressive situation. (Volnovich, 2002, p. 97)

Women participating in the occupied factories movement, the piquetero movement and the popular assemblies, have brought the trademark of feminism and the women's movement with them.

(1) They break with the assumption that only capital bosses and their technical experts know how to administer a business and make it productive, and at the same time they overcome the social expectation that they should passively wait for men to take the initiative.

(2) They destroy the system of class relations that assumes that some (the capitalists) are the owners of work who offer work to others (the female and male workers), who do not have work but who search and ask for it.

(3) They achieve reconciliation between the self-conservative aspects of the ego (to mitigate hunger) with the self-preservative aspects of the ego (to gain self respect and create solidarity). In other words, these actions permit them to eat without having to betray their identity as workers. On the contrary, they can feel proud of doing what they are doing.

These authors point out that, through their struggle, women collectively process social and individual traumata; by reinforcing alliances with other workers and reinforcing family links, they improve individual mental health. Women who have been depicted as needy and incapable people who are only fit for charitable help defy by their protagonic struggle these definitions. Struggle eliminates helplessness and, by organizing their workplace, they start attaining medical care and the medications needed for themselves and their families. They learn new trades, joining together with other sectors of the population including intellectuals, artists, and professionals; they often use the factory building to create a cultural center. Internationally renowned visual artists paint murals on the walls so that the premises can be declared of special cultural interest by the government, making it impossible for the building to be privatized, closed, or demolished.

When Volnovich and the others work with a group of women in the occupied factories, he is aware that "the struggle of women against the most damaging effects of patriarchy cannot take place without the struggle against the most damaging effects of capitalism."

Conclusion

In this chapter I have tried to provide an overview of the significant contributions of psychoanalysis to social change within the last 100 years. A whole new generation of therapists and mental health practitioners are becoming interested in psychoanalysis as a tool to study the construction of subjectivity and internal systems of representation of reality. This chapter is especially dedicated to them.

I have placed special emphasis in the developments of psychoanalysis committed to social change in Latin American and Argentina for four reasons; the first is that these developments are largely unknown to the Anglo-Saxon public; the second is that they are especially rich as they have been intertwined with the political struggles of the last 50 years; the third is that they have yielded an extraordinary wealth of theoretical new contributions to psychoanalysis, and fourth but not least is that I possess an in-depth knowledge of them derived from my first-hand experience of them. The readers are encouraged to read the original texts listed below and a good point of departure will be *From Vienna to Managua* by Marie Langer, M.D.

FURTHER READING

Bleger, J. (1963). *Psicología de la Conducta*. Editorial Universitaria de Buenos Aires.

Carpintero, E. (2004). *Las Huellas de la Memoria: psicoanálisis y salud mental en la Argentina de los años 60 y 70: tomo I: 1957–1969*. 1a ed.-Buenos Aires: Topia Editoral.

Carpintero, E. (2006). *Las Huellas de la Memoria: psicoanálisis y salud mental en la Argentina de los años 60 y 70: tomo II: 1970–2000*. 1a ed.-Buenos Aires: Topia Editoral.

Freud, S. (1921). Sexuality in the aetiology of the neuroses. In *The Standard Edition of the Complete Psychological Works of Sigmund Freud*, edn. III.

Langer, M. (1989). *From Vienna to Managua: Journey of a Psychoanalyst*. London: Free Association Books.

Petras, J., Veltmeyer, H., Volnovich, J.C. *et al.* (2002). *Produciendo Realidad Las Empresas Comunitarias*. Compiled by: Enrique Carpintero and Mario Hernández. Buenos Aires-Argentina: Topia Editorial.

Reich, W. (1961). *The Function of Orgasm*. New York.

Reich, W. (1962). *The Sexual Revolution*. Reprinted by permission of Farrar, Straus & Giroux, Inc.

Reich, W. (1963). *Character-Analysis*. 3rd edn. New York.

Reich, W. (1966). *Mass Psychology of Fascism*. New York.

Robinson, P. (1969). *The Freudian Left*. New York: Harper & Row.

Robinson, P. (1993). *Freud and his Critics*. Oxford, UK: University of California Press, Ltd.

Rozitchner, L. (1972). *Freud y los Límites del Individualismo Burgués*. Siglo xxi Editores, s.a. de c.v., Mexico.

Rozitchner, L. (1982). *Freud y el Problema del Poder*. Folios Ediciones, S.A.

Volnovich, J.C. (2003). *Psychoanalysis and Hope in the Epicenter of Despair: A View from Argentina*. Translated by Nancy Caro Hollander. http://www.healthysystem, virginia.edu/ internet/csmhi/voll3volnovich.cfm.

Volnovich, J.C. & Werthein, S. (1989). *Marie Langer: mujer, psicoanálisis, marxismo*. Editorial Contrapunto S.A.

14

A new psychiatry?

Carl I. Cohen, Sami Timimi, and Kenneth S. Thompson

If you come here to help me, then you are wasting your time. But if you come here because your liberation is bound up in mine, then let us begin.

Lily Walker, an Australian Aboriginal Women's leader

The reader of this volume will quickly grasp that there are no general agreements about the form or content of a liberatory psychiatry. This is not surprising since several of the contributors view themselves as postmodernists. Thus, "grand narratives" or universal truths and rules will be avoided. Having said that, we believe that there are some broad agreements about liberatory psychiatry. Although the authors' emphasis may be different, there are at least four themes in which the contributors to this volume are on common ground: (1) the political and psychological sphere are inseparable; (2) dominance and oppression are pervasive within the political sphere; (3) the physical and social world are inseparable; (4) there needs to be an understanding of the interactions between "the general" and "the particular." We shall review these items below.

A warning light should probably go on whenever complex concepts are combined into one word; however, Isaac Prilleltensky's notion of "psychopolitical" does capture some of the basic concerns of the writers of this volume. Namely, that the political and psychological spheres are inseparable. This means that we cannot explain the development of individuality or subjectivity apart from its political and cultural context, nor can we understand political and cultural structures without considering its psychic dimension.

Second, the contributors agree that there are problems in the political sphere, and in particular, various forms of oppression play a powerful role in preventing persons from attaining "liberation," which was defined in our introduction as "freedom from" and "freedom to." Of course, interpersonal, biological, familial, and local environmental factors may also figure in liberation. Nevertheless, at this historical moment, the writers of this volume seem to agree that the political sphere plays a dominant role worldwide in creating social and psychological

Liberatory Psychiatry: Philosophy, Politics, and Mental Health, ed. Carl I. Cohen and Sami Timimi.
Published by Cambridge University Press. © Cambridge University Press.

oppression and stymying opportunities for liberation. As a number of the authors point out, the political sphere creates direct oppressive conditions through material, legal, military, economic, and/or other social barriers to the fulfilment of self-determination, distributive justice, and democratic participation. The political sphere also helps create "psychological oppression." That is, an internalized view of self as negative and undeserving of more resources or increased participation in societal affairs. Michael Lerner (1991) has characterized this internalized situation in developed coutries as "surplus powerlessness," and Martín-Baró (1996) described a similar phenomenon among persons in the developing world.

Bruno Latour (1993) has famously underscored the inseparability of the social and physical realms, and that modernism has created an artificial dichotomy. This has important implications with respect to understanding causes of mental distress as well as for recognizing the social context of all physical (biological) explanations. For example, biological causality is often viewed as "proximal cause" of mental disorders (Link & Phelan, 1995). Consequently, genetics or neuropathological changes are seen as the cause of an illness. However, if one recognizes the inseparability of the physical and social worlds, then one must ask about "distal causes." That is, what is the social/environmental context that allows for the expression of a particular genetic trait or produces a neuropathological transformation? Moreover, although it is possible to critique and perhaps minimize the impact of the social context on scientific language and theory, we will never be able to eliminate it. Thus, the social and physical spheres are inextricably linked.

While most of the authors in this volume caution against biological reductionism in current psychiatric research and practice, we need to consider the array of possible responses to biological reductionism. These can range from simply adding social and psychological spheres to a biological perspective to a more radical vision of biology as an emergent property of matter. The latter response not only views mind but the entire living being as an emergent property. In so doing, it avoids a materialist Cartesian dualism that occurs when we divide a person into biological processes (physiological processes and structures) and thought (mind) as a different, albeit, material entity. Antonio Demascio (2003) touched upon this when he referred to the "gut feelings" that determine thinking, although he did not make the more radical leap towards suggesting that these integrative interactions are qualitatively different from mechanical processes.

Finally, each of the writers, especially as clinicians, has an interest in the concrete individual. However, in pursuing a true emancipatory agenda, they also recognize the importance of general forces – i.e., biological and social factors – that are common to or have the potential to impact on all humans. A critical piece of the agenda for liberatory psychiatry is to delineate how these general forces manifest themselves within a concrete individual, and in turn, how this individual acts on and helps transform the social and physical (biological) realms. This leads to questions such as how we can mesh the politics of being an individual in a mass society with politics of mutual interdependence and solidarity. How do we care about each other and ourselves? How do we marshall the resources of society to the benefit of all as individuals? What do we owe society for having our individual needs met? How do we pay off this debt or share it?

Psychiatry's natural territory is marginalized groups, those most vulnerable to experiencing human suffering, distress, and alienation. Thus, psychiatry should be a force for good with immense potential to contribute to the liberation and emancipation of mankind. This liberatory potential cannot be realized while psychiatry itself remains so vulnerable to being used to help maintain the potentially repressive political status quo. This book is an attempt to re-invigorate this potential ideal. In so doing, we need to ask why psychiatry has lost its liberatory ideals and its ability to analyze and intervene in a meaningful way, that includes, but goes beyond the lives of distressed individuals to look at what sort of society can help create a more humane, just and emancipatory value system that will promote human potential and liberate many more than today from mental suffering.

This book addresses a number of themes such as power/dominance, language/knowledge, class/social capital, unconscious, biology, science, ideology, consumerism/pluralism, biomedical dominance, developing countries/postcolonial legacy. This list is not exhaustive and the reader may identify additional themes. Although many of the chapters suggest different approaches towards liberation and well-being, there are often inter-connections among the themes. We have illustrated them in Fig. 14.1. For example, "language dominance" is strongly linked to power, class, ideology, postcolonial legacy, and the unconscious, but it is also related to other elements such as biology, scientific enterprise, biomedicine, and consumerism/pluralism. Thus, beneath the seemingly disparate element there are many linkages, and each element can help elucidate the others. Indeed, all the writers seem to be attempting a cross-disciplinary dialogue and reject the linear paradigms that are now dominant in psychiatry.

The authors of this book utilize a variety of theoretical approaches. Each has their strengths and weaknesses. The materialist realism approach provides the theoretical underpinnings for reintroducing biology into the project. It overcomes some of the speculative ideology found in psychoanalysis and among the Left Freudians, and allows social analyses to recognize concrete individuals within real social relations. However, there are potential problems with materialist realism's principal argument that it is possible to critically assess the social elements that are embedded in research so that we can come closer to understanding the material world. Perhaps, the two are so inextricably intertwined that this becomes a

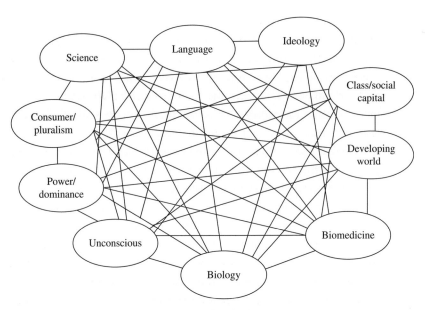

Fig. 14.1.   Themes of liberatory psychiatry addressed in the book.

hopeless task. A second problem stems from the fact that material realism is not the cosmology of the majority of the world's population. Hence, this may have implications for developing a new psychiatry in the postcolonial world.

Here, postmodernism would appear to have the upper hand with its focus on discourse and power, and local "meanings" leading to an engagement with service users and new practical models of service and psychiatric/psychotherapeutic work. On the other hand, postmodernism could be seen as neglecting important insights about the nature of economic organization of mental health, and thus has lost its "teeth" in engaging with the macro-political perspective. Moreover, postmodernism also seems to have lost sight of the concrete, physical being. In this instance, proposals for radicalizing biology as well as psychology can be potentially important in contributing to understanding how environmental influences may impact on our differential biology(s). However, one must be careful to not lapse into biological reductionism, which will invariably lead to oppressive outcomes even if we identify genes or structural abnormalities. And, as noted above, reductionism can take many forms, and how we address complexity and emergent properties at the many levels of biological being remains to be resolved.

Finally, we must also bear in mind that postmodernism's understandable aversion towards "grand narratives" may clash with many premodern systems that are built around such narratives. Perhaps, we need to explore a modified version of postmodernism – what Nicholas Gier (2000) calls "constructive postmodernism" – that allows for a melding of modernist and premodern perspectives.

The limitations of a reductionist biological perspective on the problem of human distress are easy to see. So far, this perspective has not "delivered" in the way it has in the rest of medicine – we still have no tests or markers, and no drugs or surgical procedures that effect a "cure." This does not mean that biomedical interventions can never be found to alleviate mental illness, and we also recognize that causality does not dictate cure. However, a central premise for all authors is that this failure is because mental distress is not solely a biological entity. Postmodernism has some useful analytic tools that can help us look into and open up the cracks in the assumptions that shape narrow biomedical perspectives that are currently dominant, in particular the influence of a variety of cultural discourses about normality, mental well-being, and illness. Historically, new definitions of "wellness" impose new meanings, thus creating "mental illness" and setting in motion new ideas about self and "otherness/dangerousness," which in turn lead to social exclusion, marginalization, and the like. This helpfully brings politics down to local/user group levels, as new definitions create new sites of resistance. However, this still leaves important questions about why particular cultural dynamics (such as that of medicalization) occur and what drives them at particular moments in history, and in particular settings. Answers to the "why now" and "why here" questions are aided by political and economic perspectives that frequently draw on more empirical and arguable "modernist" theoretical and analytic devices. Hence again, we see that one-sided models are too limited for our liberatory project.

In many ways the postmodern response is understandable and legitimate in relation to our current state of knowledge and how it is applied in service delivery. We have various competing frameworks of causation (and therefore treatment), each of which can claim only modest success in attaining valued outcomes. Thus, if we accept this reality rather than continually imposing our preferred meanings onto our clients, we can engage in co-constructing ways of viewing the problem that are meaningful to them. This is a *pragmatic* response, important particularly in the context of multicultural societies. Such a response might be considered "evidence based," with experience of the complexity of the world and the presence of many perspectives nested in or contradicting each other. Indeed, postmodernism can be conceptualized as a combination of the philosophical ideas expressed in the movie *Roshamon* and in Heizenberg's Uncertainty Principle, namely that: (1) there are many perspectives, each true in its way, and (2) what we think is true is always shifting before we know it.

Bill Fulford and colleagues (2003) have argued for a "new philosophy of psychiatry" that proposes that meanings as well as causes are essential to good clinical care. However, they point out that we must be cautious about swinging the balance too far the other way. That is, throwing away causality in pursuit of meanings. They also suggest that there may be a point where meaningful communication, however strange, may run out, where words and behaviors really are meaningless, and represent failures of brain processes. Although this point may not be well demarcated – e.g., late-stage dementia may be such a point – it is a researchable question.

A related concern is how do psychiatrists, especially those who seek a liberatory agenda, deal with the recognition that scientific theory and the data that it generates are not value-free but constrained by human concepts and social context? Fulford and his coauthors (2003) point out that this has both positive and negative implications. On the positive side, it makes psychiatry and medicine more hospitable for social scientists. Indeed, the contributors to this book strongly support this notion. On the negative side, there is a danger of relativizing of all knowledge – an extreme version of the postmodern stance that all perspectives are equal. However, because there is more than one way of understanding a phenomenon does not mean that all perspectives have equal weight or value. Historically though, psychiatry has been more at-risk from premature closures and exclusion of opposing viewpoints than with relativism (Fulford *et al.*, 2003).

Thus, we believe that recognizing meaning and social context shouldn't mean we stop searching for theoretically useful models. Scientific endeavors can be consistent with the liberatory psychiatry agenda. Freeman Dyson (2007) considers science an inherently subversive act because by stubbornly going where facts may lead, it is a threat to establishments of all kinds. Just like the lack of success of apparently Marxist inspired revolutions, doesn't mean Marx's insights are redundant or irrelevant. They are important causal frameworks that help us understand the nature of causal factors for human distress in many existing theories. The challenge is to develop interactive models that explore the relationship between meanings and the dynamics of the biological, psychological, and social spheres in which the person is embedded.

Several writers raised a number of specific tasks; however, in so doing, they also raised questions:

(1) What is do-able with patients and patient groups? How do we avoid excessive idealism and be pragmatic?

(2) How much can psychiatry contribute to progressive social movements? Who are our potential partner groups in this endeavor?

(3) How can, or indeed can liberatory forms of psychiatry be realized within existing institutions (such as the American Psychiatric Association, World Psychiatric Association and the Royal College of Psychiatrists)?

Perhaps the fundamental concern for liberatory psychiatry is whether it can have a constructive dialogue and engagement with mainstream institutions and yet not dilute its radicalism. How far is mainstream psychiatry with all the vested interests of individual doctors, the pharmaceutical industry, and governmental desires, willing to *seriously* engage with us?

What are the prospects for a liberatory psychiatry?

The authors of this book are most firmly unified in the belief that the current hegemonic global political system – that of neoliberal capitalism – is harmful to people and contributes to states of alienation, distress, and disenfranchisement in a myriad of ways. What the authors also seem to agree on is that current hegemonic global psychiatric systems are not succeeding in articulating scientific and/or pragmatic paths toward realization of psychiatry's liberatory goals; worse, that they are often an obstacle to achieving this.

But what of the future? Are there any islands of hope for the more radical vision of psychiatry and society that the authors in this volume are calling for, or are we doomed to continue to swim in the oceans of "revolutionary blues" that Carl Cohen's (and many other progressives') family seem to be afflicted with (see Chapter 1)?

If we are at all "right" in our proposals, then greater influence for more liberatory forms of psychiatric theory and practice relies, at least in part, on more liberatory forms of political, economic, and social organization (and arguably vice versa). Paradoxically, neoliberal globalization may provide the seeds of a renewed potentially revolutionary resistance to certain forms of capitalist domination.

The project of neoliberal globalization involves more than just that of free trade and the opening of new markets around the world. In order to achieve its ultimate aim, it seeks to export the value systems that support it. United States and other Western countries' controlled corporations dominate global communications industries. Mass media then help promote the world capitalist system by providing the necessary ideological support for the imposition of the values it requires for continuous capitalist expansion on a global scale. Thus, the commodity culture necessary for continuing market expansion penetrates all spheres of life with the creation of niche markets and the advertising of idealized and fantasy lifestyles on which to attach products. The eventual aim of such a market system is to get all cultures to submit to its logic and, by implication, to the values required for promoting continued consumption globally. As a result, McDonalds, CocaCola, Nike (and so forth) become global brands, representing more than just the product they are selling, but in addition, a set of ideals and fantasy lifestyles.

However, neither the economic or cultural flow has been all one-way. Globalization has arguably brought many aspects of non-Western cultures, from cuisine to medicinal, and from spiritual to esthetic into the mainstream in the West. The exceptions to the unidirectional neocolonial flow of economic power can also be seen with the emergence of powerful, regional economies such as those of the so-called "tiger" economies of the Far East. Thus, the center–periphery model of globalization cannot account for these other complex, overlapping and disjunctive variations that result in differing regional concerns, together with new forms of cultural hybridity and multiplicity.

Not only does globalization create the space and possibilities for reverse cultural flow and thus new emerging fusions of identities, beliefs, and practices, but, in addition, globalization can produce resistance and, in some cases, a rediscovery of the importance of certain aspects of traditional culture. For example, despite prolonged Western attempts at influencing public opinion in Arab Middle East and North Africa, attitudes have hardened against Western value systems and there has been a move to re-affirm and strengthen the regional, Muslim, identity, to the point where the so-called "war on terror" is running into serious obstacles, even within public opinion in Western capitalist countries. The rapid increase in exposure to global influences may indeed expose us to conflict between contradictory values systems. This conflict can lead to vulnerability and mental health problems, but it can also lead to innovative solutions, and new cross-cultural identities particularly within the "outsider" culture and the young of the host community.

Not only is global capitalism facing increasing resistance to the ideologies it wishes to globalize, but in addition, an increasingly visible anti-globalization movement is achieving some notable progress. In Latin America a coalition of "anti-Capitalist/anti-Imperialist" governments, such as those of Hugo Chavez in Venezuela and Evo Morales in Bolivia, is emerging, and the anti-globalization movement seems increasingly capable of providing security headaches for G8 summits, and the growing alarm about "global warming" has brought a huge international community of scientists together, warning us that our levels of consumption are unsustainable. We should be under no illusion about capitalism's tenacity in the face of challenges, and its ability to usurp any potentially radical movement, to use for its own purposes (for example, certain aspects of the feminist movement has been exploited to allow greater access for women into the "individualized" consumer culture). Nevertheless, capitalism simply has no chance of providing social justice, and the infinite "growth" on which it depends would seem to lead to either a catastrophe for mankind or it will have to at some point give way to a more redistributive solution (Kovel, 2002).

Similarly, the current hegemonic biomedical paradigm in psychiatry and psychology has many points of dissent and resistance. The collaboration that, at least in part, inspired this book, is between two groups, the *Radical Caucus* of American psychiatrists in the USA, and the *Critical Psychiatry Network* in the UK. Both groups have members who have published in several mainstream and influential journals, written several books, and have held successful, well-attended presentations at major psychiatric conferences (such as the annual conferences of the American Psychiatric Association and Royal College of Psychiatrists). Within allied professions, critical psychologists and psychotherapists have also articulated increasingly visible, political, and psychotherapeutic alternatives. For example, popular psychologist and journalist Oliver James's most recent book *Affluenza* (James, 2007) makes a similar overall point to several authors in this book. Using evidence gathered from a variety of international studies, he likens the effects of what he calls "selfish capitalism" to a virus, that spreads through the population in societies most dominated by capitalist values such as self-seeking and monetary gain, and increasing susceptibility to mental diseases such as depression and anxiety. Furthermore, the "virus" is most visible in societies with the largest levels of social inequality, and is slowly becoming a global pandemic as a result of the pressure to globalize the values of "selfish capitalism."

The question then arises of how to influence and engage positively with current "mainstream" institutions and practitioners. The dilemma about how to go about this task was illustrated in a conference attended by one of the authors (ST). In December 2005 the 5-yearly "Evolution of Psychotherapy" conference in the United States was held. This conference is billed as the world's largest psychotherapy conference with over 8000 delegates attending. At the conference, there was a sense of a profession that was angry and becoming more radicalized. We were warned that humanity was on a path to extinction with modern capitalism slowly strangling the world and corrupting and killing its citizens through adopting a value system based on greed, power, and control. The twin devils of drug companies and managed healthcare, it was claimed, were having a detrimental effect on mental health care, to the point that loneliness had become a disease called "depression," largely so that drugs can be prescribed. Delegates were encouraged to explore how our changing cultural circumstances were altering our consciousness, causing generations to become strangers to each other, and with the growth of a kind of "false consciousness" that seduces us into a world system that maintains poverty, degrades the environment, and alienates us from our neighbors – without feeling able to do anything about it. Psychotherapy, it was claimed had a role beyond that of "treatment." That is, to aid people to make the "consciousness adjustments" needed to help them as individuals and as members of communities, and to face the "false consciousness" that causes so much suffering in an increasingly selfish world (Timimi, 2006). Notwithstanding whether psychotherapy can appreciably alter the impact of the social world on individuals (Cohen, 1986), the increased recognition of these issues among psychotherapists has the potential to transform the field.

However, the psychotherapists' ability to address these sociopolitical issues is impeded by these very same economic and political dynamics that affect the people whom they treat. As the managed care system of organizing health services took hold, healthcare in the United States became organized around

Diagnostic Statistical Manual (DSM) diagnoses and in "quick fix" solutions such as medication and other less time-consuming and inexpensive methods. This modern socio-political context therefore, placed divergent demands on "psychotherapy." On the one hand, that of developing theory and practice that attempts to challenge and heal the destructive effects of rampant consumerist capitalism; on the other, that of professional survival in such a society. The latter has, of course, favored particular brands of psychotherapy, such as "Cognitive Behavior Therapy," that are more easily packaged and are more congruent with a model of psychotherapy where it is just another treatment like medication that can have treatment protocols that fit into DSM classifications, and thus are (potentially) stripped of any radical insight that may challenge the dominant socioeconomic system.

So, this then is our dilemma: If we are "too radical," we risk alienating our colleagues and our professional institutions and possibly losing our jobs, thereby making it less likely that the ideas contained in books such as this will reach the wider audience they need. On the other hand, too much compromise and we risk "fudging" the issues, making it easier for these ideas to be usurped into the mainstream, stripped of any radical potential.

Perhaps the best we can hope for at this historical moment is to keep the ideas flourishing in publications, websites, and at conferences. Economic, political, and cultural forces are constantly in flux. Therefore, theory and practice cannot stand still, and must also keep pace to reflect the changing nature of the challenges that face us. Whether, when, and the extent to which "mainstream" institutions wish to engage us, is perhaps not as important as having these alternatives well articulated, and pragmatically grounded. We do not want to see the mental health equivalent of the Iraqi invasion, when the downfall of one hegemony simply exposed a vacuum with no suitable alternative in place that was ready and willing to take the baton. Nevertheless, such a moment would only be the beginning. As Hannah Arendt (1970) recognized, "The most radical revolutionary will become a conservative the day after the revolution."

REFERENCES

Arendt, H. (1970). *New Yorker*, September, 12.

Cohen, C. I. (1986). Marxism and psychotherapy. *Science and Society*, **50**(1), 4–24.

Demasio A. (2003). *Looking for Spinoza*. Orlando, FL: Harcourt.

Dyson, F. (2007). *The Scientist as Rebel*. New York: New York Review of Books.

Fulford, B., Morris, K., Sadler, J., & Stanghellini, G. (2003). Past improbable, future possible: the renaissance in philosophy and psychiatry. In *Nature and Narrative. An Introduction to the*

New Philosophy of Psychiatry, ed. B. Fulford, K. Morris, J. Sadler, & G. Stanghellini. Oxford: Oxford University Press.

Gier, N. F. (2000). In *Spiritual Titanism: Indian, Chinese, and Western Perspectives*. New York: SUNY Press. Chapter 2.

James, O. (2007). *Affluenza*. London: Vermilion.

Kovel, J. (2002). *The Enemy of Nature: The End of Capitalism or the End of the World?* New York: Zed Books.

Latour, B. (1993). *We Have Never Been Modern*. Cambridge, MA: Harvard University Press.

Lerner, M. (1991). *Surplus Powerlessness*. Atlantic Highlands NJ: Humanities Press.

Link, B. G. & Phelan, J. C. (1995). Social conditions as fundamental causes of disease. *Journal of Health and Social Behavior*, **36**(special issue), 80–94.

Martín-Baró, I. (1996). *Writings for a Liberation Psychology*. Cambridge, MA: Harvard University Press.

Timimi, S. (2006). While you retain the power you are unlikely to challenge the assumptions that keep you powerful. *Mental Health Today*. March, 19.

Index

Note: page numbers in *italics* refer to tables. Those with 'n' suffix refer to Notes.